Principles of Neuromusculoskeletal Treatment and Management

A Guide for Therapists

D1354875

1 JUN 2024

1 JUN 2024

WITHDRAWN

Commissioning Editor: Rita Demetriou - Swanwick
Development Editor: Nicola Lally
Project Manager: Deepthi Unni and K Anand Kumar
Designer/Design Direction: Kirsteen Wright
Illustration Manager: Merlyn Harvey
Illustrator: Antbits

Principles of Neuromusculoskeletal Treatment and Management

A Guide for Therapists

Edited by

Nicola J Petty DPT MSc FMACP FHEA
Principal Lecturer, University of Brighton, UK

Foreword by

Dr Alison Rushton EdD MSc Grad Dip Phys Dip TP mILT FMACP
University of Birmingham, UK

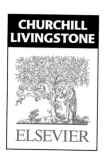

Edinburgh   London   New York   Oxford   Philadelphia   St Louis   Sydney   Toronto   2011

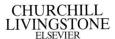

First edition 2004
Second edition 2012
   Reprinted 2013, 2014

ISBN 978-0-7020-5309-2

British Library Cataloguing in Publication Data
A catalogue record for this book is available from the British Library

Library of Congress Cataloging in Publication Data
A catalog record for this book is available from the Library of Congress

Notices

ELSEVIER your source for books,
journals and multimedia
in the health sciences

www.elsevierhealth.com

Working together to grow
libraries in developing countries

www.elsevier.com | www.bookaid.org | www.sabre.org

 ELSEVIER   BOOK AID International   Sabre Foundation

The
Publisher's
policy is to use
**paper manufactured
from sustainable forests**

Printed in China

Contents

List of contributors

Kieran Barnard MSc BSc(Hons) MCSP MMACP
Extended Scope Physiotherapist, West Sussex Primary
Care Trust, Horsham, UK

Laura Finucane MSc BSc(Hons) MCSP MMACP HPC Reg
Consultant Musculoskeletal Physiotherapist,
Physiotherapy Department, East Surrey Hospital,
Redhill, UK

Karen McCreesh MSc(Manip Ther) BPhysio MMACP MISCP
Lecturer, Department of Physiotherapy, University of
Limerick, Limerick, Ireland

Ann Moore PhD FCSP FMACP CertEd DipTp FHEA
Director Clinical Research Centre for Health Professions,
University of Brighton, Eastbourne, UK

Chris Murphy MSc MCSP MMACP PGCert
PhysioUK, Epsom, Surrey, UK

Anne O'Connor MSc BSc
Senior Therapist, Department of Physiotherapy,
University of Limerick, Limerick, Ireland

Nicola J Petty DPT MSc GradDipPhys FMACP FHEA
Principal Lecturer, School of Health Professions,
University of Brighton, Eastbourne, UK

Colette Ridehalgh MSc BSc(Hons) MMACP
Senior Lecturer, School of Health Professions,
University of Brighton, Eastbourne, UK

Foreword

This text is unique in providing a review and synthesis of knowledge informing clinical decisions in the treatment and management of patients presenting with neuromusculoskeletal problems. The focus of the original edition is maintained, to explore the interaction of different tissues (joint, muscle and nerve) and their integrity within the neuromusculoskeletal system; recognising the functional and dysfunctional interdependence of these tissues.

It barely seems 7 years since the publication of the first edition of this text. Since then, the research into neuromusculoskeletal therapy has increased dramatically to further inform our clinical practice. A key illustration of this is through our developing understanding of musculoskeletal pain and its implications for us clinically. Its main strength is that the text logically develops an in-depth analysis of the theoretical rationale underpinning treatment and management interventions and systematically conducts an exploration of the existing evidence in support of these possible interventions. In this edition, Nicola Petty takes an editorial role and has invited experienced clinicians and academics to review and write each chapter. The clinical experience of the contributors is explicitly used to ensure the application of the content to practice situations. The inclusion of work from a comprehensive range of authors who are already recognised for their work clinically is effectively synthesised to further challenge our current practice. Many of the points made are therefore thought-provoking, and will stimulate wider reading.

An effective introduction provides the context for the text and an overview of the following chapters. The previous edition's section on assessment now sits within the companion text, but the previous chapters focused to function and dysfunction, and principles of treatment for joint, muscles and nerves are continued. A new chapter focused to the principles of managing pain is a valuable addition. The final chapter on the principles of patient management is maintained to synthesise the preceding chapters and to remind us of the complexity of our clinical context for decision making when treating and managing patients. The international definition of Orthopaedic Manual Therapy (neuromusculoskeletal) from the International Federation of Orthopaedic Manipulative Physical Therapists (IFOMPT), illustrates this complexity and highlights the factors that are integral to patient management and central to this text.

"Orthopaedic Manual Therapy is a specialised area of physiotherapy / physical therapy for the management of neuromusculoskeletal conditions, based on clinical reasoning, using highly specific treatment approaches including manual techniques and therapeutic exercises.

Orthopaedic Manual Therapy also encompasses, and is driven by, the available scientific and clinical evidence and the biopsychosocial framework of each individual patient".
(IFOMPT, 2004)

The effective educational perspective of the text provides a framework for the practice of a clinician without being prescriptive. It facilitates application of the principles to the individual patient within the patient centred and evidence based framework of practice illustrated in the IFOMPT definition.

The development over the past 7 years of physiotherapy (and allied neuromusculoskeletal professions) research and its dissemination has contributed to the greatest change in this text, with the contributors updating current theories and knowledge through use of the new evidence. This is illustrated in the review of each previous chapter and through pain as an example of rapid development leading to a new chapter. This new chapter provides a useful chronological overview of our developing understanding of pain enabling us to evaluate existing theories, pain mechanisms, and empirical evidence and thereby provide a framework for treating pain.

The first text was innovative in synthesising literature from all components of neuromusculoskeletal practice – the obvious clinical sciences, but also, the important components of the process of clinically reasoned patient management. This updated text continues to strive to present best current practice to assist the decision making of neuromusculoskeletal clinical practitioners as we move through the next decade of development. The synthesis that this text provides is of unique value for beginning or existing clinicians who are seeking to base their management decisions on contemporary knowledge whilst also understanding the challenges that this premise provides. Readers will be able to select additional reading from the reference lists included to further inform their depth of understanding in key areas. The text encourages criticality of our existing understanding and the developing empirical evidence that underpins treatment and management strategies. While it states that criticality of research has not been included, this critically reflective stance is encouraged in readers. In addition, the text will be a useful resource for researchers and students who have a research component to their programmes, as it effectively collates existing evidence to identify gaps in the literature that require our further consideration and investigation.

The value of this text to us is inherently captured through the following quotation:

"Books are the quietest and most constant of friends; they are the most accessible and wisest of counsellors, and the most patient of teachers".

Charles W Eliot (1834 - 1926), author of 'The Happy Life', 1896, and President of Harvard University.

Alison Rushton

Preface

This new edition has been updated in a variety of ways. The book has been improved by the involvement and contribution of a number of key clinicians and academics who bring specialised knowledge and expertise in the field of neuromusculoskeletal treatment and management. A number of contributors are members of the Manipulation Association of Chartered Physiotherapists (MACP) and as such hold a recognised postregistration qualification in neuromusculoskeletal physiotherapy.

A number of years ago, it was planned to merge this book with the companion text entitled *Neuromusculoskeletal Examination and Assessment*. Feedback from users indicated it would be better to keep them separate. However, to enhance the way each book complements the other, new editions of both books have been prepared at the same time; it has been a busy year!

Contributors worked with chapters from the previous edition of this book, editing the text, adding new sections and updating the references. The chapter on assessment has moved out to the companion examination and assessment textbook and this has allowed space for a colleague to write a new chapter on pain. I am grateful, not only for the valuable input each contributor has made to the text, but also for the energy and enthusiasm to complete the job under tight timescales.

A number of people have been involved in this new edition. In particular in relation to Chapters 4 and 5, thanks go to Mary McAllister for her expert knowledge on exercise prescription and Helen Lindfield for her proof-reading and guidance. Thanks also go to Elsevier and in particular Anand Kumar, Deepthi Unni, Nicola Lally, Rita Demetriou-Swanick and Sarena Wolfaard for their guidance and support throughout the publishing process.

Clinical expertise and patient-centred care require a critical understanding of the theory and research knowledge underpinning treatment and management strategies. This text seeks to present this knowledge to the reader in a clear and straightforward fashion, so that understanding is enhanced. A delightful side-effect for some readers may be the realisation of how wonderfully made (Psalm 139 v14) the neuromusculoskeletal system is.

Nicola J Petty
Eastbourne 2010

Introduction

Nicola J Petty

The aim of this book is to make explicit the underlying principles behind the treatment and management of patients with neuromusculoskeletal disorders. It has been written as a companion text to the examination and assessment of the neuromusculoskeletal system (Petty 2011).

This chapter aims to help the reader understand how the information has been laid out, by giving a brief résumé of what is contained within each chapter.

Chapter 2 provides key information on the anatomy, biomechanics, physiology and movement of joint structures, and, on the basis of this summary of joint function, classifies and discusses common clinical presentations of joint dysfunction. Using this classification of dysfunction, Chapter 3 provides the principles underpinning joint treatment.

Chapter 4 provides key information on the anatomy, biomechanics and physiology of muscle, and, from this summary of muscle function, classifies and discusses common clinical presentations of muscle dysfunction. Using this classification of dysfunction, Chapter 5 provides the principles underpinning muscle treatment.

Chapter 6 provides key information on the anatomy, biomechanics, physiology and movement of nerve, and, from this summary of nerve function, classifies and discusses common clinical presentations of nerve dysfunction. Using this classification of dysfunction, Chapter 7 provides the principles underpinning nerve treatment.

In this text, a 'joint treatment' is defined as a 'treatment to effect a change in joint'; that is, the intention of the clinician is to produce a change in a joint, and therefore it is described as a joint treatment.

Similarly, where a technique is used to effect a change in a muscle, it will be referred to as a 'muscle treatment', and where a technique is used to effect a change in a nerve, it will be referred to as a 'nerve treatment'. Thus, techniques are classified according to which tissue the clinician is predominantly attempting to affect. What is emphasised throughout the text is the impossibility of affecting only one tissue in isolation; treatment will always affect all three tissues.

Treatment is very often aimed to relieve pain and, for this reason, Chapter 8 provides information related to the management of pain.

However, treatment of an individual patient is not simply the physical treatment of joint, muscle and nerve to relieve pain and other symptoms. The patient is a person with mind and spirit, as well as body, as is the clinician. This potent combination creates a complex therapeutic relationship, which defies a simple cause-and-effect analysis of our therapeutic interaction. Chapter 8 discusses these issues and provides an overview of the principles of managing patients with neuromusculoskeletal disorders.

Thus, readers who would like to learn more about the principles of treatment and management of patients with joint disorders would be advised to read Chapters 2, 3, 8 and 9, with muscle disorders Chapters 4, 5, 8 and 9, and with nerve disorders Chapters 6, 7, 8 and 9.

In terms of content, it may be helpful to make some general comments here. Anatomy, biomechanics, physiology and pathology textbooks provide general information that is often articulated in a straightforward manner; textbooks often aim to enhance broad understanding of the reader. In contrast, articles published in scientific journals often awaken the reader to a more complex and uncertain view of the subject. Anatomy journals, for example, describe variations in joint architecture, muscle attachments and nerve pathways, demonstrating the uniqueness of individuals. So while anatomy textbooks describe what is generally true, they do not describe what is particularly true for any one individual. This has important implications for clinical practice. Each individual patient presenting for treatment may not have the anatomical structure that has been described in textbooks. The same might be said of biomechanics, physiology and pathology texts. The content of this textbook is no different; it provides general information on joint, nerve and muscle function and dysfunction, and may not be directly applicable to an individual patient.

Much of what is known about the neuromusculoskeletal system of the human body is based on animal research studies. While in general it may be assumed that the findings would be similar in the human body, it cannot be assumed to be identical.

Our knowledge of the neuromusculoskeletal system is far from complete. Research often focuses on one area, which is then assumed to reflect other similar areas. For example, the quadriceps muscle group has been used to investigate the principles of muscle strengthening and the cat knee joint has been used to investigate the behaviour of joint afferent activity during movement. The research provides knowledge of one area, and indirect knowledge of other similar areas. So, for example, the behaviour of joint afferent activity in the cat is presumed to be similar to that of the human, and is presumed to reflect afferent activity in other joints. These are logical and reasonable assumptions to make, but we must be aware that we are making these assumptions.

One final point is that research articles are used widely within the text to support or refute arguments. Details of the research carried out and a critical evaluation of the research are not provided in the text, as this would limit the flow of the arguments. Readers are encouraged to refer to these articles so that their own understanding is enhanced. For those completing degree level study, reference to the original article will be vital.

Reference

Petty, N.J., 2011. Neuromusculoskeletal
examination and assessment:
a handbook for therapists, fourth ed.
Elsevier, Edinburgh.

Function and dysfunction of joint

2

Anne O'Connor   Karen McCreesh

CHAPTER CONTENTS

In this text, the term 'joint' refers to both the intra-articular and periarticular structures. The function of the neuromusculoskeletal system is to produce movement. This is dependent on each component of the system, that is, normal function of joint, nerve and muscle. This interrelationship is depicted in Figure 2.1, which shows a theoretical model originally devised to describe stability of the spine (Panjabi 1992a) but which is applicable to the entire neuro-musculoskeletal system. Similarly, the stability of the knee joint has been described as 'a complex systematic sensory–motor synergy which includes the ligaments, antagonistic muscle pair (flexors and extensors), bones, and sensory mechanoreceptors in the ligaments, joint capsule, and associated muscles' (Solomonow et al. 1987). This description could equally be applied to all peripheral joints, so, while this chapter is concerned with the function of joints, it is important to highlight that the joint does not function in isolation but in a highly interdependent way with muscle and nerve. For a joint to function optimally there must be normal functioning of the relevant muscles and nerves.

Some examples of how joint, nerve and muscle function together to stabilise joints may help to highlight this close relationship. Anatomically, ligament is often not a separate distinctive tissue but blends together with muscle to form a unified stability system (Strasmann et al. 1990). For example, in the spine the supraspinous ligament and the superficial part of the interspinous ligament form the attachment of longissimus thoracis pars thoracis (Adams et al. 2002). In the lumbar spine, multifidus blends with the zygapophyseal joint capsule (Yamashita et al. 1996), in the shoulder supraspinatus and teres minor blend with the glenohumeral joint capsule and at the knee biceps femoris fuses with the lateral collateral ligament (Williams et al. 1995). So, anatomically, ligament and muscle appear to function together.

Stability of a joint is a function of joint stiffness (Panjabi 1992b), and this is provided not only by the joint capsule but also by skin, muscle and tendon. The relative contribution of these tissues has been estimated in the wrist of the cat, with the joint capsule providing 47% of joint stiffness, muscle 41%, tendon 10% and skin 2% (Johns & Wright 1962). In the human lumbar spine, a number of the ligaments are considered too weak to contribute significantly to joint stiffness

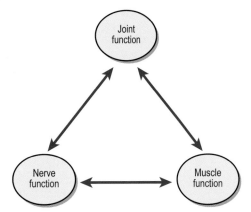

Figure 2.1 • Interdependence of the function of joint, nerve and muscle for normal movement (after Panjabi 1992a, with permission). Normal function of the neuromusculoskeletal system requires normal function of joint, nerve and muscle.

and are regarded as transducers serving a proprioceptive function (Panjabi 1992a; Adams et al. 2002). During lumbar spine flexion and extension, muscle has been found to augment segmental stability (Panjabi et al. 1989; Wilke et al. 1995). There is substantial evidence throughout the body that stability of joints is enhanced by muscle (Perry et al. 1975; Pope et al. 1979; Shoemaker & Markolf 1982; Louie et al. 1984; Walla et al. 1985; McGill & Norman 1986; Solomonow et al. 1986, 1987; Louie & Mote 1987; Panjabi et al. 1989; Knatt et al. 1995; Wilke et al. 1995; Phillips et al. 1997; Hortobagyi & DeVita 2000).

The nervous system underpins this joint stability function of muscle. In the upper limb, stimulation of afferents in the medial ligament of the elbow causes activation of the muscles overlying this ligament (flexor carpi radialis, flexor carpi ulnaris, flexor digitorum profundus and flexor digitorum superficialis and pronator teres). This is thought to be a protective reflex to avoid excessive ligamentous tension (Phillips et al. 1997). In the lower limb, in the anaesthetised cat, passive ankle dorsiflexion causes activation of mechanoreceptors in the posterior joint capsule which produces a reflex facilitation of gastrocnemius and inhibition of tibialis anterior; similarly, passive plantarflexion causes activation of mechanoreceptors in the anterior joint capsule which produces facilitation of tibialis anterior and inhibition of gastrocnemius (Freeman & Wyke 1967a). In the lumbar spine, the supraspinous ligament contains mechanoreceptors which, when stimulated, cause a reflex contraction of the multifidus muscle; this is thought to improve

spinal stability (Indahl et al. 1995, 1997; Solomonow et al. 1998). Collectively, this research clearly links the interdependent relationship of joint, nerve and muscle in providing joint stability.

Joint function

The previous section has highlighted the complex, interdependent nature of joint muscle and nerve. This should be borne in mind when reading the next section on aspects of joint function. Aspects of joint function that will be discussed are:

* classification of joints
* anatomy, biomechanics and physiology of joints
* nerve supply of joints
* classification of synovial joints
* joint movement
* biomechanics of joint movement.

A joint is the junction between two or more bones, and the function of a joint is to permit limited movement and to transfer force from one bone to another (Nigg & Herzog 1999).

Classification of joints

Joints can be classified as either synarthrosis (not synovial) or diarthrosis (synovial) (Norkin & Levangie 1992). Synarthrosis joints are further divided into fibrous and cartilaginous joints (Figure 2.2).

Fibrous joints can be further subdivided into suture joints, as in the joints of the skull, gomphosis joints, as in the joints between a tooth and the mandible or maxilla, and a syndesmosis joint between the shaft of the radius and ulna (Figure 2.3). As the name suggests, in each type of joint fibrous tissue unites the joint surfaces and, as a result, only a small amount of movement is possible.

Cartilaginous joints can be further subdivided into symphysis, as in the symphysis pubis and the interbody joint (two vertebral bodies and the intervening disc) in the vertebral column (Figure 2.3), and synchondroses, as in the first chondrosternal joint. In this type of joint, fibrocartilage or hyaline cartilage directly unites the bone and, again, only a small amount of movement is possible.

Diarthrosis or synovial joints are characterised by having no tissue uniting each end of the bone; rather, a joint space exists, thus allowing movement to occur. Synovial joints are characterised by a fibrous joint capsule lined with a synovial membrane, the

Figure 2.2 • Classification of synarthrosis joints (Norkin & Levangie 1992).

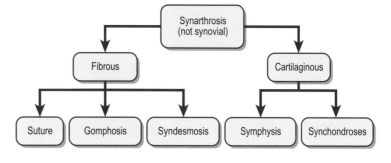

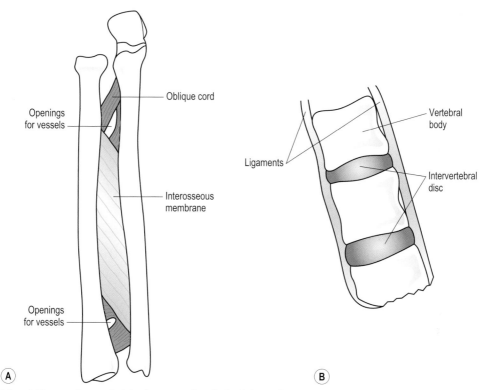

Figure 2.3 • **A** The syndesmosis joint between the shaft of the radius and ulna; the fibrous interosseous membrane unites the two bones (from Palastanga et al. 2002, with permission). **B** The symphysis joint between the vertebral bodies in the spine (from Palastanga et al. 2002, with permission).

bone end being covered by hyaline cartilage with a film of synovial fluid. Fat pads lie within the synovial membrane, filling the irregularities and potential spaces within the joint, and ligaments and tendons lie either within or adjacent to the joint. There may be a meniscus, for example in the knee joint, fibroadipose meniscoids in the zygapophyseal joints, a labrum in the glenohumeral or hip joints, an intervertebral disc in the spinal column and in some cases bursae within the joint. Figure 2.4 identifies the features of two synovial joints, one with an intra-articular disc and one without.

Anatomy, biomechanics and physiology of joint tissues

Ligaments

Ligaments may be:

- named parallel bundles of the outer fibrous capsule
- intra-articular, as in the cruciate ligaments of the knee, the ligamentum teres of the hip and the intra-articular ligament of the costovertebral joint
- periarticular, as in the lateral collateral ligament of the knee.

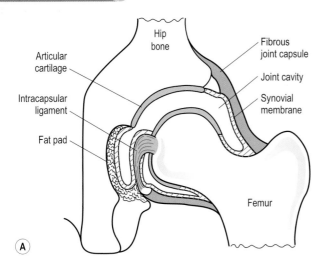

Figure 2.4 • Two synovial joints (from Palastanga et al. 2002, with permission). A Hip joint. B Temporomandibular joint with an intra-articular disc.

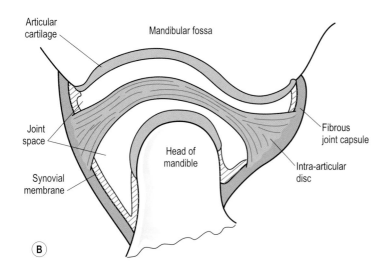

Ligaments consist of 70% water and 30% solids, with the solids made up of 70–80% collagen, 3–5% elastin and the remainder a ground substance (Akeson et al. 1987; Nordin & Frankel 1989; Stanish 2000). Ligaments attach directly to bone, that is, there is an abrupt well-defined area of attachment, with a clear demarcation of ligament and bone (Woo et al. 1988). The ligament in direct attachments has a superficial layer blending with the periosteum and a larger, deep layer inserting directly into the bone via a layer less than 1 mm thick of fibrocartilage (Cooper & Misol 1970; Woo et al. 1988). Sometimes, ligament attaches rather more indirectly, such that there is a more gradual and less distinct area of attachment (Woo et al. 1988). Similar to direct attachments, the ligament has a superficial and deep layer. The superficial layer this time provides the predominant attachment, blending with the periosteum and bone via Sharpey's fibres (Woo et al. 1988), while the deep layer attaches directly to the bone.

The collagen fibres in ligament are arranged in parallel bundles which have an undulated or 'crimping' appearance under the microscope (Frank & Shrive 1999; Stanish 2000) when they are relaxed. The ligament buckles under compression, and so it is only the stretching of ligament with tensile loading that is functionally important (Panjabi & White 2001). The crimping gives some slack to the ligament during minimal tensile loading (longitudinal stretching), and as it straightens out it provides some resistance (Threlkeld 1992; Frank & Shrive 1999). Figure 2.5 demonstrates the change in fibre alignment during lengthening of a typical ligament.

The strength of connective tissue to tensile loading can be depicted on a force (or load)–displacement curve, shown in Figure 2.6. The load or force is plotted against the stretch or deformation. In both load–displacement and stress–strain curves, the slope of the curve is the modulus of elasticity and is a measure of the 'stiffness' of the ligament (Panjabi & White 2001). It can be seen in Figure 2.6 that very little force is initially required to deform the ligament, a region referred to as the 'toe' region (Threlkeld 1992) or 'neutral zone' (Panjabi & White 2001). Stiffness then increases, so that greater force is required to deform the ligament; this region is referred to as the elastic zone (Panjabi & White 2001). Forces within the elastic zone will result in no permanent change in length; as soon as the force is released the tissue returns to its pre-load shape and size (Panjabi & White 2001). The neutral zone and elastic zone fall within the normal physiological range of forces and deformation on ligament during everyday activities (Nordin & Frankel 1989).

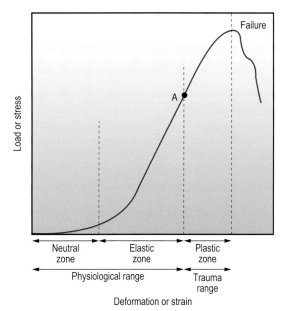

Figure 2.6 • Load (or force)–displacement curve or stress–strain curve of connective tissue (after Panjabi & White 2001, with permission). The physiological range is divided into an initial neutral zone followed by an elastic zone. Further force causes trauma and enters the plastic zone. Point A is the junction between the elastic and temporary displacement, and the plastic and permanent displacement. This point is known as the yield stress and is the minimum stress necessary to cause a residual strain in the material.

Figure 2.5 • A typical force–displacement curve for a ligament (after Frank & Shrive 1999, with permission). I, toe region where the collagen is crimped (schematic representation); II, linear region where the collagen is straightened out; III, microfailure; IV, failure region.

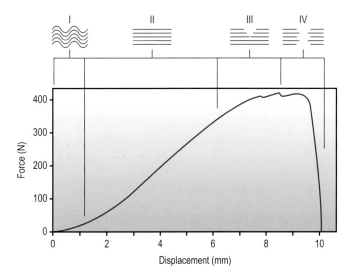

Towards the end of a joint's physiological range the force and deformation may be sufficient to cause micro-trauma of individual collagen fibres and bundles and to produce a permanent elongation of the connective tissue (Threlkeld 1992). A rough guide to the amount of force required to cause a permanent change in length has been estimated to be between 224 and 1136 N (Threlkeld 1992), with microfailure of connective tissue beginning at approximately 3% elongation and macrofailure at approximately 8% (Noyes et al. 1983). The point at which there is permanent deformation is termed the 'yield stress', and the region beyond this point is known as the plastic zone (Panjabi & White 2001). A further increase in force will lead to trauma and eventually failure of the ligament, i.e. a strain injury.

The progressive failure of the human anterior cruciate ligament of the knee can be seen in the force–displacement curve in Figure 2.7. The early part of the curve relates to clinical testing of the anterior drawer test for the knee. During normal functional activities, forces occur within the physiological loading zone. Greater forces than this result in micro-failure, injury and eventually failure of the ligament. Figure 2.8 depicts various force–displacement curves for other ligaments in the body. It can be readily seen that there are quite large variations between ligaments, reflecting differences in function.

If the strength of a ligament is to be compared with another tissue, then a stress–strain curve can be drawn, where stress is the force per unit area (measured in Pa or N/m^2) and strain is the percentage change in length (from the resting length). The stress–strain tensile properties of ligament compared with bone, cartilage, muscle and nerve are shown in Table 2.1. The stress–strain curve of collagen, of which ligament is mostly composed, is shown in Figure 2.6.

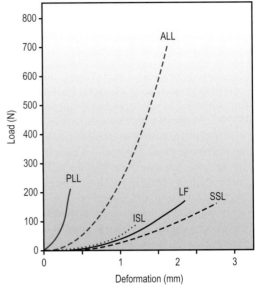

Figure 2.8 • Load–displacement curves for various spinal ligaments (from Panjabi & White 2001, with permission). The slope of the curve of the posterior longitudinal ligament (PLL) is greatest, demonstrating greatest stiffness. Stiffness values gradually lessen with the anterior longitudinal ligament (ALL), interspinous ligament (ISL), ligamentum flavum (LF) and finally supraspinous ligament (SSL).

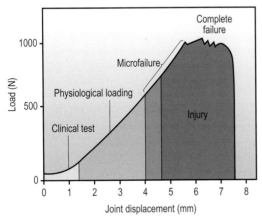

Figure 2.7 • Load (or force)–displacement curve or stress–strain curve of connective tissue (from Nordin & Frankel 1989, with permission). The force–displacement curve during the anterior drawer test is depicted in the early toe region, with physiological loading in the linear region, followed by eventual microfailure and complete failure.

Table 2.1 Tensile properties of ligament compared with bone, cartilage, muscle and nerve (Panjabi & White 2001)

Tissue	Stress at failure (MPa)	Strain at failure (%)
Ligament	10–40	30–45
Cortical bone	100–200	1–3
Cancellous bone	10	5–7
Cartilage	10–15	80–120
Tendon	55	9–10
Muscle (passive)	0.17	60
Nerve roots	15	19

Ligaments are viscoelastic, that is, they have time-dependent mechanical properties. These properties affect the behaviour of ligaments to movement and forces and are therefore important principles for clinicians. They can be summarised as:

• elastic nature
• viscous nature
• creep phenomena
• stress relaxation
• load-dependent
• hysteresis.

The elastic nature means that ligaments will stretch and return to their original shape like an elastic band. The viscous nature means that ligaments will gradually elongate over a period of time, when a constant force is applied. The ability of ligaments to elongate gradually with a constant force (or load) is known as creep and is depicted in Figure 2.9 (Panjabi & White 2001). The magnitude of the force is below the linear region of the load–displacement curve. The phenomenon of stress relaxation means that ligaments undergo load (or stress) relaxation. When the deformation is kept constant (Figure 2.9), the force (or stress) within ligament decreases over time (Panjabi & White 2001).

Ligaments share load-dependent properties, that is, the stress–strain (or load–displacement) curve depends on the rate of loading. When the ligament is loaded quickly it will be stiffer and will deform less than when it is loaded more slowly (Figure 2.10). This is relevant when applying therapeutic force, as a slower rate will result in less resistance and more movement. The additional effect of having

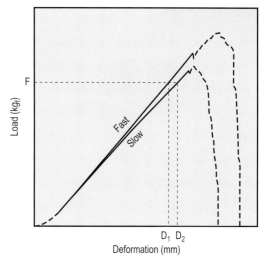

Figure 2.10 • Ligament is load-dependent. It can be seen that a given force (F) applied quickly will produce a certain deformation (D_1), and if applied more slowly will produce a greater deformation (D_2) (after Noyes et al. 1974, with permission).

load-dependent properties is that the failure point of the ligament will be higher with a higher loading rate; in other words, the ligament will be stronger and less likely to rupture when the force is applied at a faster rate.

Ligaments demonstrate the phenomenon of hysteresis, which is the energy loss during loading and unloading (Figure 2.11). The unloading curve lies below the loading curve and reflects a greater energy expenditure on loading than the energy regained during unloading. This results in a loss of energy

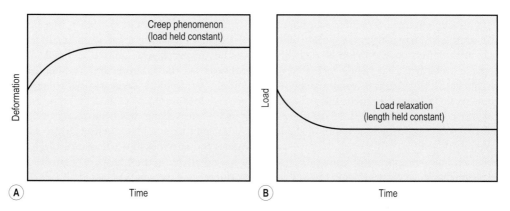

Figure 2.9 • Creep and load relaxation (from Nordin & Frankel 1989, with permission). A Creep is the increase in deformation that occurs when a constant load is applied over time. B Load relaxation is the decrease in stress within a ligament when a constant force is applied over a period of time.

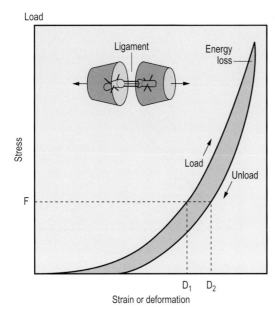

Figure 2.11 • Loading and unloading curves to indicate hysteresis (after Panjabi & White 2001, with permission). The shaded area depicts the loss of energy with deformation and is a measure of hysteresis. The unloading curve does not return to the same point on the strain or deformation axis; there is an increase in length as a result of the application of load. For a given force (F) there is a lengthening from the loading curve (D_1) to the unloading curve (D_2).

at 30% elongation with a stress of 13 MPa (Noyes & Grood 1976). Ageing causes changes in collagen and elastin which result in reduced compliance of ligamentous structures, thus making them more susceptible to injury. This effect can be reduced or retarded to an extent by exercise (Menard 2000).

Fibrous joint capsules and synovial membranes

The outer layer of a fibrous capsule is composed of dense irregular and regular fibrous tissue and completely surrounds the bone ends, attaching into the periosteum of the bone. Where the fibrous tissue is arranged in regular fashion, in parallel bundles, it is referred to as a named ligament. Fibrous capsules have a poor blood supply but are highly innervated. They are often reinforced by adjacent ligamentous and musculotendinous structures. The inner layer of the fibrous capsule forms the synovial membrane, which is composed of areolar connective tissue and elastic fibres, and is highly vascularised.

Articular cartilage

Articular cartilage is white dense connective tissue covering the bone ends of synovial joints and is between 1 and 5 mm in thickness. The function of articular cartilage is to distribute load, minimise friction of opposing joint surfaces and provide shock absorption from impact forces (Mow et al. 1989; Nigg 2000). It is composed largely of water, chondrocytes, collagen and proteoglycans, and it contains no blood or lymph vessels or nerve supply in normal joints. It obtains nutrients from synovial fluid, and during movement nutrients are pumped through the cartilage (O'Hara et al. 1990). The permeability of articular cartilage is greatest on its surface and least in the deeper layers (Shrive & Frank 1999), and depends on the compressive loading (Mow et al. 1984). Permeability decreases with increased compressive loading (Mow et al. 1989). Cyclic loading of joints, as in walking, has been found to increase the pumping of large solutes such as growth factors, hormones and enzymes into articular cartilage – although it has no effect on the transport of small solutes such as glucose and oxygen (O'Hara et al. 1990).

Microscopically, articular cartilage has a layered appearance. The most superficial layer is densely packed with collagen fibrils which are oriented parallel to the articular surface. This arrangement is thought to help resist shear forces at the joint (Shrive &

known as hysteresis loss (Panjabi & White 2001). It can also be seen that hysteresis produces an elongation of the tissues. If the force applied is less than the yield stress, then the elongation will be temporary, and if it is the same, or greater, than the yield stress the elongation will be permanent.

A ligament is stiffest in its central area and less stiff at its attachment site. So when a ligament is stretched, most lengthening occurs at the site of least resistance, at the insertion site (Woo et al. 1988).

The tensile strength of a ligament is increased with exercise (Stanish 2000). Exercise causes an increase in the cross-sectional area of ligament and an increase in the collagen content (Tipton et al. 1970) as well as increased strength at the attachment site of the ligament (Woo et al. 1988).

The biomechanical properties of ligaments change with age; ligaments in younger subjects (16–26 years of age) have two to three times greater strength and stiffness than those in subjects of more than 60 years of age (Noyes & Grood 1976). In a younger age group, ligament fails after 44% elongation and a stress of 37 MPa, while in an older population failure occurs

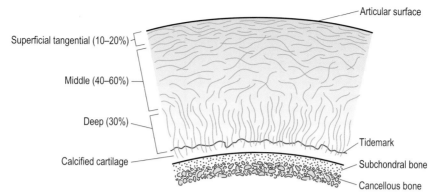

Articular surface

Superficial tangential (10–20%)

Middle (40–60%)

Deep (30%)

Tidemark

Calcified cartilage

Subchondral bone

Cancellous bone

Figure 2.12 • Longitudinal section of articular cartilage demonstrating the varied orientation of collagen fibrils in the superficial, middle and deep layers (after Mow et al. 1989, with permission).

Frank 1999). The middle layer is characterised by the collagen fibrils being further apart, and the deepest layer has fibrils lying at right angles to the articular surface (Figure 2.12). The collagen fibrils in this layer cross the interface between the articular cartilage and the underlying calcified cartilage beneath, a region known as the tidemark. This arrangement anchors the cartilage to the underlying bone.

The orientation of the collagen fibres in the different layers is considered to enhance the tissue's ability to distribute tensile loading across the articular surface (Askew & Mow 1978; Nigg 2000). Collagen fibrils are able to resist high tensile forces; the fibres collapse on compressive forces (Figure 2.13). Most of the water in articular cartilage is closely associated with the collagen fibrils which, together with the proteoglycans, create a fluid-filled matrix that has the mechanical characteristics of a solid object (Mow et al. 1989).

Articular cartilage, like ligamentous tissue, is viscoelastic. It therefore has an elastic and viscous nature, displaying creep, stress relaxation and hysteresis, and has a sensitivity to the rate of loading.

The behaviour of articular cartilage to compressive and tensile loading is discussed below.

Compressive loading of articular cartilage

The compressive properties of articular cartilage depend on which layer is tested; the deepest layer is the stiffest because of its higher proteoglycan content (Shrive & Frank 1999). The creep response of articular cartilage when a constant compressive force is applied is due to exudation of fluid (Figure 2.14). The rate of fluid loss reduces over time until the compressive stress within the cartilage equals the applied compressive load so that equilibrium is reached. At this point the compressive load is resisted by the matrix of collagen and proteoglycan.

The stress relaxation of articular cartilage is shown in Figure 2.15. A compressive force is applied to the cartilage until a specific amount of deformation is reached; the force is then held constant. During the initial compression phase the stress within the cartilage increases (to point B), but, once the force is held constant, there is a gradual reduction in stress

Figure 2.13 • Mechanical properties of collagen fibrils (from Mow et al. 1989, with permission). A Resistance to tension. B Resistance to compression.

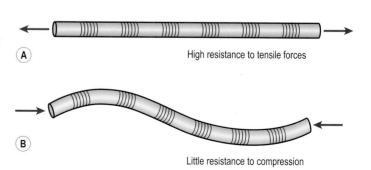

(A)   High resistance to tensile forces

(B)   Little resistance to compression

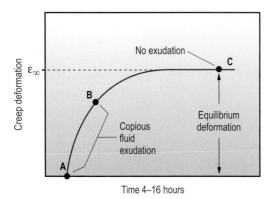

Figure 2.14 • Creep response of articular cartilage with a constant compressive load (after Mow et al. 1989, with permission).

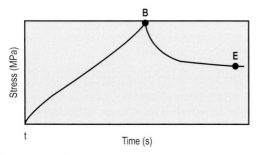

Figure 2.15 • Stress relaxation of articular cartilage with a constant rate of compression. Point B is the maximum stress within the tissue, followed by the gradual reduction in stress until equilibrium is reached at point E. (After Mow et al. 1989, with permission.)

(from point B to point E). Point E indicates the point where equilibrium is reached.

Articular cartilage demonstrates the phenomenon of hysteresis with cyclic compressive loading (Figure 2.16). The unloading curve lies below the loading curve and reflects a greater energy expenditure on loading than the energy regained during unloading. Hysteresis produces a reduction in cartilage thickness.

The stress–strain curve of articular cartilage is dependent on the rate of loading: the faster the rate of loading, the stiffer the articular cartilage becomes and the less deformation occurs; with slower rates of loading the articular cartilage is more compliant and there is greater deformation (Shrive & Frank 1999).

Synovial fluid

Synovial fluid contains surface-active phospholipid (SAPL), which is adsorbed as the outermost layer of articular cartilage (Hills & Monds 1998). The term 'adsorb' refers to how the articular cartilage holds

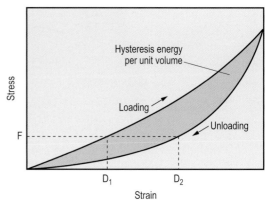

Figure 2.16 • Hysteresis in articular cartilage. The energy expenditure on loading is greater than the energy regained during unloading; the area between the curves depicts the energy loss or hysteresis energy (after Shrive & Frank 1999, with permission). For a given force (F) there is a reduction in thickness from the loading curve (D_1) to the unloading curve (D_2).

SAPL to its surface to form a thin film. This film creates, in engineering terms, boundary lubrication, which prevents the adjacent articular surfaces contacting each other and reduces friction during movement, even under high loading (Hills 1989, 1995). SAPL has also been shown to have antiwear properties (Hills 1995). SAPL has been found to be deficient in osteoarthritic joints (Hills & Monds 1998) and this reduction causes increased resistance to joint movement (Hills & Thomas 1998), a commonly reported clinical phenomenon.

Movement of the joint increases the production of synovial fluid (Levick 1983) and helps to distribute synovial fluid over the articular cartilage (Levick 1984). The flow of synovial fluid into the joint cavity depends, to some extent, on the intra-articular fluid pressure and on the removal of fluid via the synovial lymphatic system (Levick 1984). Intra-articular fluid pressure depends on a large number of factors, including the volume of fluid, rate of change of volume, joint angle, age of the person and muscle action (Levick 1983). Joint movement is also required to remove fluid via the synovial lymphatic system. Lack of movement will reduce the removal of synovial fluid and so will result in an increase in intra-articular volume and pressure. Moderate amounts of movement will increase both the volume of synovial fluid and also the removal of fluid via the lymphatic system. Excessive movement causes a greater increase in the volume of synovial fluid than the removal of fluid, resulting in increased intra-articular volume and pressure (Levick 1984).

Synovial joint lubrication

A variety of mechanisms are thought to ensure that synovial joints are able to maintain almost friction-free movement under a variety of functional activities. The mechanisms are taken from engineering principles of joint lubrication and include boundary and fluid lubrication.

Boundary lubrication

SAPL is adsorbed as the outermost layer of articular cartilage (Hills & Monds 1998). This layer prevents the adjacent articular surfaces contacting each other and reduces friction during movement, even under high loading (Hills 1989, 1995).

Fluid lubrication

A thin film of lubricant separates the adjacent articular surfaces. There are three mechanisms: hydrodynamic lubrication, squeeze film lubrication and elastohydrodynamic lubrication. Fluid film lubrication is thought to operate under low loads and high speeds (Nordin & Frankel 1989).

Hydrodynamic lubrication occurs when the articular surfaces do not lie parallel and then one articular surface slides on the other. A wedge of viscous fluid provides a lifting pressure to support the load (Figure 2.17).

Squeeze film lubrication occurs when the two articular surfaces move towards each other – the fluid pressure between them increases and helps to support the load (Figure 2.18).

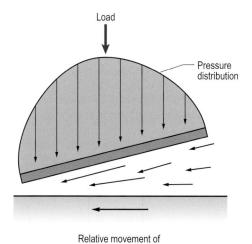

Figure 2.17 • Hydrodynamic lubrication (from Nordin & Frankel 1989, with permission).

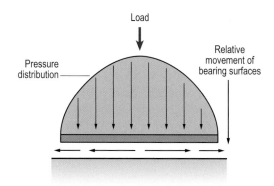

Figure 2.18 • Squeeze film lubrication (from Nordin & Frankel 1989, with permission).

These two mechanisms are related to the nature of the fluid and the shape and position of the joint surfaces. An additional mechanism is related to the fact that articular cartilage is not rigid and is termed elastohydrodynamic lubrication (Nordin & Frankel 1989). The fluid pressures developed from the above two mechanisms cause deformation of the articular surface, which increases its surface area. This increases the time taken for the fluid to be squeezed out and therefore enhances the ability to withstand load.

Fat pads

Fat pads are generally considered to be space fillers or cushions in synovial membrane, in the potential spaces or irregularities of synovial joints. They may enhance joint lubrication (Williams et al. 1995). At the elbow, for example, there are a number of fat pads, including one in the olecranon, coronoid and radial fossae and the trochlear notch (Williams et al. 1995). In the lumbar spine, fat pads in the zygapophyseal joints extend through the joint capsule to the superior articular recess where they are displaced during spinal movement (Bogduk 1997).

Menisci and meniscoids

Fibrocartilage menisci are found in the temporomandibular, knee and sternoclavicular joints. The menisci in the knee joint increase the congruence between the articular surfaces of the femur and tibia, distribute weight-bearing forces, act as shock absorbers and reduce friction (Norkin & Levangie 1992; Palastanga et al. 2002). The medial meniscus is innervated (apart from the inner third) by mechanoreceptors and free nerve endings, with greatest density at the anterior and posterior horns (Albright et al. 1987). The greater density at the horns is thought to enable proprioceptive feedback at the extreme of joint range (Albright et al. 1987). The same arrangement has been found in the temporomandibular joint, with greatest density of mechanoreceptors at the anterior and posterior margins of the intra-articular disc (Zimny & St Onge 1987). Fibroadipose meniscoids in the zygapophyseal joints are thought to protect the joint by preventing articular surface apposition during movement and by reducing friction (Bogduk 1997).

Bursae

Bursae are sacs made of connective tissue lined by a synovial membrane and filled with fluid similar to synovial fluid. A bursa acts as a cushion to reduce friction. Bursae can be found between skin and bone, between muscle and bone, tendon and bone, and ligament and bone. Some named bursae include the subacromial bursa, lying between acromion and the glenohumeral joint capsule, and the psoas bursa, lying between the tendon of psoas and the pubis and hip joint capsule (Williams et al. 1995).

Labra

Two joints in the human body contain a labrum: the glenohumeral joint and the hip joint. They form a fibrocartilaginous wedge-shaped rim around the glenoid and acetabular fossae, respectively. They deepen the articulating socket and may aid lubrication of the joints (Williams et al. 1995).

Intervertebral disc

Intervertebral discs comprise an outer ring of thick fibrous cartilage, the annulus fibrosis, which contains the gelatinous inner core, the nucleus pulposus, with the superior and inferior cartilaginous end-plates completing the structure.

Discs are vulnerable to injury, particularly in spinal flexion and rotation (Gordon et al. 2001), which can lead to annular tears and end-plate fracture and subsequent herniation of annular material. Degenerative changes cause a loss of hydration, reduction in disc height, neural ingrowth and a loss of ability to resist compressive load – this can shift greater load-bearing to the facet joints, predisposing them to arthritic change (Fujiwara et al. 1999).

Nerve supply of joints

Most of the components of joints, such as capsule, ligament, articular disc, meniscus and fat pad, are innervated; in fact the only structure that is not innervated is the avascular articular cartilage (Messner 1999).

The nerve endings in joint can be classified into four types:

1. Ruffini end-organs
2. pacinian corpuscles
3. Golgi endings
4. free nerve endings.

Ruffini end-organs

These are encapsulated (covered in a capsule) type I nerve endings that lie around collagen fibres and are stimulated by displacement of collagen (Figure 2.19). They are low-threshold, static and dynamic mechanoreceptors, supplied by Aβ fibres (or group II afferents). They signal static joint position, direction, amplitude and velocity of joint movement and change in intra-articular pressure (Messner 1999). Activation of Ruffini end-organs has been found to affect the tone of the overlying muscle directly (Freeman & Wyke 1967a). Ruffini end-organs innervate the posterior capsule of the cat knee joint, almost exclusively, and are extremely sensitive to a change in capsule stretch (Fuller et al. 1991). For this reason they are thought to signal the limit of knee extension (Grigg & Hoffman 1982).

Pacinian corpuscles

These are encapsulated, low-threshold, type II mechanoreceptors (Freeman & Wyke 1967b), supplied by Aβ fibres (or group II afferents) (Figure 2.19). They are stimulated by dynamic movement, signalling the start and end of a movement, deceleration and acceleration and a change in stress applied to the tissue in which they occur (Messner 1999). Some are stimulated mainly by compression (Clark 1975; Grigg et al. 1982), while others are stimulated by tensile loading (Clark 1975; Grigg et al. 1982; Grigg 1994). In the cat they are stimulated throughout knee joint movement, particularly during end-range and combined movements (Clark 1975; Krauspe et al. 1992). Activation of pacinian corpuscles directly affects the tone of the overlying muscle (Freeman & Wyke 1967a).

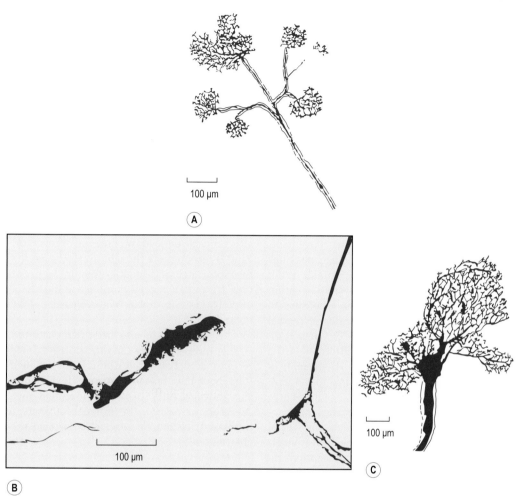

Figure 2.19 • Three types of nerve ending. A Ruffini end-organs (type I). B Pacinian corpuscles (type II). C Golgi endings (type III). (From Skoglund 1956, with permission.)

Golgi endings

These are encapsulated, high-threshold type II mechanoreceptors (Figure 2.19) that signal extreme ranges of movement (Zimny 1988). They are supplied by Aβ fibres (or group III afferents).

Free nerve endings

Free nerve endings do not have a capsule. There are two types of free nerve ending: type IVa and type IVb (Messner 1999). Type IVa nerve endings are associated with blood vessels and have a vasomotor function. Type IVb nerve endings lie between the collagen and elastic fibres of the connective tissue in which they occur. Both type IVa and type IVb nerve endings signal pain and are therefore classed as nociceptors.

The axon may be a myelinated A fibre or an unmyelinated C fibre with a lower conduction velocity.

Afferent fibres can be classified according to their conduction velocity as I or Aα, II or Aβ, III or Aδ and IV or C fibres (Palastanga et al. 2002). These nerve endings have been identified in the limbs, spine, costovertebral joints and temporomandibular joints in both humans and animals (Wyke & Polacek 1975). Fresh amputated human knees revealed innervation by a variety of the encapsulated and free nerve endings (Kennedy et al. 1982). Encapsulated nerve endings were found in the joint capsule, posterior cruciate ligament and the outer surface of the menisci. Free nerve endings have been found throughout the joint tissues, including the collateral ligaments, joint capsules, synovia, cruciate ligaments, infrapatellar fat pad and the outer surface of the menisci (Kennedy et al. 1982). Interestingly, in the human cervical spine group III nerve endings have not been identified; the zygapophyseal joint contains types I, II and IV nerve endings only (Wyke 1970). Type I is found in the superficial layer of the joint capsule, type II in the deeper layer of the joint capsule and fat pads and type IV throughout the joint capsule, fat pads and walls of blood vessels (Wyke & Polacek 1975).

The various descriptive names for each type of nerve ending, along with its function, position and afferent nerve, are given in Table 2.2.

In the cat, free nerve endings are continuous with group III and IV axons, or afferents (Heppelmann et al. 1990). In the cat knee joint group III and IV afferents have a limited response to joint movement, with rather more response to end-range positions (Clark & Burgess 1975; Schaible & Schmidt 1983; Krauspe et al. 1992). There is a large variation within any one animal, and also variation according to whether the afferent is in the posterior or medial articular nerve (Clark & Burgess 1975; Grigg et al. 1986). While the group III and IV afferents in the medial articular nerve and the group III afferents in the posterior articular nerve respond to movement, group IV afferents in the posterior articular nerve respond only to noxious input, suggesting a nociceptive function (Grigg et al. 1986). While group III and IV afferents respond to movement, their sensitivity is low, suggesting a limited role in proprioception and perhaps more of a nociceptor role (Schaible & Schmidt 1983; Grigg 1994). Group III and IV afferents are sensitised in the presence of joint inflammation (Coggeshall et al. 1983; Schaible & Schmidt 1985; Grigg et al. 1986), suggesting that they may have a proprioceptive function (Ferrell 1980).

Effect of joint afferent activity on muscle

Joint afferent activity directly affects overlying muscle activity. Passive dorsiflexion of an anaesthetised cat ankle joint causes activation of mechanoreceptors in the posterior joint capsule, which produces a reflex facilitation of gastrocnemius motor neurones and inhibition of tibialis anterior (Freeman & Wyke 1967a). Similarly, passive plantarflexion causes activation of mechanoreceptors in the anterior joint capsule, which facilitates tibialis anterior and inhibits gastrocnemius (Freeman & Wyke 1967a). Thus, when the joint capsule is put on a stretch, the mechanoreceptors cause activation of muscle that would, on contraction, reduce this stretch, and

inhibition of the muscle that would increase the stretch. The mechanoreceptors stimulated were slowly adapting type I fibres which are activated during the ankle movement and continue to be active once the movement has stopped, and rapidly adapting type II fibres which are activated only during the ankle movement. The type III fibres in the ankle ligaments and the type IV fibres distributed throughout the capsule, ligaments, fat pad and blood vessels are not activated during passive ankle movements (Freeman & Wyke 1967a). In the cervical spine, activation of type I, II and IV receptors affects not only the muscles around the neck but also the muscles around the eye and the mandible (Wyke & Polacek 1975).

The mechanism by which joint mechanoreceptors affect muscle depends on the type of receptor. Type I and II receptors are thought to affect muscle via the fusimotor neurone–muscle spindle loop, whereas type III and IV receptors influence muscle activity directly via the alpha motor neurone (Wyke & Polacek 1975).

The converse has also been demonstrated, that is, that muscle activity can directly affect mechanoreceptor activity (Ferrell 1985). In the cat knee joint, it has been found that, at extreme flexion and extension positions, and with passive movement, mechanoreceptor activity can be influenced (increased or decreased) by muscle contraction around the knee (Ferrell 1985).

Effect of joint afferent activity on pain

Stimulation of the joint mechanoreceptors causes a reduction in transmission of nociceptor activity from the free nerve endings (Wyke 1970). It has been suggested that it is only type I afferent discharge that effects the transmission of pain (Wyke & Polacek 1975).

From Table 2.2 it can be seen that type I, II and III nerve endings are supplied by Aβ fibres, while type IV nerve endings are supplied by group Aδ and C fibres.

The nerve supply to the skin is also relevant, as this will be involved in any joint movement. Details of skin sensation can be found under nerve function in Chapter 6.

Classification of synovial joints

While all synovial joints share the features described above, they vary a great deal in terms of the shape of the articular surfaces and subsequent movement that occurs.

Table 2.2 Nerve endings and afferents supplying joints (Freeman & Wyke 1967b; Wyke 1970; Kennedy et al. 1982; Albright et al. 1987; Zimny & St Onge 1987; Strasmann & Halata 1988; Zimny 1988; Messner 1999; Palastanga et al. 2002)

Type of nerve ending	Descriptive name for nerve ending	Function	Position	Afferent nerve
Type I	Ruffini endings Golgi–Mazzoni endings Meissner corpuscles Spray-type endings Basket endings Ball-of-thread endings Bush-like endings	Low-threshold slowly adapting static and dynamic mechanoreceptors – signal static joint position, changes in intra-articular pressure and direction, amplitude and velocity of joint movement	Joint capsule (superficial layer) Ligaments Meniscus Articular disc	Aβ fibre, myelinated, diameter 5–10 μm or group II afferent
Type II	Pacinian corpuscle Krause's Endkörperchen Vater'schen Körper Vater–pacinian corpuscle Modified pacini(an) corpuscle Simple pacinian corpuscle Paciniform corpuscle Golgi–Mazzoni body Meissner corpuscle Gelenknervenkörperchen Corpuscle of Krause Club-like ending Bulbous corpuscle Corpuscula nervosa articularia	Low-threshold rapidly adapting dynamic mechanoreceptors – signal beginning and end of movement, deceleration and acceleration, change in vibration or stress	Joint capsule (deeper layer) Ligaments Meniscus Articular disc Fat pads Synovium	Aβ fibre, myelinated diameter 8–12 μm or group II afferent
Type III	Golgi endings Golgi–Mazzoni corpuscles	High-threshold very slowly adapting mechanoreceptors – signal extreme ranges of movement or when there is considerable stress	Ligaments Meniscus Articular disc	Aβ fibre, myelinated diameter 13–17μm Group II axons
Type IVa	Free nerve terminals	High-threshold, non-adapting pain receptors	Joint capsule (superficial and deep layers) Ligaments Meniscus Articular disc Fat pads	C fibre, unmyelinated, diameter 1–2 μm and thinly myelinated A fibre, diameter 2–4 μm Type III and IV axons
Type IVa	Free nerve endings	High-threshold, non-adapting pain receptors	Articular blood vessels	Aδ fibre, myelinated diameter 2–5 μm Group II/III axons
Type IVb	Free nerve endings	Vasomotor function	Articular blood vessels	C fibre, unmyelinated diameter <2 μm Group IV axons

Joint surfaces can be classified as flat, ovoid and sellar (MacConaill 1966):

- Flat is where the articular surfaces are flat, or plane, although no surface is completely flat.
- Ovoid is where the articular surfaces are wholly concave or wholly convex.
- Sellar is where the articular surfaces are concave in one plane and convex in another.

Synovial joints are classified as gliding, hinge, pivot, ellipsoidal, saddle and ball and socket (Figure 2.20):

1. Gliding joints include intercarpal and intertarsal joints, zygapophyseal joints in the cervical and thoracic spine, patellofemoral and the costotransverse and costovertebral joints in the lower ribs. The articular surfaces are more or less flat (MacConaill 1953), and, as the name suggests, simple gliding or translational movement can occur.

2. Hinge joints include tibiofemoral, humeroulnar, ankle and interphalangeal joints in the hand and foot. One articular surface is convex and the other concave, allowing rotational flexion and extension movement.

3. Pivot joints include the atlantoaxial and the superior radioulnar joints. One articular surface is round and sits within a ring formed partly by bone and partly by ligament. Rotational movement is around the longitudinal axis of the bone, producing, for example, in the forearm, pronation and supination.

4. Condyloid or ellipsoidal joints include the radiocarpal joint and the metacarpophalangeal joints. One articular surface is oval and the other elliptical; movement can occur in two planes. For example, at the radiocarpal joint, there is both flexion and extension and radial and ulnar deviation.

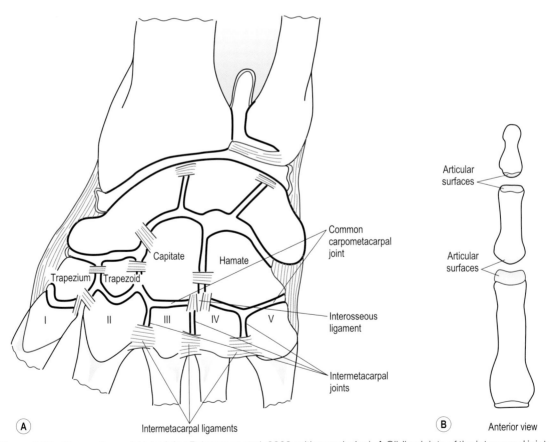

Figure 2.20 • Types of synovial joint (after Palastanga et al. 2002, with permission). A Gliding joints of the intercarpal joints at the wrist. B Hinge: interphalangeal joints.

(Continued)

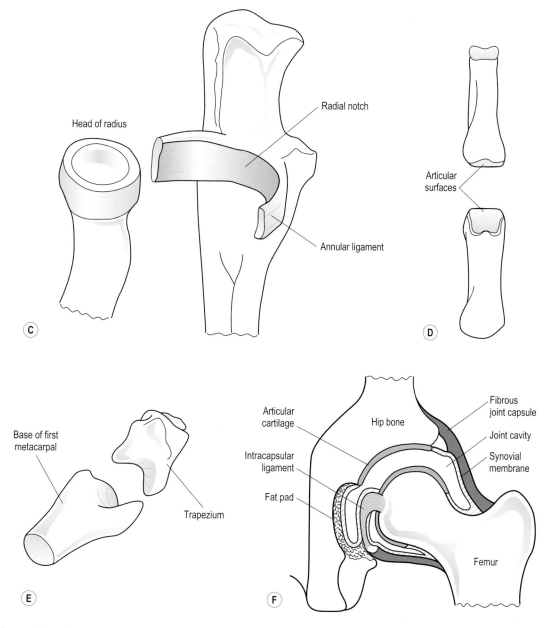

Figure 2.20—Cont'd • C Pivot: superior radioulnar joint. D Condyloid: metacarpophalangeal joint of the thumb. E Saddle: carpometacarpal of the thumb. F Ball and socket: hip joint.

5. Saddle joints include the first carpometacarpal joint, pisotriquetral joint and lumbar zygapophyseal joints (MacConaill 1953). The shape of the articular surfaces is like the saddle on a horse: each articular surface is reciprocally concave in one plane and convex in another, sometimes referred to as sellar (MacConaill

1953). Like the condyloid joints, movement occurs in two planes, allowing flexion and extension and abduction and adduction.

6. Ball and socket joints include the glenohumeral and hip joints. One articular surface is shaped like a ball and the other articular surface is shaped as a hand, which holds the ball. Movement occurs in three planes of movement, allowing flexion and extension, abduction and adduction, and medial and lateral rotation.

Joint movement

The study of the movement of joint surfaces is termed arthrokinematics. The type of movement at a joint surface can be classified as slide, roll, or spin:

- Slide or glide is a pure translation of one surface on another.
- Roll is when the bone rolls or rotates over the articular surface as a wheel rolls along the ground.
- Spin is pure rotation; it occurs at the humeroulnar joint during pronation and supination and at the hip and glenohumeral joint during flexion and extension (MacConaill 1966).

The movement that occurs at a plane (or gliding) joint is slide or glide, but at all the other types of joint (hinge, pivot, condyloid, saddle, ball and socket) movement is a combination of slide with roll or spin.

Movement at a joint is further complicated by conjunct rotation, where a secondary rotation occurs during a rotational movement. For example, during flexion of the elbow and the knee joint, there is lateral rotation of the humerus and femur, respectively (MacConaill 1966).

At any joint, there is potentially six degrees of freedom (Figure 2.21), which can be described in terms of movement in a plane, or according to the axis of movement (Oliver & Middleditch 1991). Movements according to the plane of movement are:

- rotation and translation in the sagittal plane
- rotation and translation in the coronal plane
- rotation and translation in the horizontal plane.

During lumbar spine flexion, for example, there is at each spinal level a combination of anterior sagittal rotation and anterior sagittal translation; during extension there is posterior sagittal rotation and posterior sagittal translation. The amount of sagittal rotation and translation at each segmental level during lumbar spine flexion and extension has been measured using three-dimensional radiographic analysis (Pearcy et al. 1984). At each level, there is 8–13° anterior sagittal rotation and 1–3 mm anterior sagittal translation; during extension there is 1–5° posterior sagittal rotation and 1° posterior sagittal translation (Pearcy et al. 1984). During lateral flexion, there is

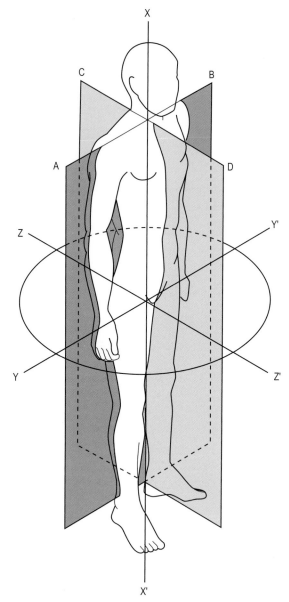

Figure 2.21 • Planes of the body and axes of movement. AB is the coronal plane, CD is the sagittal plane and the horizontal circle surrounding the person depicts the horizontal plane; XX' is the vertical axis, YY' is the frontal axis and ZZ' is the sagittal axis. (From Oliver & Middleditch 1991, with permission.)

approximately 3–10° of lateral rotation and 1–2 mm of lateral translation in the frontal plane, and during rotation approximately 2–3° rotation and 1–2 mm of translation in the horizontal plane (Pearcy & Tibrewal 1984).

Joint glide during physiological movements

Movement at a joint is a combination of roll or spin with a glide or translation; for example, during elbow flexion, the radial head rotates around the capitulum of the humerus and translates (that is, slides) anteriorly. During knee flexion, non-weight-bearing, the tibia rotates posteriorly around the femur and slides posteriorly. Because movement consists of both a roll or spin and a glide, the axis of movement constantly changes and is referred to as the instantaneous axis of rotation. Table 2.3 identifies, for each joint movement, the direction of the bone translation.

The direction in which the bone glides (or translates) depends upon the shape of the moving articular surface (Figure 2.22) (MacConaill 1966; Kaltenborn 1989). When the joint surface of the moving bone is concave, the glide usually occurs in the same direction as the bone is moving so that, with flexion on the knee joint (in non-weight-bearing), posterior glide of the tibial condyles occurs on the femoral condyles. When the joint surface is convex, the glide is usually in the opposite direction to the bone movement so that, with ankle dorsiflexion, there is a posterior glide of the talus on the inferior tibia and fibula. There is some evidence to suggest that this rule may not be valid in relation to movement of the glenohumeral joint (Brandt et al. 2007).

Another consideration is the relative size of the articular surfaces; for example, at the glenohumeral joint the head of the humerus has a much larger surface area than the glenoid cavity. The effect of this is that the head of the humerus, as it rolls, would run out of articular surface on the glenoid. This is overcome by a glide and also by accompanying movement of the scapula, during humeral movements (Norkin & Levangie 1992).

The examples given above refer to peripheral joints. The spinal joints follow the same principles but are worth describing separately here. Each spinal segmental level, between C2 and S1, consists of an interbody joint (two vertebral bodies and the intervening intervertebral disc) and two zygapophyseal joints (Oliver & Middleditch 1991), functionally a triad joint. The shape and direction of the articular surface of the zygapophyseal joints influence the gliding movement available at that segmental level (Table 2.4). The shape and direction of the articular surfaces vary throughout the spine (Table 2.5 and Figure 2.23).

Table 2.3 Direction of bone translation during active physiological movements

Movement	Translation
Glenohumeral	
Flexion	Anterior and superior
Extension	Posterior and inferior
Abduction	Inferior
Elbow: humeroulnar	
Flexion	Anterior
Extension	Posterior
Elbow: radiohumeral	
Flexion	Anterior
Extension	Posterior
Forearm: superior radioulnar	
Pronation	Posterior
Supination	Anterior
Forearm: inferior radioulnar	
Pronation	Anterior
Supination	Posterior
Wrist: proximal row of carpus on radius and ulnar	
Flexion	Posterior
Extension	Anterior
Radial deviation	Medial
Ulnar deviation	Lateral
Thumb: base of first metacarpal on trapezium	
Flexion	Anterior
Extension	Posterior
Abduction	Medial
Adduction	Lateral
Hip	
Flexion	Posterior
Extension	Anterior
Abduction	Medial
Adduction	Lateral
Knee, non-weight-bearing	
Flexion	Posterior
Extension	Anterior
Ankle, non-weight-bearing talus on tibia and fibula	
Dorsiflexion	Posterior
Plantarflexion	Anterior

The upper cervical spine, C0/C1 (between the occiput and atlas) and C1/C2 (between C1 and the axis) are, anatomically, rather different from the rest of the spine. The superior articular facets of C1 are concave and face upwards and medially;

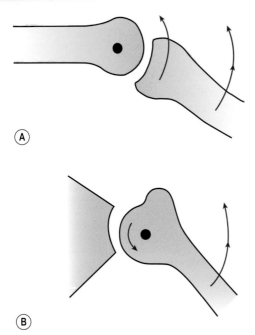

Figure 2.22 • Movement of articular surfaces during physiological movements. The single arrow depicts the direction of movement of the articular surface and the double arrow depicts the physiological movement. **A** With knee extension (non-weight-bearing), the concave articular surface of the tibia slides superiorly on the convex femoral condyles. **B** With shoulder elevation through abduction, the convex articular surface of the humerus slides inferiorly on the concave glenoid cavity. (From Kaltenborn 1989, with permission).

in addition, the lines of the two facets, when viewed superiorly, converge anteriorly (Figure 2.24A). The occipital condyles are reciprocally shaped. The shape of the facets at C0/C1 facilitates flexion and extension movement. As the head rotates forwards on C1, the occipital condyles slide (or translate) in a posterior direction, following the above principle of a convex surface moving on a concave surface (Figure 2.24B). With extension of the head on C1, the occipital condyles slide in an anterior direction.

The superior articular facets of C2 are large, oval and convex, and they lie in an anteroposterior direction. They face superiorly and laterally (Figure 2.25A). The inferior articular facets of C1 are reciprocally shaped. The shape of the facets at C1/C2 facilitates rotation. With rotation to the right, the right inferior facet of C1 glides posteriorly and slightly downwards (Figure 2.25B). The posterior movement produces the rotation movement, and the downward (inferior) movement produces a right

lateral flexion movement. Thus, at this segmental level, rotation to the right is accompanied by ipsilateral (right) lateral flexion. During flexion, the inferior facets of C1 glide backward on the superior facets of C2. During extension, the inferior facets of C1 glide forward.

In the cervical spine (C3–C7 levels) the superior articular facets are oval and flat and face upwards and backwards (Figure 2.23). During cervical spine flexion, the inferior articular facets of each cervical vertebra slide upward and forward on the superior articular facets of the vertebra below. For example, the inferior facets of C5 slide upward and forward on the superior facets of C6. On extension the reverse occurs throughout the cervical spine, so, for example, at C5/6, the inferior facets of C5 slide downward and backward on the superior facets of C6.

On right lateral flexion, the left inferior articular facets of each cervical vertebra slide upward and forward on the vertebra below, and on the righthand side the inferior articular facets slide downward and backward. If we consider the movement of the left inferior articular facets during the movement of right lateral flexion, the upward movement produces the right lateral flexion movement and the forward movement produces a right rotation movement. Thus, in the cervical spine, right lateral flexion is accompanied by right (ipsilateral) rotation.

On cervical rotation to the right, the left inferior articular facets at each cervical level glide upward, forward and laterally on the superior facet of the vertebra below (Figure 2.26). Once again, the opposite movement occurs on the other side: the right inferior articular facets glide downward, backward and medially on the vertebra below. On the left side, the forward movement (of the left inferior articular facet) produces the right rotation movement, and the upward movement produces a right lateral flexion movement. Thus, in the cervical spine, right rotation is accompanied by right (ipsilateral) lateral flexion. In summary, then, cervical lateral flexion is accompanied by ipsilateral rotation, and rotation is accompanied by ipsilateral lateral flexion.

In the thoracic spine the flat, triangular superior articular facets face backward and slightly upward and lateral (Figure 2.23). During thoracic flexion, the inferior articular facets at each level glide essentially upward, with some forward translation (Figure 2.27). On thoracic extension, the inferior articular facets glide downward with some backward translation. On left lateral flexion, the right inferior articular facets glide upward and slightly forward;

Table 2.4 Glide of inferior articular facets during physiological movements of the spine. Movement in parentheses denotes minimal amount of movement

	Flexion	Extension	Left lateral flexion	Right lateral flexion	Left rotation	Right rotation
C2–C7						
Left inferior articular facet	Upward Forward	Downward Backward	Downward Backward	Upward Forward	Downward Backward medial	Upward Forward lateral
Right inferior articular facet	Upward Forward	Downward Backward	Upward Forward	Downward Backward	Upward Forward lateral	Downward Backward medial
T1–T12						
Left inferior articular facet	Upward (Forward)	Downward (Backward)	Downward (Backward)	Upward (Forward)	Medial	Lateral
Right inferior articular facet	Upward (Forward)	Downward (Backward)	Upward (Forward)	Downward (Backward)	Lateral	Medial
L1–S1						
Left inferior articular facet	Upward (Forward)	Downward (Backward)	Downward (Backward)	Upward (Forward)		
Right inferior articular facet	Upward (Forward)	Downward (Backward)	Upward (Forward)	Downward (Backward)		

Table 2.5 Shape and direction of the superior articular surfaces of the zygapophyseal joints in the spine

Spinal level	Shape of superior facets	Direction of superior facets	Movement facilitated by direction of facets
C1	Concave	Upwards and medial	Flexion and extension
C2	Large, oval, convex	Upwards and lateral	Rotation
C2–C7	Oval, flat	Upwards and backwards	All directions
T1–T12	Triangular, flat	Backwards, slightly upwards and lateral	Rotation Lateral flexion
L1–L5	Concave	Backwards and medial	Flexion, extension, lateral flexion

the upward movement produces the lateral flexion, the forward movement produces a rotation movement to the left (ipsilateral). The left inferior articular facets glide in a reciprocal manner, that is, they glide downward and slightly backward. On rotation to the left, the right inferior articular facets glide laterally, while the left inferior articular facets glide medially. The combination of rotation and lateral flexion movements in the thoracic spine is not as straightforward as in the cervical spine. The coupled movements vary in different regions of the thoracic spine. At T2, lateral flexion is accompanied by ipsilateral rotation, whereas at T6 and T11 lateral flexion can be accompanied by ipsilateral rotation or contralateral rotation; the direction varies with individuals (White 1969).

In the lumbar spine, the superior articular facets are concave, facing backwards and medially (Figure 2.23). During lumbar flexion, the inferior articular facets glide upward and forward. On extension,

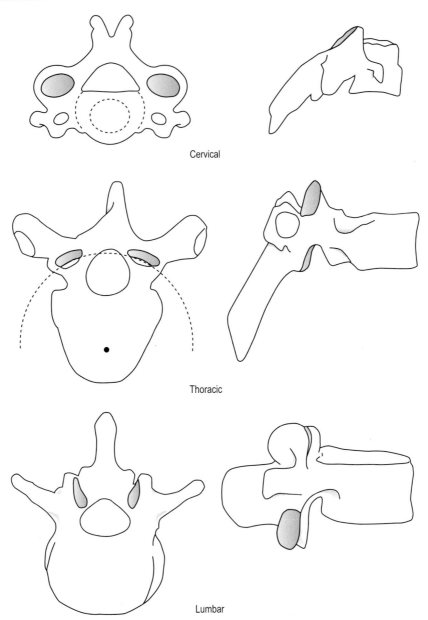

Cervical

Thoracic

Lumbar

Figure 2.23 • Direction of articular surfaces in cervical, thoracic and lumbar spine (from Palastanga et al. 2002, with permission). The superior articular facets of the cervical vertebrae face upwards and backwards, those of the thoracic vertebrae backwards and laterally, and those of the lumbar vertebrae backwards and medially.

the inferior articular facets glide downward and backward (Figure 2.28). The movement of the articular facets during lateral flexion is less clear. With lateral flexion, there may be ipsilateral or contralateral rotation (Pearcy & Tibrewal 1984). On lumbar rotation to the left (moving the trunk), the inferior articular facet on the right glides anteriorly and laterally to impact onto the superior articular facet of the vertebra below. The left inferior articular facet glides in a posterior and medial direction, so there is gapping of the joint space. Rotation of the lumbar spine from L1 to L4 is accompanied by contralateral lateral flexion, whereas rotation at L5/S1 is accompanied by ipsilateral lateral flexion (Pearcy & Tibrewal 1984).

Normal function of any synovial joint, then, requires the moving bone to rotate and translate.

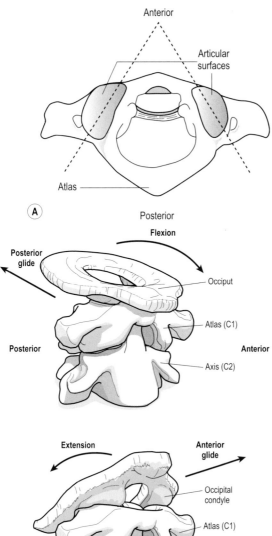

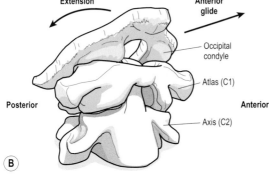

Figure 2.24 • A Superior surface of atlas (from Palastanga et al. 2002, with permission). Superior articular facets of C1 are concave and face upwards and medial. The lines of the two facets, when viewed superiorly, converge anteriorly. B Flexion and extension at the C0/C1 joint (after Edwards 1999, with permission). During flexion the occipital condyles glide posteriorly whereas during extension they glide anteriorly.

Each of these movements, rotation and translation, if normal, would be full-range, symptom-free, and with normal through-range and end-range resistance; normal muscle and nerve function is assumed. In the examination of a patient, normal rotation and translation is examined during active and passive physiological movements, and normal translation is examined during accessory movements; this is described in detail elsewhere (Maitland et al. 2001; Petty 2011).

A knowledge of the normal rotation and translation of bone during movement of a joint is important when attempting to restore normal joint function. Some examples may highlight this. The examples assume that the patient is lying prone with the spine in a neutral position. To facilitate an increase in cervical flexion at the C4/5 level, a central posteroanterior force with a cephalad inclination could be used on the C4 spinous process. This accessory movement will also enhance extension at the C3/4 segmental level. In the same way, to facilitate cervical lateral flexion or rotation to the right at the C4/5 level, a unilateral posteroanterior pressure with a cephalad inclination could be applied on the left C4 articular pillar. This accessory movement would also enhance ipsilateral lateral flexion and rotation at the C3/4 level.

In the thoracic spine, similar accessory movements could be used; the major difference is the greater downward obliquity of the middle four spinous processes, which would require the force to be in a more cephalad direction than in the cervical spine and possibly also positioning into flexion to achieve an enhancement of thoracic flexion.

In the lumbar spine, there have been quite a number of studies investigating the effect of a central posteroanterior mobilisation force to L3 or L4, in terms of stiffness and movement. Stiffness of a posteroanterior mobilisation has been found to:

- vary widely between asymptomatic subjects (Lee & Svensson 1993)
- increase with increased speed of application of the force (Lee & Evans 1992)
- increase with increased muscle activity (Lee et al. 1993; Shirley et al. 1999)
- increase in patients with low-back pain (Latimer et al. 1996)
- increase from cephalad to caudad: L5 is stiffest, then L4, then L3 (Edmondston et al. 1998)
- vary with the position of the spine: it is increased in flexion (32%) and in extension (12%) compared with neutral (Edmondston et al. 1998).

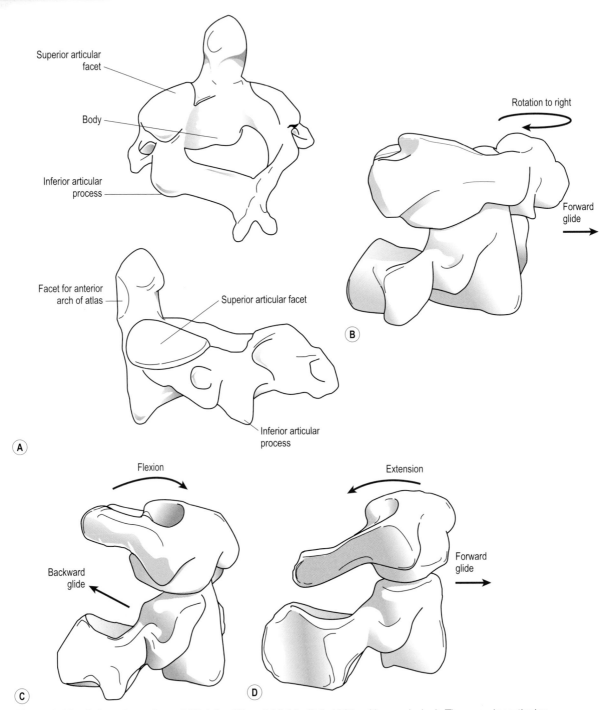

Figure 2.25 • **A** Superior surface of C2 (after Oliver & Middleditch 1991, with permission). The superior articular facets of C2 are large, oval and convex and face superiorly and laterally. **B** Rotation to the right at the C1/2 joint. The right inferior facet of C1 glides posteriorly and slightly downwards, while the left inferior facet of C1 glides anteriorly and slightly upwards (after Edwards 1999, with permission). **C** Flexion at the C1/2 joint: the inferior facets of C1 glide backward on the superior facets of C2. **D** Extension at the C1/2 joint: the inferior facets of C1 glide forward on the superior facets of C2.

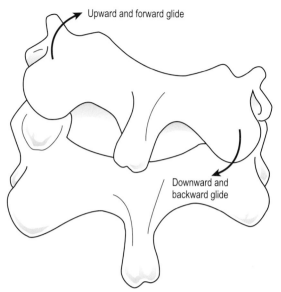

Figure 2.26 • Cervical rotation to the right is accompanied by lateral flexion to the right (after Oliver & Middleditch 1991, with permission). The left inferior articular facet glides upward and forward, while the right inferior articular facet glides downward and backward.

In terms of movement that occurs with a central posteroanterior pressure to L3 or L4, the following have been found:

- a generalised extension movement from T8 to S1 (Lee & Svensson 1993)
- more movement at the caudad level than at the cephalad level, apart from L5 (Lee & Evans 1992)

- a sustained central posteroanterior mobilisation results in a greater displacement and more generalised movement throughout the spine than an oscillatory movement (Lee & Svensson 1993)
- an increasing displacement over time with a sustained posteroanterior force, with nearly 70% of creep occurring in the first 30 seconds (Lee & Evans 1992).

The biomechanical nature of the posteroanterior force means that the composite tissues of the spine, as a whole, behave like viscoelastic tissues. For example, the displacement achieved when applying a posteroanterior force depends on the rate and time of loading. All of this research has focused on one or two levels of the lumbar spine and so the findings cannot be transferred directly to other types of spinal accessory movement or to different regions of the spine. However, it does provide, in a general sense, the biomechanical effects of spinal accessory movements.

Another concept is that of close pack and loose pack position of a joint. Close pack is where there is maximal congruency of joint surfaces, maximal tension in the joint capsule and ligaments, and least joint play; it is usually found at the extreme of range. Loose pack is any position other than close pack, where the joint capsule and ligaments are relatively slack and there is some joint play. Joint play is the amount of slack, or give, in the joint.

Knowledge of the close-packed and loose-packed positions of a joint helps with determining which

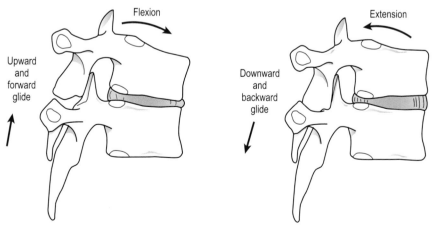

Figure 2.27 • Flexion and extension movements in the thoracic spine (after Palastanga et al. 2002, with permission). During flexion the inferior articular facets glide upward and slightly forward, and on extension the inferior articular facets glide downward and slightly backward.

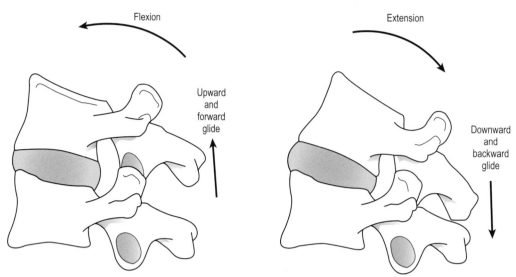

Figure 2.28 • Flexion and extension in the lumbar spine (after Palastanga et al. 2002, with permission). During lumbar flexion the inferior articular facets glide upward and forward, while on extension they glide downward and backward.

joint movements cause compression and which cause distraction of the adjacent articular surfaces. The position of the joint at the time of injury can ultimately predict the injury that occurs. For example, in a close-packed position, the application of force is likely to lead to a bony injury, as, in this position, the congruency of the adjoining bones enables the force to be taken up through the bone rather than the supporting ligaments/capsular structures, e.g. a Colles fracture sustained by a fall on the outstretched hand and the wrist joint in extension. With the wrist in flexion, a loose-packed position, it is more likely that a capsular or ligamentous injury will occur as the force of impact is taken up by the supporting soft-tissue structures. In the lower limb, for example, an anterior cruciate ligament tear may be sustained with the knee in a flexed and rotated position (Hertling & Kessler 2006a).

Biomechanics of normal joint movement

The normal function of most joints is to allow full-range movement of the adjacent bones. As the bones move towards the end-range of joint movement, resistance to movement increases (Wright & Johns 1961; Nigg & Herzog 1999) as the surrounding joint capsule, ligaments and muscles become taut (Wright & Johns 1961), eventually causing movement to stop. This is a protective mechanism so that the joint does not sublux or dislocate. Force–displacement curves from physiological movements at the knee and at the finger are shown in Figure 2.29, while curves from accessory movements of the lumbar spine, knee and shoulder are shown in Figure 2.30; these curves identify the increasing resistance from the beginning of range to the end of range.

End-feel

Different joints are limited by different structures at the end of a particular range of movement. For example, elbow extension is limited by bony opposition of the olecranon process of the ulna in the olecranon fossa, knee flexion is limited by soft-tissue opposition between the calf and the thigh, and wrist flexion is limited by the wrist dorsal ligaments as well as the bony configuration of the carpus. This resistance at the end of range of a joint movement and when felt by a clinician is referred to as end-feel. End-feel varies for different movements in different joints, whether pathology is present or not. It is used in clinical assessment of joint movement. The testing of end-feel can be performed for both physiological and accessory movements.

Classification of end-feel as normal or pathological is based on the ability to interpret the movement occurring at the joint, in conjunction with anatomical knowledge and the point in the range at which the resistance is felt. End-feel can be normal or indicative of pathology, and therefore requires interpretation by an experienced clinician.

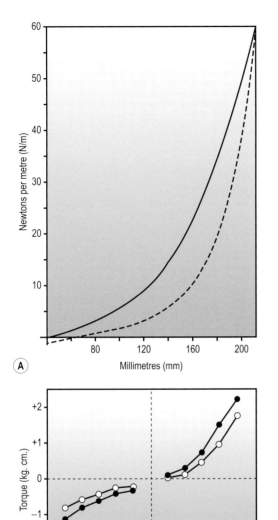

(A) Millimetres (mm) / Newtons per metre (N/m)

(B) Extension   Displacement (radian)   Flexion
● Total
○ Elastic

Figure 2.29 • Force–displacement curves for physiological movements. **A** The last 20–30° of passive knee extension (from Tindle 1987, with permission). The dotted line depicts the unloading curve and, where it crosses the x-axis, demonstrates the increase in length. **B** Finger metacarpophalangeal flexion and extension (after Wright & Johns 1961, with permission).

- Capsular end-feel: a firm, leathery feeling (Cyriax 1982; Kaltenborn 1989; Kesson & Atkins 2004; Hertling & Kessler 2006b), considered normal when felt at the end of some ranges of movement, e.g. lateral rotation of the shoulder/hip. It is considered

abnormal when felt early in the range, and may be indicative of early degenerative changes in a joint.

- Bony end-feel: occurs normally at end-range when there is bony apposition of approximating surfaces, e.g. full-range elbow extension. This end-feel is considered abnormal when occurring before expected end-range and may indicate degenerative change or malunion of an intra-articular fracture.

- Soft-tissue end-feel: a soft feeling at the end of range occurs when muscular tissue is approximated, as in elbow flexion and knee flexion. It may be considered abnormal if joint range of motion is restricted due to muscle hypertrophy (Cyriax 1982; Kaltenborn 1989; Hertling & Kessler 2006b).

- Ligamentous end-feel: this is a firm end-feel with no appreciable give, and may be felt when applying an abduction/adduction force to an extended knee. Any notable give may be due to ligamentous damage.

Abnormal end-feel may be categorised as follows:

- Hard end-feel: seen in capsular and degenerative pathology. End-feel is harder than expected and/ or occurs earlier in the range (Kesson & Atkins 2004; Hertling & Kessler 2006b).

- Springy end-feel: often occurs in the presence of a loose body; full range of joint movement is not achieved and an abnormal 'bouncy' feeling is experienced by the clinician at the end of the available range (Kesson & Atkins 2004).

- Muscle spasm end-feel: often occurs with pain; end-feel is that of an abrupt stop to movement, often with visible muscle contraction present as a 'guarding' mechanism to prevent further movement.

- Empty end-feel: rare, but of high clinical significance. The sensation is described as 'empty' as the examiner experiences no resistance to continuation of movement, but the patient halts the movement due to severe pain. Interpretation of this response must be treated with caution but may be indicative of neoplasm, fracture, septic arthritis or acute bursitis.

Functional movement

While movement at an individual joint can occur, functional activities often involve movement throughout the limb. For example, in standing, when a person bends at the knees this will be accompanied by hip flexion and ankle dorsiflexion. This predictable

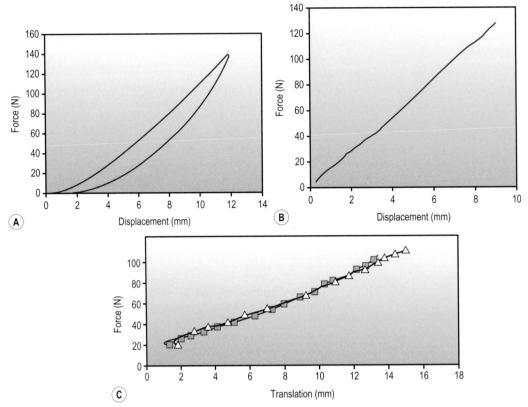

Figure 2.30 • Force–displacement curves for accessory movements. **A** Central posteroanterior glide to L3, loading and unloading curves (from Petty et al. 2002, with permission). **B** Anteroposterior glide on the tibia with the knee in slight flexion (from Petty et al. 2002, with permission). **C** Posteroanterior to the glenohumeral joint in 90° abduction and in neutral, internal and external rotation (from McQuade et al. 1999, with permission).

movement pattern can be referred to as a closed kinematic chain, a term used in engineering for linkages that make up a system. In contrast, the unpredictable movement patterns that can occur in the upper limb (and the lower limb when not weight-bearing) can be termed an open kinematic chain. The concept of open and closed kinematic chains is useful in that it highlights that movement involves a number of joints, and rarely does a joint move in isolation. Furthermore, these patterns are used in clinical practice in varying stages of rehabilitation to mimic normal functional movement.

Proprioception

Joint stability occurs through the integration of dynamic and mechanical restraints (Richie 2001;

Myers et al. 2006). Dynamic restraints pertain to the joint capsule, ligaments, bony anatomy and intra-articular pressures while mechanical restraints include muscle activation and the force produced from this muscle activity. These dynamic and mechanical restraints are mediated by the sensorimotor system, which includes sensory, motor, central integration and processing components. When functioning optimally, this provides a feedforward/feedback system, where mechanical restraints provide neural feedback to the central nervous system. This in turn provides feedback to the dynamic restraints (Richie 2001; Myers et al. 2006).

Proprioception is part of this system and forms the afferent feedback from joint and soft-tissue mechanoreceptors, present in muscle, ligaments, joint capsule and fascia, through mechanical and dynamic restraints. Proprioception, by definition, is a perception of position and movement gained from skin, joint and muscle receptors (Strasmann et al. 1990; Grigg 1994). It has three main components: joint position sense, kinaesthesia and sensation of force. Damage to the joint, ligaments, muscle or skin can affect this feedback system and thus cause a loss of proprioception which may ultimately lead to muscle, joint and/or nerve dysfunction.

Joint dysfunction

Just as the function of joints depends on the function of muscles and nerves, so dysfunction of joints can lead to dysfunction in muscles and nerves. They are dependent on each other in both normal and abnormal conditions, and this relationship is depicted in Figure 2.31. The following examples explore how joint dysfunction is often accompanied by muscle and/or nerve dysfunction.

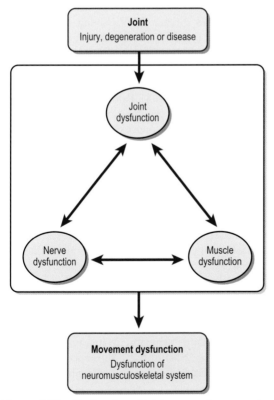

Figure 2.31 • Dysfunction of joint can produce muscle and/or nerve dysfunction.

Joint pathology and muscle/nerve dysfunction

There is overwhelming evidence that pathology in a joint can lead to weakness of the overlying muscle and deficits in neuromuscular control (Hurley 1997; Myers & Lephart 2000). This has been demonstrated in the knee in the presence of a variety of pathologies: rheumatoid arthritis (deAndrade et al. 1965); osteoarthritis (deAndrade et al. 1965; Hurley & Newham 1993; Hurley 1997); ligamentous knee injuries (Kennedy et al. 1982; Newham et al. 1989; Hurley et al. 1992, 1994; Snyder-Mackler et al. 1994; DeVita et al. 1997; Urbach & Awiszus 2002) and following meniscectomy (Stokes & Young 1984; Shakespeare et al. 1985; Hurley et al. 1994; Suter et al. 1998); in the elbow in the presence of rheumatoid arthritis (Hurley et al. 1991); and in the glenohumeral joint in the presence of anterior dislocation (Keating & Crossan 1992). The inhibition of muscle is thought to be due to inhibitory (Iles et al. 1990; Suter & Herzog 2000; Torry et al. 2000) or abnormal (Hurley et al. 1991; Hurley & Newham 1993) input from joint afferents. Thus, joint pathology leads to altered nervous system activity, which leads to altered muscle activity.

Joint immobilisation and muscle/nerve dysfunction

Joint immobilisation can also have a negative effect on muscular and neural function. Joint immobilisation for 3 weeks has been shown to cause a reduced maximal voluntary contraction of the muscle around the joint, and a decrease in the maximal firing rate of motor neurones supplying muscle (Seki et al. 2001; Kazuhiko & Hiroshi 2007). Thus, immobilisation of a joint leads to muscle weakness and altered nervous system activity.

Joint instability and muscle/nerve dysfunction

Joint instability and ligament insufficiency have been shown to alter nervous system activity, which leads to altered muscle activity. Ligamentous insufficiency at the elbow joint (Glousman et al. 1992) and glenohumeral joint (Glousman et al. 1988) has been found to alter muscle activity over the elbow and shoulder region, respectively, when throwing. In the lower limb, anterior cruciate ligament deficiency has been found to alter electromyographic (EMG) activity of quadriceps and hamstring muscle groups during knee movement (Solomonow et al. 1987) and gait (Berchuck et al. 1990). A cycle of events leading to dysfunction in ligament, muscle and nerve is shown in Figure 2.32 (Kennedy et al. 1982). Thus, ligamentous injury leads to altered nervous system activity, which leads to altered muscle activity, altered neuromuscular control and altered proprioception.

Proprioceptive deficits have been identified in human arthritic conditions, and are attributed to reduced activity of the joint, local muscle atrophy (Cuomo et al. 2005) and the presence of pain, where increased nociceptor activity causes a reduction in proprioception (Safran et al. 2001) and joint swelling. Although it was previously thought that swelling had a negative influence on proprioception, it is now believed that the loss of proprioception in the presence of swelling is more likely to be due to the nature of the fluid contents or the length of time the effusion is present, e.g. arthritic conditions (McNair et al. 1995; Palmieri et al. 2003).

It has also been hypothesised that loss of proprioceptive mechanisms either due to age or due to decreased muscle mass may initiate or accelerate arthritic damage through its effect on a joint's dynamic and mechanical restraints. This is well acknowledged in the literature, where ligamentous injury such as damage to the anterior cruciate ligament can affect postural control in both the injured

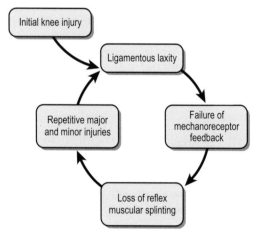

Figure 2.32 • A proposed cycle of progressive knee instability following an initial ligament injury (from Kennedy et al. 1982, with permission).

and uninjured side (Lysholm et al. 1998; Ageberg 2002), muscle fatigue can adversely affect joint proprioception (Blasier et al. 1993; Voight et al. 1996) and joint damage, such as in arthritic conditions, may evoke abnormal articular afferent information, causing subsequent loss of muscle activation (Hurley 1997) and altered neuromuscular control (Myers & Lephart 2000). Problems with muscle activation are also reported following joint injury and proprioceptive loss and can contribute to recurrent instability problems, through suppressed reflexive activation and slow coactivation patterns from muscles with stabilising roles (Myers et al. 2006).

Joint nociception and muscle dysfunction

Joint nociceptor activity directly affects muscle activity. Pain around the knee causes a nociceptive flexor withdrawal response: hip and knee flexion and ankle dorsiflexion. There is increased alpha motor neurone excitability of the muscles to produce this movement (Stener & Peterson 1963) and reciprocal inhibition of the knee extensors (Stener & Peterson 1963; Stener 1969; Young et al. 1987). For example, pressure or tension on a partially ruptured medial collateral ligament results in increased activity of sartorius and semimembranosus (knee flexors), with inhibition of vastus medialis (extensor) (Stener & Petersen 1963). Pain over the lateral femoral epicondyle leads to inhibition of the vastus medialis and lateralis, both knee extensors (Stener 1969), and pain from the lumbar zygapophyseal joint causes increased activity of the hamstring muscle group (Mooney & Robertson 1976). Nociceptor activity is thought to influence muscle activity via the alpha motor neurone (Wyke & Polacek 1975). Interestingly, activation of type I, II and IV receptors in the zygapophyseal joints of the cervical spine has more widespread effects than just the muscles around the neck; it also influences the muscles around the eye and mandible (Wyke & Polacek 1975).

Joint nociceptor activity can enhance joint dysfunction. In rats with inflammatory arthritis, joint nociceptors have been found to release substance P, and postganglionic sympathetic neurones to release catecholamines; both of these substances exacerbate joint inflammation (Levine et al. 1985b; Basbaum & Levine 1991).

Conversely, dysfunction in muscle is thought to lead to joint dysfunction. For example, abnormal eccentric force of quadriceps muscle is thought to be a contributing factor in anterior knee pain (Hughston et al. 1984), and muscle weakness may make a joint more vulnerable to injury (Stokes & Young 1984; Young et al. 1987; Keating & Crossan 1992). For example, quadriceps muscle weakness is thought to alter knee joint loading which may, in the long term, lead to osteoarthritis in the joint (Brandt 1997; Felson & Zhang 1998). Thus, joint dysfunction may occur as a result of a muscle dysfunction and this sequence of events is outlined in Figure 2.33.

Classification of joint dysfunction

The description of joint dysfunction flows directly from the description of normal joint function. The function of a joint is to transfer force from one bone to another and to permit limited movement (Nigg & Herzog 1999). Some joints, such as the sacroiliac joint, transmit very high forces and have hardly any movement, whereas other joints, such as the glenohumeral joint, transmit less force and have a large range of movement. The movement available at a joint includes physiological and accessory movements. The signs and symptoms of joint dysfunction are directly related to these functions, that is, there may be one or more of the following: reduced range of joint movement (hypomobility), increased range of joint movement (hypermobility), altered quality of movement or production of symptoms. A particular mix of these signs and symptoms occurs with a ligamentous sprain, and for clarity this is discussed in a separate section at the end of this chapter. Box 2.1 highlights these characteristics of joint function and dysfunction.

The signs and symptoms of joint dysfunction include reduced range of joint movement (hypomobility), increased range of joint movement

Box 2.1

Characteristics of joint dysfunction

Hypomobility or hypermobility
Altered quality of movement
Production of symptoms

(hypermobility), altered quality of movement and production of symptoms. These signs and symptoms can occur in isolation or in any combination.

Hypomobility

There may be hypomobility of one or more accessory movements and/or hypomobility of one or more physiological movements. It seems reasonable to suggest that if there is a reduced range of translation this will affect, to some degree, the range of rotation of the bone. In the same way, if there is a reduced range of rotation movement, this will affect the range of translation movement.

Limited range of accessory or physiological movement is often associated with an altered quality of movement. This is most commonly increased resistance to movement or production of symptoms; these are depicted in Figure 2.34.

Traumatised or pathological tissues, which may produce a physical resistance to further movement, include intra-articular structures, such as joint capsule, a torn meniscus or a loose body, and periarticular structures such as ligament, muscle or nerve overlying the joint. Each joint has its own unique range and resistance to movement owing to its particular intra-articular and periarticular arrangement. In the upper and lower limbs, the clinician compares the left and right side to determine normality for the patient, comparing the range of movement and the through-range and

Figure 2.33 • Effect of joint damage and/or immobilisation on muscle and nerve tissue (Reproduced, with permission, from Stokes M, Young A 1984 Clinical Science 67:7–14. © The Biochemical Society and the Medical Research Society.).

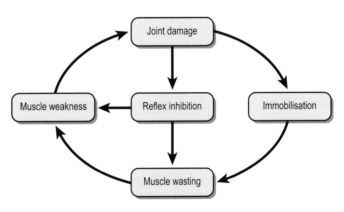

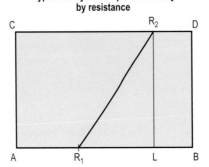

Hypomobility limited predominantly by resistance

Resistance is first felt (R_1) between ¼ and ½ range and increases to limit range (R_2) just beyond ¾ range (L)

Figure 2.34 • Movement diagram of hypomobility due to resistance or production of symptoms, where L is the limit of range, R_1 is the first point of resistance felt by the examiner, R_2 is the maximum intensity of resistance which limits further movement, P_1 is the point in the range where pain is first felt and P_2 is the maximum intensity of pain which limits further movement.

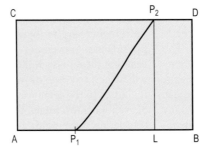

Hypomobility limited predominantly by pain

Pain is first felt (P_1) between ¼ and ½ range and increases to limit range (P_2) just beyond ¾ range (L)

end-range resistance to movement (Petty 2011). A comparison is made and the clinician judges any difference, while bearing in mind that range of movement varies from side to side in normal asymptomatic subjects. Where there is no other side with which to compare, as with central posteroanterior pressures of the vertebrae, the clinician can compare movement at adjacent levels, but again bearing in mind that there are normal differences in the range of movement at different segmental levels (Oliver & Middleditch 1991).

Limited range of accessory or physiological movements may be caused by the production of symptoms. Symptoms can be any sensation felt by the patient and can include pain, ache, pulling, pins and needles, numbness, a sense of something crawling along the skin, as well as apprehension by the patient to move further into range.

Hypomobility can be more fully appreciated by exploring the effects of immobilisation on joint structures, as this produces the most profound joint hypomobility.

Immobilisation

Knowledge of the effects of immobilisation on joint tissue has come about largely from research on animals, where it is possible to control the environment carefully, immobilise the joint, and then identify the changes that have occurred. Human joints undergo the same effects as the animal joint described below (Enneking & Horowitz 1972), and so this research aids our understanding of the effect of joint immobilisation in humans.

The timescales involved with rat knee joint immobilisation on the joint space, articular cartilage and subchondral bone are summarised in Table 2.6 (Evans et al. 1960). Within 15 days there is connective tissue filling the joint space and the formation of adhesions between the connective tissue and the articular cartilage. At 1 month there is atrophy of the opposing articular cartilage, and at 2 months the formation of dense adhesions, more widespread atrophy and ulceration of the articular cartilage and erosion of subchondral bone. All the knees investigated following immobilisation had reduced range of movement and joint stiffness due to the connective tissue and adhesion formation in the joint space (Evans et al. 1960).

The detailed effect of immobilisation on joint capsule, synovial membrane, ligament and articular cartilage has also been investigated. The fibrils within the joint capsule and synovial membrane have been

Table 2.6 Effect of immobilisation on joint

Tissue	Time (Evans et al. 1960)	Effect	Study
Joint space	15 days; well established at 1 month	Fibrofatty connective tissue appears within the joint space	Evans et al. 1960
Adhesions	15 days; dense at 2 months	Adhesions between the fibrofatty connective tissue and the articular cartilage	Evans et al. 1960
Articular cartilage	1 month 2 months 2 months	Atrophy of opposing articular cartilage Atrophy of unapposing cartilage Ulceration of articular cartilage	Evans et al. 1960
Subchondral bone	2 months 2 months	Under an area of articular cartilage lesion proliferation of very vascular connective tissue Erosion of subchondral bone	Evans et al. 1960
Synovial membrane		Reduced ability of fibres to glide	Akeson et al. 1987
Joint capsule		Reduced ability of fibres to glide	Akeson et al. 1987

found to have a reduced ability to glide (Akeson et al. 1987). The ligament undergoes alterations in its water and glycosaminoglycans content, degradation in collagen synthesis, increase in collagen cross-links after 9 weeks, bone resorption at the bone–ligament junction, reduced stiffness and increased extensibility of the ligament and a reduction in load to failure (Box 2.2). The substantial change in the load–displacement curve of the rabbit femur–medial collateral ligament–tibia complex, after 9 weeks of immobilisation, compared with a control group is depicted in Figure 2.35 (Woo et al. 1988). The structural and mechanical effects of immobilisation and remobilisation of the bone–ligament–bone complex are depicted in Figure 2.36 (Woo et al. 1987).

The detailed changes of articular cartilage following immobilisation (Box 2.3) include reduced proteoglycan synthesis, softening of the articular cartilage, softening and reduced thickness, adhesions to the fibrofatty connective tissue in the joint space, and pressure necrosis where adjacent surfaces are in contact with chondrocyte death (Vanwanseele et al. 2002).

The position in which the joint is immobilised is important in determining the rate of the tissue changes. If a joint is immobilised in full flexion (Salter & Field 1960) or in a position where there is continuous compression of adjacent articular surfaces (Salter & Field 1960), degeneration of the articular cartilage can occur within 6 days, rather than 30 days (Box 2.3). With prolonged

Box 2.2

Effect of immobilisation on ligament

Effect on ligament	Author
Decrease in water content and glycosaminoglycan level in collagen at 9 weeks	Akeson et al. 1973
Initially an increase in collagen synthesis and degradation then a decrease in synthesis and degradation of collagen by 3 months	Amiel et al. 1983 Tipton et al. 1970
Increase in collagen cross-links at 9 weeks	Akeson et al. 1977
Decrease in cross-sectional area	Tipton et al. 1970
Increase in osteoclastic activity at the bone–ligament junction, causing an increase in bone resorption in that area	Woo et al. 1987
Reduced stiffness	Akeson et al. 1987
Increased extensibility	Akeson et al. 1987
Reduction in load to failure and reduction in energy-absorbing capabilities	Woo et al. 1987

immobilisation over 1 year, the ligaments and joint capsule contract, the joint space becomes obliterated with fibrous connective tissue and ossification occurs where the articular surfaces contact each other (Baker et al. 1969; Enneking & Horowitz 1972).

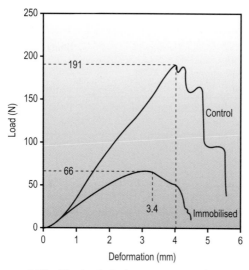

Figure 2.35 • The load–displacement curve of the rabbit femur–medial collateral ligament–tibia complex after 9 weeks of immobilisation compared with a control group (Reprinted with permission from Woo S, Buckwalter J. Injury and repair of the Musculoskeletal Soft Tissues. Rosemont, IL: American Academy of Orthopedic Surgeons, 1988.).

Hypermobility

Joint hypermobility is a condition in which synovial joints move excessively beyond normal limits, even after age, gender and race are taken into account (Grahame 2003). Joint hypermobility may be inherited (Ferrell et al. 2004) or acquired through years of training or stretching (Grahame 2003). In many cases it causes no symptoms and in some cases is considered advantageous in areas such as the performing arts. It is important to note that the presence of joint hypermobility with symptoms is given the term

Box 2.3

Effect of immobilisation on articular cartilage (Vanwanseele et al. 2002)

Decrease in proteoglycan synthesis
Softening of articular cartilage
Decreased thickness of articular cartilage
Adherence of fibrofatty connective tissue to cartilage surfaces
Pressure necrosis at points of cartilage–cartilage contact
Chondrocyte death

benign joint hypermobility syndrome (BJHS) but symptom-free presentation of joint hypermobility is simply referred to as joint hypermobility (Murray & Woo 2001; Simmonds & Keer 2007). BJHS refers to the existence of physical signs and symptoms in persons with generalised joint laxity in the absence of systemic rheumatological disease (Aktas et al. 2008). These hypermobility symptoms are considered in conjunction with other clinical signs and symptoms using a validated scoring system known as the Revised (Brighton 1998) Criteria for the Diagnosis of BJHS (Grahame et al. 2000). For those individuals who do have symptoms, these may include soft-tissue injury, arthralgias, myalgias, widespread pain, joint stiffness, clunking, popping, subluxations, dislocations, instability, as well as paraesthesiae, tiredness, faintness, feeling unwell, flu-like symptoms, skin fragility and laxity (Grahame 2003; Simmonds & Keer 2007).

As mentioned it is also possible for a person to experience joint hypermobility without the accompanying symptoms listed in the previous section. There may be hypermobility of one or more accessory movements and/or physiological movements

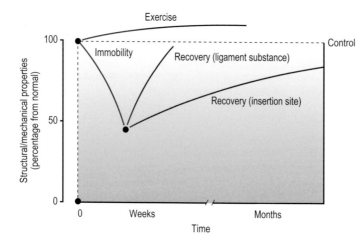

Figure 2.36 • The structural and mechanical properties of bone–ligament–bone complex following immobilisation and recovery (from Woo et al. 1988, with permission of the American Academy of Orthopaedic Surgeons).

in one or more joints. This increased range of motion may cause an increase in the range of translation of the joint surfaces or, conversely, an increase in translation may cause an increase in range of motion. This type of hypermobility may be inherited or may be due to injury/recurrent injury causing symptoms of increased joint range on active or passive testing.

Joint instability

Joint instability may be due to a deficit in the ligamentous, muscular and/or neural functioning around a joint. Instability refers to a significant reduction in the spine's ability to maintain the intervertebral neutral zones within their normal physiological boundaries, thus avoiding pain, deformity and neurological damage (Panjabi 1992a). This definition was put forward to describe instability of the vertebral column; however, it can be extended to include any joint. Instability may be further described as mechanical or functional in nature. Mechanical instability refers to laxity of a joint due to instability of the ligamentous tissues which support the joint (Hertel 2000). Functional instability refers to a subjective feeling of instability which can occur due to joint movement occurring outside voluntary control but not necessarily exceeding the physiological range of motion (Tropp et al. 1985). This is hypothesised to be due to the damage of the mechanoreceptors within the ligamentous structures following injury, which causes a reduction in perception of movement and particularly changes in direction (Tropp et al. 1985; Hughes & Rochester 2008). The relationship between the two is unclear, although mechanical instability can cause functional instability over time (Richie 2001).

Instability can occur in any region of the spine, but may be more common in the cervical and lumbar regions due to the anatomical arrangement of the joints, particularly in the cervical spine, which may predispose to instability owing to the large range of movement available. Instability of the spine occurs when the size of the neutral zone increases, causing uncontrolled or unstable movement patterns with an altered quality of movement, which the stabilising subsystems are unable to control (Panjabi 1992a; Olsen & Joder 2001). The causes of the increase in the neutral zone size include degenerative change and/or mechanical injury (Panjabi 1992a). As no clinical or diagnostic tests have been found to produce valid and reliable results for this condition, diagnosis can be challenging and requires careful interpretation by an experienced clinician (Cook et al. 2005). In a study by Cook et al. (2005) undertaken among physiotherapists, there was general agreement that the diagnosis of clinical cervical spine instability would be considered when symptoms such as reduced tolerance to prolonged static postures, fatigue, decreased ability to hold head up, improvement of symptoms with external support, frequent acute attacks and sharp pain triggered by quick movements were reported. Physical examination findings, including poor muscular control, poor muscle recruitment and dissociation of cervical movement, increased joint play on manual testing and poor-quality movement patterns including hingeing/ pivoting were reported as the most common physical signs that would lead a clinician to consider this diagnosis. Although this reporting is useful, there is still a lack of evidence on which to base decision-making regarding this condition.

As in hypomobility, the clinician makes a judgement that a joint has more movement than 'normal', which may be based on comparing sides or, in the spine, comparing adjacent levels. The presence of increased range of accessory and/or physiological movement may be associated with an altered quality of movement and can be associated with symptoms.

Altered quality of joint movement

Quality of movement includes instability, increased or decreased resistance to movement, poor control of movement, the presence of joint noise such as a clunk or crepitus, excessive effort or reluctance of the patient to move; in short, it is anything considered to be abnormal either by comparison with the other side or from the clinician's experience of what is 'normal'. Altered quality of movement can occur in an otherwise normal joint; for example, muscle weakness will cause active movement to be perceived as greater effort for the patient – there is altered quality of movement with no dysfunction of the joint. Altered quality of movement can be associated with altered joint range; often hypomobility is associated with increased resistance with or without production of symptoms, and hypermobility with reduced resistance and production of symptoms.

Altered quality of movement has been shown to occur with some pathologies. For example, patients with anterior shoulder instability have been found to have abnormal anterior glide of the humeral head on the glenoid cavity during arm movements (Howell et al. 1988). The joint lubricant in synovial fluid, SAPL, has been found to be deficient in osteoarthritic joints (Hills & Monds 1998) and this reduction causes increased resistance to joint movement (Hills & Thomas 1998).

Production of symptoms

Symptoms from joint dysfunction are most commonly a pain or an ache. Other symptoms include soreness, pulling and apprehension by the patient to move further into range. Symptoms can come on at any point, or increase through the joint range of movement and/or at the end of the range of joint movement. Sometimes a symptom is felt only during a part of the range, that is, through a particular arc of the movement, and if the symptom is pain it is then commonly referred to as an 'arc or catch of pain'. This would be documented, for example, as 'active shoulder abduction 120–140° produces lateral shoulder pain'. More commonly, symptoms are produced some time during the range and increase to the limit of range. The symptom may be sufficiently intense to be the cause of the limitation in range, depicted as P_2 on a movement diagram (Figure 2.37), or may reach a particular intensity at the limit of range (P'). Symptoms may be produced in a joint with 'normal', hypomobile or hypermobile range

of movement, with or without altered quality of movement. For further information on movement diagrams see Petty (2011).

Nociception and pain

Most of the tissues that make up a joint (capsule, ligament, articular disc, meniscus and fat pad) are innervated; in fact, the only structure that is not innervated is the avascular articular cartilage (Messner 1999). The nociceptors in joint are type IV free nerve endings and have been found throughout the joint tissues. In the knee, for example, they have been found in the collateral ligaments, joint capsule, synovium, cruciate ligaments, infrapatellar fat pad and the outer surface of the menisci (Kennedy et al. 1982). All of these tissues are therefore capable of being a source of pain. The type IV fibres that signal pain can be an unmyelinated meshwork, usually associated with blood vessels, or unmyelinated free nerve terminals lying between the collagen and elastic fibres of the connective tissue in which they lie (Messner 1999). These fibres are supplied by myelinated Aδ and unmyelinated C fibres.

Nociceptors in joint tissues can be activated by a noxious mechanical force or chemical stimulus

Pain limiting movement

Pain is first felt at ¼ range and increases to limit range (P_2) to ¾ range (L). Resistance is first felt at ½ range and increases to about 5/10 at limit of range

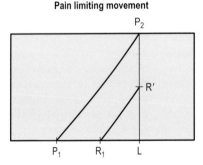

(A)

Figure 2.37 • Movement diagram depicting A P_2 with some resistance and normal range, and B P' and resistance limiting movement.

Resistance limiting movement

Resistance is first felt at ½ range and increases to limit range (R_2) to ¾ range (L). Pain is first felt at ¼ range and increases to about 3/10 at limit of range (where 0 is no pain and 10 is maximum pain ever felt by patient)

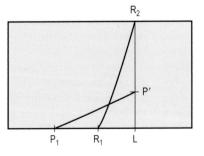

(B)

(Jessell & Kelly 1991). The effect of nociceptor activity by a mechanical or chemical stimulus alters the physiology of the nociceptor itself; in this way the nociceptor is plastic, that is, it changes. This increased sensitivity of nociceptors leads to a decreased pain threshold and increased pain to suprathreshold stimuli – changes collectively referred to as primary hyperalgesia. If a stimulus is applied which would normally not provoke pain, such as joint movement or light touch, and pain is provoked, this is termed allodynia (Raja et al. 1999). In addition, mechanoreceptors in adjacent uninjured tissue develop the ability to evoke pain, a phenomenon known as secondary hyperalgesia (Raja et al. 1999). This is thought to be due to an increase in the responsiveness of second-order nociceptor neurones in the spinal cord which become activated by mechanoreceptor activity, a response known as central sensitisation (Raja et al. 1999).

Because joint nociceptors are activated by a noxious mechanical force or chemical stimulus (Jessell & Kelly 1991), the pain from joint can be classified as mechanical or chemical nociceptive pain (Gifford 1998).

Mechanical pain occurs where certain movements stress injured tissue, increasing the mechanical deformation and activation of nociceptors; other movements reduce the stress on injured tissue, reducing the mechanical deformation and activation of nociceptors (Box 2.4). Thus, with mechanical pain, there are particular movements which aggravate and ease the pain, sometimes referred to as 'on/off pain'. The magnitude of the mechanical deformation may be directly related to the magnitude of nociceptor activity; this has been found in the skin of the cat where greater forces cause greater nociceptor activity (Garell et al. 1996).

Chemical nociceptive pain can be produced by the chemicals released as a result of inflammation, ischaemia or activity of the sympathetic nervous system (Gifford 1998).

Inflammation releases noxious chemicals into the tissues; these chemicals induce or sensitise activity of the nociceptors (Dray 1995; Levine & Reichling 1999), that is, hyperalgesia. It has been proposed that resting pain, pain with movement and pain on local pressure over a joint associated with joint inflammation are caused largely by sensitisation of group III and group IV fine articular afferents (Schaible & Schmidt 1985). Prostaglandin E_2 has been identified in inflamed tissue, and this is known to sensitise fine articular afferents (Schaible & Schmidt 1988). Experimentally induced knee joint inflammation of

---

Box 2.4

The effect of acute pain on respiratory, cardiovascular, gastrointestinal and genitourinary systems, and endocrine and metabolic function (Cousins & Power 1999)

Body system	Effect of acute pain
Respiratory	Splinting of abdominal and thoracic muscles
	Grunting on expiration
	Small tidal volume
	Rapid respiratory rate
Cardiovascular	Increased heart rate
	Increased blood pressure
	Increased cardiac output
	Decreased blood flow in the limbs
Gastrointestinal and genitourinary	Increased intestinal secretions
	Increased smooth-muscle tone
	Reduced intestinal motility
	Urinary retention
	Nausea, vomiting
Endocrine and metabolic function	Altered metabolic rate

---

the cat results in a spontaneous discharge from free nerve endings, increased frequency of discharge and reduced threshold for activation by movement (Coggeshall et al. 1983; Schaible & Schmidt 1985; Grigg et al. 1986). In the rat, some joint afferents and some nociceptors have been found to contain proinflammatory chemicals (Levine et al. 1985a, b; Salo & Theriault 1997); this suggests that mechanoreceptors and nociceptors may contribute to the development of joint inflammation (Levine et al. 1985a, b; Holzer 1988).

The effect of joint inflammation on the dorsal horn of the spinal cord has also been investigated. Experimental inflammation in rat and cat ankle and knee joints has been found to cause spontaneous release of substance P, in the dorsal horn of the spinal cord, and this release is increased with passive movements of the inflamed joint (Oku et al. 1987; Schaible et al. 1990). This may account, at least in part, for the increase in pain when an inflamed joint is passively moved.

Clinical features of inflammatory pain (Box 2.4) are: redness, oedema and heat, acute pain and tissue damage, a close relationship of stimulus response and pain, a diurnal pattern with pain and stiffness worst at night and, in the morning, signs of neurogenic inflammation (redness, swelling or symptoms in the neural zone) and a beneficial effect of anti-inflammatory medication (Butler 2000).

In the cat, it has been demonstrated that knee joint inflammation causes an increased sensitivity of alpha and gamma motor neurones in the hamstring muscles to local pressure and to knee flexion and extension movements (Proske et al. 1988). The number of stimulated alpha motor neurones increased, while some gamma motor neurones were stimulated and others were inhibited. The authors consider this to be part of the flexor reflex pattern, with the inhibitory effect on some gamma motor neurones facilitating co-contraction, so that the knee is held in a position of maximum comfort (Proske et al. 1988).

Ischaemic nociceptive pain is caused by a lowered pH (acidosis) in tissues, which stimulates nociceptor activity (Steen et al. 1995). Lowered pH level is frequently related to both painful ischaemic conditions and painful inflammatory conditions (Steen et al. 1995). Clinical features of ischaemic pain are thought to be: symptoms produced after prolonged or unusual activities, rapid ease of symptoms after a change in posture, symptoms towards the end of the day or after the accumulation of activity, a poor response to anti-inflammatory medication and sometimes absence of trauma (Butler 2000).

In the presence of tissue injury or inflammation, the sympathetic nervous system activity can maintain the perception of pain or enhance nociception in inflamed tissue. Sympathetically maintained pain can occur with complex regional pain syndromes and may play a part in chronic arthritis and soft-tissue trauma (Raja et al. 1999). In rats with inflammatory arthritis, postganglionic sympathetic neurones have been found to release catecholamines, a substance that exacerbates joint inflammation (Levine et al. 1985a, b; Basbaum & Levine 1991).

Clinicians must also be aware of the possibility of joint infection, referred to as septic arthritis, which can occur in both natural and artificial joints. A number of possible organisms (bacterial, fungal or viral) can be responsible and possible associated factors are recent surgery or injection, human immunodeficiency virus (HIV) infection, immune deficiency, intravenous drug use or pre-existing systemic inflammatory arthritis. Local signs of inflammation will be present as well as systemic signs such as fever and chills.

The commonest symptom from a joint is pain. The perception of pain occurs in the central nervous system and is multidimensional, including sensory, physiological, affective, cognitive, behavioural and sociocultural factors. Almost all the tissues that make up joint, except for the articular cartilage, contain nociceptors and can therefore be a potential source of pain. Joint nociceptors are sensitive to mechanical deformation and chemical irritation and can thus produce mechanical or chemical nociceptive pain. Chemical irritation may be due to inflammation, ischaemia or sympathetic nervous system activity.

It should be noted that the information given here has focused on pain from joint tissue only. Clearly, pain may be felt from a number of tissues, including the skin, muscle and nerve overlying the joint. Muscle pain is discussed in Chapter 4, pain from skin and nerve is discussed in Chapter 6, and Chapter 8 provides a broad overview of pain.

Pain referral areas

Some generalisation can be made about the pattern of pain referral from bone, joint, capsule and ligaments. In general, pain does not usually cross the midline of the spine (Kellgren 1939; Cloward 1959), although this has been observed in some individuals (Hockaday & Whitty 1967; Mooney & Robertson 1976). Pain from more superficial tissue, regardless of whether that tissue is bone, joint or ligament, gives rise to more localised pain; deeper tissue gives rise to more diffuse pain that may be referred in a segmental distribution (Kellgren 1939, 1977; Inman & Saunders 1944). Pain from skin is the most localised and accurate (Inman & Saunders 1944), which would seem to make sense because it is the interface between the body and the world around. Because pain from bone, joint, capsule and ligament is diffuse and widespread, the area of a patient's pain will not directly relate to the source of the patient's symptom. For example, pain from the hip joint can produce anterior thigh pain without any pain actually over the joint (Grieve 1994).

The segmental distribution may be related to a dermatome or sclerotome (Figure 2.38). Dermatomes describe the segmental innervation of the skin, and sclerotomes the segmental innervation of bone (Inman & Saunders 1944). These charts provide a generalised segmental supply of skin and bone and are used clinically to interpret pain referral areas. However, there is such a wide variation of these areas between individuals that they are considered invalid (Hockaday & Whitty 1967; McCall et al. 1979).

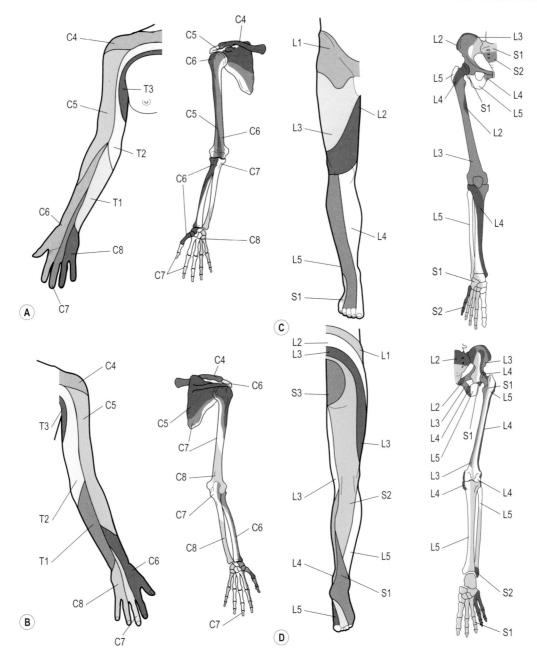

Figure 2.38 • Dermatomes and sclerotomes. In the upper and lower limbs: A anterior view; B posterior view. In the lower limbs: C anterior view; D posterior view. (From Inman & Saunders 1944, with permission).

Dermatome and sclerotome charts, therefore, need to be considered as a guideline for clinical practice.

Bone. The sensitivity of the various tissues to producing pain differs, with periosteum having the greatest sensitivity, followed by ligaments, joint capsules, tendons, fascia and finally muscle tissues (Inman & Saunders 1944). The sensitivity of the joint capsule and ligamentous tissue varies, and is greatest where it attaches to the periosteum (Inman & Saunders 1944). Superficial irritation of periosteum produces pain over the area, while deep irritation of periosteum causes more of a diffuse pain, which may be referred (Kellgren 1939). Some distributions of pain from the periosteum of the lumbar spine and the scapula are given in Figure 2.39.

Ligaments

The pattern of pain referral from provocative injection of saline into the interspinous ligament has been explored by a number of workers (Kellgren 1939; Inman & Saunders 1944; Hockaday & Whitty 1967). If the interspinous ligament is injected in the midline, pain is felt bilaterally, and if slightly to one side, pain is felt only on that side (Kellgren 1939), although occasionally injection on one side produces bilateral pain (Hockaday & Whitty 1967). The pattern of ache and deep tenderness felt by three subjects for each interspinous ligament from the C4/5 level to the sacrum is shown in

Figure 2.40. In a similar study with 28 subjects, it was found that referral to the arms was rare, with most pain felt around the posterior trunk (Hockaday & Whitty 1967). Two examples from injection of the interspinous ligament at C7/T1 and at T6/7 are shown in Figure 2.41. While there was consistency in the response on different occasions for any one individual, there was a large variation between individuals (Hockaday & Whitty 1967).

Joints

The pattern of pain referral from the cervical interbody joint has been explored with cervical discography (Cloward 1959; Holt 1964; Klafta & Collis 1969). This involves a provocative injection of radioopaque solution into the outer and middle parts of the intervertebral disc. Stimulation of the disc in

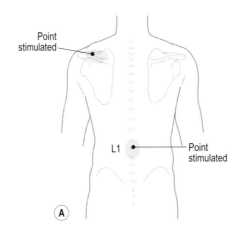

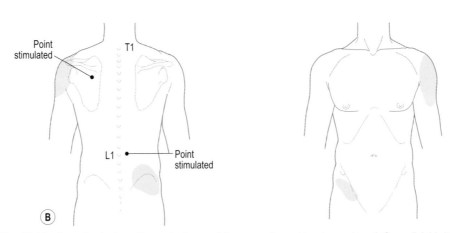

Figure 2.39 • Distribution of pain from the periosteum of the scapula and lumbar spine. A Superficial irritation of tip of scapula and L1 lamina. B Deep irritation of spine and infraspinous fossa of scapula. (Reproduced with permission, from Kellgren J H 1939 Clinical Science 4:35–46. © The biochemical Society and the medical Research Society (http://www.clinsci.org)).

the midline produced bilateral pain, and stimulation on one side produced unilateral pain (Cloward 1959). While there was variation between individuals, a consistent pattern of more caudad cervical levels producing more caudad thoracic pain was apparent (Cloward 1959). The pattern of pain referral from the anterior aspect of the disc differs from the pain referral from the posterior aspect (Figure 2.42). When the posterior aspect of the disc was stimulated, the pain was more intense and more widespread (Cloward 1959). Provocation to the left of the midline on the posterior aspect of C4/5 produced pain over the base

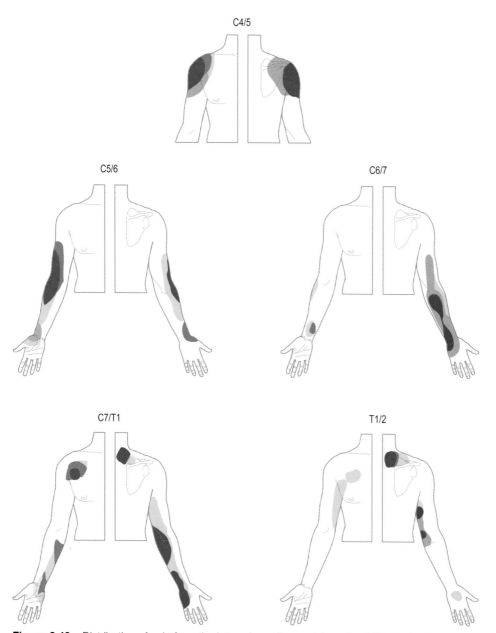

Figure 2.40 • Distribution of pain from the interspinous ligament from the C4/5 level to the sacrum (Reproduced with permission, from Kellgren J H 1939 Clinical Science 4:35–46. © The biochemical Society and the medical Research Society (http://www.clinsci.org)).

(Continued)

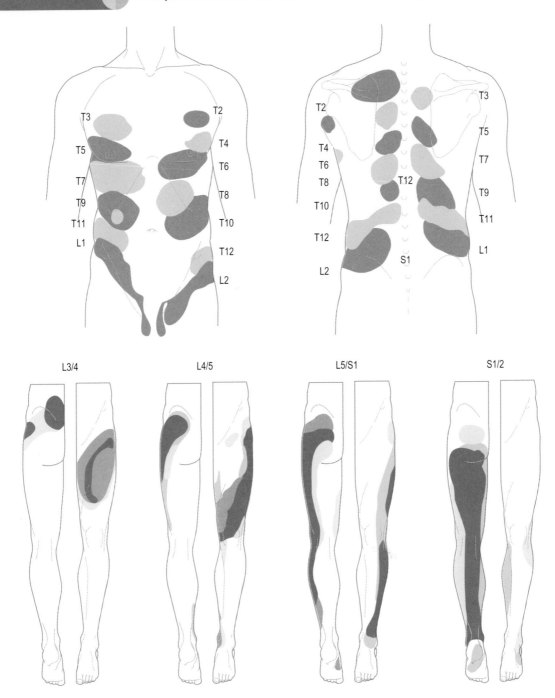

Figure 2.40 • —Cont'd

of the neck and top of the shoulder (Cloward 1959). These pain referral areas, however, were not substantiated by a similar study a few years later (Holt 1964). In 50 asymptomatic subjects, injection at each level between C3/4 and C7/T1 failed to produce any consistent pattern of pain referral (Holt 1964). The use of discography to identify the intervertebral disc as the source of the patient's symptoms is, however, limited (Holt 1964; Klafta & Collis 1969). For discs with degeneration or protrusion, injection

Figure 2.41 • A–D Distribution of hyperalgesia and pain from the interspinous ligament from C7/T1 and T6/7 (after Hockaday & Whitty 1967, with permission of Oxford University Press).

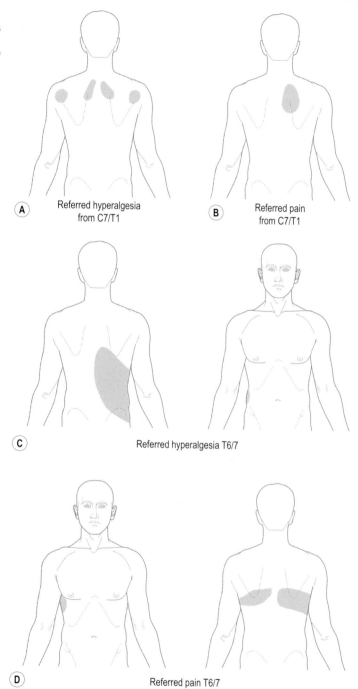

A   Referred hyperalgesia
from C7/T1

B   Referred pain
from C7/T1

C   Referred hyperalgesia T6/7

D   Referred pain T6/7

reproduced the patient's symptoms in only 20% or 30% of cases respectively (Klafta & Collis 1969). Interscapular pain, as well as chest pain, arm pain and occipital headaches, was found to be associated with C4/5, C5/6 and C6/7 disc pain (Brodsky 1985).

Pain arising from the lumbar zygapophyseal joints has been investigated by injection of saline into the joint cavity (Mooney & Robertson 1976; McCall et al. 1979). The extent of referral into the leg was dependent on the degree of irritation, greater

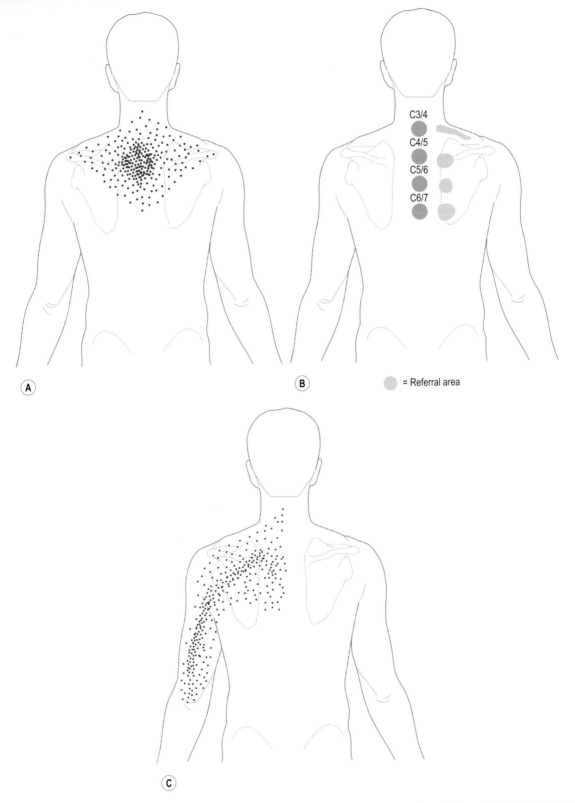

Figure 2.42 • **A** Referred pain from the anterior aspect of the cervical intervertebral discs between C3/4, C4/5, C5/6 and C6/7 (after Cloward 1959, with permission). **B** Referred pain from the posterior aspect and midline of the cervical intervertebral discs between C3/4, C4/5, C5/6 and C6/7. The midline dots indicate the area of referred pain from provocation of the midline of the disc, while the shaded areas to the right indicate the area of referred pain from provocation to the right of midline. **C** Referred pain from provocation to the left of midline at C5/6 and C6/7.

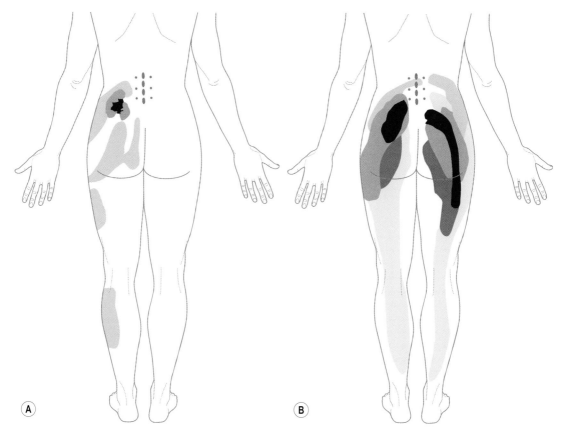

Figure 2.43 • Distribution of pain following saline injection into the zygapophyseal joints of **A** left L4/5 and L5/S1 levels of asymptomatic subjects, and **B** all three levels – L3/4, L4/5 and L5/S1 – of chronic low-back pain patients. (After Mooney & Robertson 1976, with permission.)

amounts of saline causing more distal symptoms (Mooney & Robertson 1976). Saline injection into the L4/5 and L5/S1 zygapophyseal joints of five asymptomatic subjects and 15 patients suffering chronic low-back pain is shown in Figure 2.43. Similar results in asymptomatic subjects were found with injection at the L1/2 and L4/5 zygapophyseal joints (McCall et al. 1979). Interestingly, the areas of referred pain from L1/2 and L4/5 are close and even overlap (Figure 2.44) – which makes interpretation of this information in the clinical field difficult. This is compounded by the fact that patients diagnosed with zygapophyseal joint pain with anaesthetic blocks have no clinical features in common (Schwarzer et al. 1994). So, while zygapophyseal joints can theoretically be a source of pain, clinicians are unable to identify this joint on the basis of a patient's clinical pain presentation.

Information on pain from the sacroiliac joint has been explored in 10 asymptomatic subjects by radiopaque injection into the joint (Fortin et al. 1994a).

Pain was felt fairly locally around the posterior superior iliac spine (Figure 2.45). In a further study, it was found that this area of referral could not be used to identify accurately patients with sacroiliac joint pain (Fortin et al. 1994b).

Pain arising from joints in the upper or lower limb tends to be localised around the joint. This localisation is greatest in the distal joints of the hand and foot, while the hip and shoulder can refer pain in a more segmental distribution (Kellgren 1939). Referral of pain from the tibiofemoral joint by provocation of the medial collateral ligament, lateral and posterior joint capsule is shown in Figure 2.46 (Kellgren 1939).

Joint injury: ligament tear and healing

Ligaments can tear in the middle region by avulsion of bone and, more rarely, at the insertion site (Woo et al. 1988). Untreated ligaments have been shown

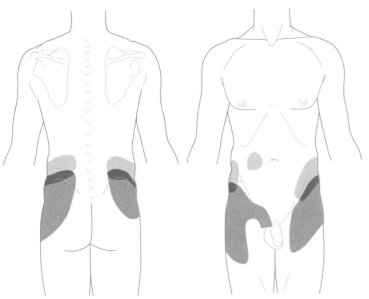

Figure 2.44 • Distribution of pain following injection of saline into the L1/2 (lighter shading) and L4/5 (darker shading) zygapophyseal joint (after McCall et al. 1979, with permission).

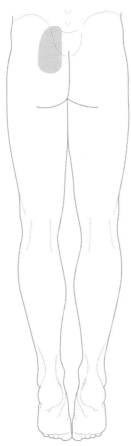

Figure 2.45 • Distribution of pain from the sacroiliac joint (after Fortin et al. 1994a, with permission).

Posterior   Anterior

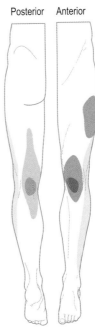

Figure 2.46 • Referred pain from the knee: from medial collateral ligament – horizontal hatching; lateral joint capsule – stippling; posterior joint capsule – vertical hatching (reproduced, with permission, from Kellgren 1939. © The Biochemical Society and the Medical Research Society).

to repair by scar tissue formation that is inferior to the original ligamentous tissue (Frank et al. 1983). The natural repair process of ligamentous tissue has been observed in rabbit knees by experimentally transecting the medial collateral ligament (Frank et al. 1983). Granulation tissue bridged the gap between the ligament ends within 10 days, with hypertrophy at 3 weeks. Remodelling then occurred so that the ligament looked normal by 14 weeks. Normal ligamentous tissue is made up of type I collagen; ligamentous scar tissue, however, consists of type III collagen, giving the ligament less stiffness and strength than before the injury (Woo & Akeson 1987). In the skin, maturation causes a gradual reduction in the type III collagen (Forrest 1983); however, in ligaments even after 40 weeks, there are still significant amounts of type III collagen (Woo & Akeson 1987). Healing can be considered to occur in three stages: an inflammatory response lasting approximately 72 hours, a proliferation phase lasting several weeks and finally the remodelling and maturation phase, which can take 1–2 years (Vicenzino et al. 2002). The reader is directed to the numerous pathology textbooks for further information on inflammation and healing.

Following a joint sprain, such as a sprained ankle with a tear of the lateral ligament, the dysfunction is more localised to specific movements. Typically, with a lateral ligament sprain, the movements of the foot which cause tension on the lateral ligament are limited in range and may give rise to pain. So the movement dysfunction, in this case, is hypomobility due to resistance and pain produced by plantarflexion, inversion and perhaps anteroposterior and posteroanterior glides of the talus.

Joint effusion may accompany a joint injury and, if excessive, can impair synovial nutrition (Jayson & Dixon 1970a). Knee joint pressure is generally greatest in extension and is reduced at about 30° flexion, which corresponds to the position of ease that a patient often finds in a swollen joint (Jayson & Dixon 1970b).

Common joint dysfunctions seen clinically are hypomobility limited by resistance or pain, hypermobility with and without symptoms such as pain and proprioceptive deficits, altered quality of movement and the production of symptoms. Joint dysfunction does not exist in isolation. Not only may there be a number of movements affected at any one joint, and a number of joints affected, but muscle and nerve tissue will also, to some degree, always be involved.

References

Adams, M.A., Bogduk, N., Burton, K., et al., 2002. The biomechanics of back pain. Churchill Livingstone, Edinburgh.

Ageberg, E., 2002. Consequences of a ligament injury on neuromuscular function and relevance to rehabilitation using the anterior cruciate ligament-injured knee as model. J. Electromyogr. Kinesiol. 12, 205–212.

Akeson, W.H., Woo, S.L-Y., Amiel, D., et al., 1973. The connective tissue response to immobility: biochemical changes in periarticular connective tissue of the immobilized rabbit knee. Clin. Orthop. Relat. Res. 93, 356–362.

Akeson, W.H., Amiedl, D., Mechanic, G.L., et al., 1977. Collagen cross-linking alterations in joint contractures: changes in the reducible cross-links in periarticular connective tissue collagen after nine weeks of immobilization. Connect. Tissue Res. 5, 15–19.

Akeson, W.H., Amiel, D., Abel, M.F., et al., 1987. Effects of immobilization on joints. Clin. Orthop. Relat. Res. 219, 28–37.

Aktas, I., Ofluoglu, D., Albay, T., 2008. The relationship between benign joint hypermobility syndrome and carpal tunnel syndrome. Clin. Rheumatol. 27, 1283–1287.

Albright, D.J., Zimny, M.L., Dabezies, E., 1987. Mechanoreceptors in the human medial meniscus. Anat. Rec. 218, 6A–7A.

Amiel, D., Akeson, W.H., Harwood, F.L., et al., 1983. Stress deprivation effect on metabolic turnover of the medial collateral ligament collagen, a comparison between nine- and 12-week immobilization. Clin. Orthop. Relat. Res. 172, 265–270.

Askew, M.J., Mow, V.C., 1978. The biomechanical function of the collagen fibril ultrastructure of articular cartilage. J. Biomech. Eng. 100, 105–115.

Baker de, W.C., Thomas, T.G., Kirkaldy-Willis, W.H., 1969. Changes in the cartilage of the posterior

intervertebral joints after anterior fusion. J. Bone Joint Surg. 51B (4), 736–746.

Basbaum, A.I., Levine, J.D., 1991. The contribution of the nervous system to inflammation and inflammatory disease. Can. J. Physiol. Pharmacol. 69, 647–651.

Blasier, R.B., James, E.C., Laura, J.H., 1993. Shoulder proprioception: effect of joint laxity, joint position, direction of motion, and muscle fatigue. Orthop. Rev. 23, 45–50.

Bogduk, N., 1997. Clinical anatomy of the lumbar spine and sacrum, third ed. Churchill Livingstone, New York.

Brandt, K.D., 1997. Putting some muscle into osteoarthritis. Ann. Intern. Med. 127 (2), 154–156.

Brandt, C., Sole, G., Krause, M.W., et al., 2007. An evidence-based review on the validity of the Kaltenborn rule as applied to the glenohumeral joint. Man. Ther. 12 (1), 3–11.

Brodsky, A.E., 1985. Cervical angina, a correlative study with emphasis on the use of coronary arteriography. Spine 10 (8), 699–709.

Butler, D.S., 2000. The sensitive nervous system. Noigroup, Adelaide.

Clark, F.J., 1975. Information signaled by sensory fibers in medial articular nerve. J. Neurophysiol. 38, 1464–1472.

Clark, F.J., Burgess, P.R., 1975. Slowly adapting receptors in cat knee joint: can they signal joint angle? J. Neurophysiol. 38, 1448–1463.

Cloward, R.B., 1959. Cervical discography: a contribution to the etiology and mechanism of neck, shoulder and arm pain. Ann. Surg. 150, 1052–1064.

Coggeshall, R.E., Hong, K.A.H.P., Langford, L.A., et al., 1983. Discharge characteristics of fine medial articular afferents at rest and during passive movements of inflamed knee joints. Brain Res. 272, 185–188.

Cook, C., Brismée, J.M., Fleming, R., et al., 2005. Identifiers Suggestive of Clinical Cervical Spine Instability: A Delphi Study of Physical Therapists. Phys. Ther. 85 (9), 895–906.

Cooper, R.R., Misol, S., 1970. Tendon and ligament insertion: a light and electron microscopic study. J. Bone Joint Surg. 52A (1), 1–20.

Cousins, M., Power, I., 1999. Acute and postoperative pain. In: Wall, P.D., Melzack, R. (Eds.), Textbook of pain, fourth ed. Churchill Livingstone, Edinburgh, pp. 447–491.

Cuomo, F., Birdzell, M.G., Zuckerman, J.D., 2005. The effect of degenerative arthritis and prosthetic arthroplasty on shoulder proprioception. J. Shoulder Elbow Surg. 14 (4), 345–348.

Cyriax, J., 1982. Textbook of orthopaedic medicine – diagnosis of soft tissue lesions, eighth ed. Baillière Tindall, London.

deAndrade, J.R., Grant, C., Dixon St., A. J., 1965. Joint distension and reflex muscle inhibition in the knee. J. Bone Joint Surg. 47A (2), 313–322.

DeVita, P., Hortobagyi, T., Barrier, J., et al., 1997. Gait adaptations before and after anterior cruciate ligament reconstruction surgery. Med. Sci. Sports Exerc. 29 (7), 853–859.

Dray, A., 1995. Inflammatory mediators of pain. Br. J. Anaesth. 75, 125–131.

Edmondston, S.J., Allison, G.T., Gregg, C.D., et al., 1998. Effect of position on the posteroanterior stiffness of the lumbar spine. Man. Ther. 3 (1), 21–26.

Edwards, B.C., 1999. Manual of combined movements, second ed. Butterworth-Heinemann, Oxford.

Enneking, W.F., Horowitz, M., 1972. The intra-articular effects of immobilization on the human knee. J. Bone Joint Surg. 54A (5), 973–985.

Evans, E.B., Eggers, G.W.N., Butler, J.K., et al., 1960. Experimental immobilization and remobilization of rat knee joints. J. Bone Joint Surg. 42A (5), 737–758.

Felson, D.T., Zhang, Y., 1998. An update on the epidemiology of knee and hip osteoarthritis with a view to prevention. Arthritis Rheum. 41 (8), 1343–1355.

Ferrell, W.R., 1980. The adequacy of stretch receptors in the cat knee joint for signalling joint angle throughout a full range of movement. J. Physiol. 299, 85–99.

Ferrell, W.R., 1985. The response of slowly adapting mechanoreceptors in the cat knee joint to tetanic contraction of hind limb muscles. Q. J. Exp. Physiol. 70, 337–345.

Ferrell, W.R., Tennant, N., Sturrock, R.D., et al., 2004. Amelioration of symptoms by enhancement of proprioception in patients with joint hypermobility syndrome. Arthritis Rheum. 50, 3323–3328.

Forrest, L., 1983. Current concepts in soft connective tissue wound healing. Br. J. Surg. 70, 133–140.

Fortin, J.D., Dwyer, A.P., West, S., et al., 1994a. Sacroiliac joint: pain referral maps upon applying a new injection/ arthrography technique, part I: asymptomatic volunteers. Spine 19 (13), 1475–1482.

Fortin, J.D., Aprill, C.N., Ponthieux, B., et al., 1994b. Sacroiliac joint: pain referral maps upon applying a new injection/arthrography technique, part II: clinical evaluation. Spine 19 (13), 1483–1489.

Frank, C.B., Shrive, N.G., 1999. Ligament. In: Nigg, B.M., Herzog, W. (Eds.), Biomechanics of the musculo-skeletal system, second ed. John Wiley, Chichester, pp. 107–126.

Frank, C., Woo, S.L.-Y., Amiel, D., et al., 1983. Medial collateral ligament healing: a multidisciplinary

assessment in rabbits. Am. J. Sports Med. 11 (6), 379–389.

Freeman, M.A.R., Wyke, B., 1967a. Articular reflexes at the ankle joint: an electromyographic study of normal and abnormal influences of ankle joint mechanoreceptors upon reflex activity in the leg muscles. Br. J. Surg. 54 (12), 990–1001.

Freeman, M.A.R., Wyke, B., 1967b. The innervation of the knee joint. An anatomical and histological study in the cat. J. Anat. 101 (3), 505–532.

Fujiwara, A., Tamai, K., Yamato, M., et al., 1999. The relationship between facet joint osteoarthritis and disc degeneration of the lumbar spine: an MRI study. Eur. Spine J. 8 (5), 396–401.

Fuller, M.S., Grigg, P., Hoffman, A.H., 1991. Response of joint capsule neurons to axial stress and strain during dynamic loading in cat. J. Neurophysiol. 65 (6), 1321–1328.

Garell, P.C., McGillis, S.L.B., Greenspan, J.D., 1996. Mechanical response properties of nociceptors innervating feline hairy skin. J. Neurophysiol. 75 (3), 1177–1189.

Gifford, L., 1998. Pain. In: Pitt-Brooke, J., Reid, H., Lockwood, J., Kerr, K. (Eds.), Rehabilitation of movement, theoretical basis of clinical practice. W B Saunders, London, pp. 196–232.

Glousman, R., Jobe, F., Tibone, J., et al., 1988. Dynamic electromyographic analysis of the throwing shoulder with glenohumeral instability. J. Bone Joint Surg. 70A (2), 220–226.

Glousman, R.E., Barron, J., Jobe, F.W., et al., 1992. An electromyographic analysis of the elbow in normal and injured pitchers with medial collateral ligament insufficiency. Am. J. Sports Med. 20 (3), 311–317.

Gordon, S., Yang, K.H., Mayer, P., et al., 2001. Mechanism of disc rupture: a preliminary report. Spine 16 (4), 450–456.

Grahame, R., 2003. Hypermobility and hypermobility syndrome. In: Keer, R., Grahame, R. (Eds.), Hypermobility syndrome – recognition and management for physiotherapists. Butterworth-Heinemann, London.

Grahame, R., Bird, H.A., Child, A., et al., 2000. The revised (Brighton 1998) criteria for the diagnosis of benign joint hypermobility syndrome. J. Rheumatol. 27, 1777–1779.

Grieve, G.P., 1994. Referred pain and other clinical features. In: Boyling, J.D., Palastanga, N. (Eds.), Grieve's modern manual therapy, the vertebral column, second ed. Churchill Livingstone, Edinburgh, pp. 271–292.

Grigg, P., 1994. Peripheral neural mechanisms in proprioception. J. Sport Rehabil. 3, 2–17.

Grigg, P., Hoffman, A.H., 1982. Properties of Ruffini afferents revealed by stress analysis of isolated sections of cat knee capsule. J. Neurophysiol. 47 (1), 41–54.

Grigg, P., Hoffman, A.H., Fogarty, K.E., 1982. Properties of Golgi–Mazzoni afferents in cat knee joint capsule, as revealed by mechanical studies of isolated joint capsule. J. Neurophysiol. 47 (1), 31–40.

Grigg, P., Schaible, H.G., Schmidt, R.F., 1986. Mechanical sensitivity of group III and IV afferents from posterior articular nerve in normal and inflamed cat knee. J. Neurophysiol. 55 (4), 635–643.

Heppelmann, B., Messlinger, K., Neiss, W.F., et al., 1990. Ultrastructural three-dimensional reconstruction of group III and group IV sensory nerve endings ('free nerve endings') in the knee joint capsule of the cat: evidence for multiple receptive sites. J. Comp. Neurol. 292, 103–116.

Hertel, J., 2000. Functional instability following lateral ankle sprain. Sports Med. 29, 361–371.

Hertling, D., Kessler, R.M., 2006a. Arthrology. In: Hertling, D., Kessler, R. (Eds.), Management of common musculoskeletal disorders: physical therapy, principles and methods. Lippincott, Williams and Wilkins, Philadelphia, pp. 27–52.

Hertling, D., Kessler, R., 2006b. Assessment of musculoskeletal disorders and concepts of management. In: Hertling, D., Kessler, R.M. (Eds.), Management of common musculoskeletal disorders: physical therapy principles and methods. Lippincott, Williams and Wilkins, Philadelphia, pp. 61–107.

Hills, B.A., 1989. Oligolamellar lubrication of joints by surface active phospholipid. J. Rheumatol. 16 (1), 82–91.

Hills, B.A., 1995. Remarkable anti-wear properties of joint surfactant. Ann. Biomed. Eng. 23, 112–115.

Hills, B.A., Monds, M.K., 1998. Deficiency of lubricating surfactant lining the articular surfaces of replaced hips and knees. Br. J. Rheumatol. 37, 143–147.

Hills, B.A., Thomas, K., 1998. Joint stiffness and 'articular gelling': inhibition of the fusion of articular surfaces by surfactant. Br. J. Rheumatol. 37, 532–538.

Hockaday, J.M., Whitty, C.W.M., 1967. Patterns of referred pain in the normal subject. Brain 90 (3), 481–495.

Holt, E.P., 1964. Fallacy of cervical discography: report of 50 cases in normal subjects. J. Am. Med. Assoc. 188 (9), 799–801.

Holzer, P., 1988. Local effector functions of capsaicin-sensitive sensory nerve endings: involvement of tachykinins, calcitonin gene-related peptide and other neuropeptides. Neuroscience 24 (3), 739–768.

Hortobagyi, T., DeVita, P., 2000. Muscle pre- and coactivity during downward stepping are associated with leg stiffness in aging. J. Electromyogr. Kinesiol. 10, 117–126.

Howell, S.M., Galinat, B.J., Renzi, A.J., et al., 1988. Normal and abnormal mechanics of the glenohumeral joint in the horizontal plane. J. Bone Joint Surg. 70A (2), 227–232.

Hughes, T., Rochester, P., 2008. The effects of proprioceptive exercise and taping on proprioception in subjects with functional ankle instability: a review of the literature. Phys. Ther. Sport 9, 136–147.

Hughston, J.C., Walsh, W.M., Puddu, G., 1984. Patellar subluxation and dislocation, vol. 5. W B Saunders, Philadelphia.

Hurley, M.V., 1997. The effect of joint damage on muscle function, proprioception and rehabilitation. Man. Ther. 2 (1), 11–17.

Hurley, M.V., Newham, D.J., 1993. The influence of arthrogenous muscle inhibition on quadriceps rehabilitation of patients with early, unilateral osteoarthritic knees. Br. J. Rheumatol. 32, 127–131.

Hurley, M.V., O'Flanagan, S.J., Newham, D.J., 1991. Isokinetic and isometric muscle strength and inhibition after elbow arthroplasty. J. Orthop. Rheumatol. 4, 83–95.

Hurley, M.V., Jones, D.W., Wilson, D., et al., 1992. Rehabilitation of

quadriceps inhibited due to isolated rupture of the anterior cruciate ligament. J. Orthop. Rheumatol. 5, 145–154.

Hurley, M.V., Jones, D.W., Newham, D.J., 1994. Arthrogenic quadriceps inhibition and rehabilitation of patients with extensive traumatic knee injuries. Clin. Sci. 86, 305–310.

Iles, J.F., Stokes, M., Young, A., 1990. Reflex actions of knee joint afferents during contraction of the human quadriceps. Clin. Physiol. 10, 489–500.

Indahl, A., Kaigle, A., Reikeras, O., et al., 1995. Electromyographic response of the porcine multifidus musculature after nerve stimulation. Spine 20 (24), 2652–2658.

Indahl, A., Kaigle, A., Reikeras, O., et al., 1997. Interaction between the porcine lumbar intervertebral disc, zygapophysial joints, and paraspinal muscles. Spine 22 (24), 2834–2840.

Inman, V.T., Saunders DeC, J.B.M., 1944. Referred pain from skeletal structures. J. Nerv. Ment. Dis. 99, 660–667.

Jayson, M.I.V., Dixon St., A.J., 1970a. Intra-articular pressure in rheumatoid arthritis of the knee. II. Effect of intra-articular pressure on blood circulation to the synovium. Ann. Rheum. Dis. 29, 266–268.

Jayson, M.I.V., Dixon St., A.J., 1970b. Intra-articular pressure in rheumatoid arthritis of the knee. III. Pressure changes during joint use. Ann. Rheum. Dis. 29, 401–408.

Jessell, T.M., Kelly, D.D., 1991. Pain and analgesia. In: Kandel, E.R., Schwartz, J.H., Jessell, T.M. (Eds.), Principles of neural science, third ed. Elsevier, New York, pp. 385–399.

Johns, R.J., Wright, V., 1962. Relative importance of various tissues in joint stiffness. J. Appl. Physiol. 17, 824–828.

Kaltenborn, F.M., 1989. Manual mobilization of the extremity joints: basic examination and treatment, fourth ed. Olaf Norlis Bokhandel, Oslo.

Kazuhiko, S.K.T., Hiroshi, Y., 2007. Reduction in maximal firing rate of motoneurons after 1-week immobilization of finger muscle in human subjects. J. Electromyogr. Kinesiol. 17, 113–120.

Keating, J.F., Crossan, J.F., 1992. Evaluation of rotator cuff function following anterior dislocation of the shoulder. J. Orthop. Rheumatol. 5, 135–140.

Kellgren, J.H., 1939. On the distribution of pain arising from deep somatic structures with charts of segmental pain areas. Clin. Sci. 4, 35–46.

Kellgren, J.H., 1977. The anatomical source of back pain. Rheumatol. Rehabil. 16 (3), 3–12.

Kennedy, J.C., Alexander, I.J., Hayes, K.C., 1982. Nerve supply of the human knee and its functional importance. Am. J. Sports Med. 10 (6), 329–335.

Kesson, M., Atkins, E., 2004. Clinical diagnosis. In: Kesson, M., Atkins, E. (Eds.), Orthopaedic medicine: a practical approach. Elsevier, London.

Klafta, L.A., Collis, J.S., 1969. The diagnostic inaccuracy of the pain response in cervical discography. Cleve. Clin. Q. 36, 35–39.

Knatt, T., Guanche, C., Solomonow, M., et al., 1995. The glenohumeral-biceps reflex in the feline. Clin. Orthop. Relat. Res. 314, 247–252.

Krauspe, R., Schmidt, M., Schaible, H.G., 1992. Sensory innervation of the anterior cruciate ligament. J. Bone Joint Surg. 74A (3), 390–397.

Latimer, J., Lee, M., Adams, R., et al., 1996. An investigation of the relationship between low back pain and lumbar posteroanterior stiffness. J. Manipulative Physiol. Ther. 19 (9), 587–591.

Lee, R., Evans, J., 1992. Load-displacement–time characteristics of the spine under posteroanterior mobilisation. Aust. J. Physiother. 38, 115–123.

Lee, M., Svensson, N.L., 1993. Effect of loading frequency of the spine to lumbar posteroanterior forces. J. Manipulative Physiol. Ther. 16 (7), 439–446.

Lee, M., Esler, M.A., Mildren, J., et al., 1993. Effect of extensor muscle activation on the response to lumbar posteroanterior forces. Clin. Biomech. 8, 115–119.

Levick, J.R., 1983. Joint pressure–volume studies: their importance, design and interpretation. J. Rheumatol. 10, 353–357.

Levick, J.R., 1984. Blood flow and mass transport in synovial joints. In: Renkin, E.M., Michel, C.C. (Eds.), Handbook of physiology section 2: the cardiovascular system volume IV: microcirculation, part 2. American Physiological Society, Bethesda, Maryland, pp. 917–947.

Levine, J.D., Reichling, D.B., 1999. Peripheral mechanisms of inflammatory pain. In: Wall, P.D., Melzack, R. (Eds.), Textbook of pain. fourth ed. Churchill Livingstone, Edinburgh.

Levine, J.D., Dardick, S.J., Basbaum, A.I., et al., 1985a. Reflex neurogenic inflammation. 1. Contribution of the peripheral nervous system to spatially remote inflammatory responses that follow injury. J. Neurosci. 5 (5), 1380–1386.

Levine, J.D., Moskowitz, M.A., Basbaum, A.I., 1985b. The contribution of neurogenic inflammation in experimental arthritis. J. Immunol. 135 (2), 843s–847s.

Louie, J.K., Mote, C.D., 1987. Contribution of the musculature to rotatory laxity and torsional stiffness at the knee. J. Biomech. 20 (3), 281–300.

Louie, J.K., Kuo, C.Y., Gutierrez, M.D., et al., 1984. Surface EMG and torsion measurements during snow skiing: laboratory and field tests. J. Biomech. 17 (10), 713–724.

Lysholm, M., Ledin, T., Odkvist, L.M., et al., 1998. Postural control – a comparison between patients with chronic anterior cruciate ligament insufficiency and healthy individuals. Scand. J. Med. Sci. Sports 8 (6), 432–438.

MacConaill, M.A., 1953. The movements of bones and joints, 5. The significance of shape. J. Bone Joint Surg. 35B (2), 290–297.

MacConaill, M.A., 1966. The geometry and algebra of articular kinematics. Biomed. Eng. (1), 205–211.

Maitland, G.D., Banks, K., English, K., et al., 2001. Maitland's vertebral manipulation, sixth ed. Butterworth-Heinemann, Oxford.

McCall, I.W., Park, W.M., O'Brien, J.P., 1979. Induced pain referral from posterior lumbar elements in normal subjects. Spine 4 (5), 441–446.

McGill, S.M., Norman, R.W., 1986. Partitioning of the L4–L5 dynamic moment into disc, ligamentous, and muscular components during lifting. Spine 11 (7), 666–678.

McNair, P., Marshall, R.N., Maguire, K., et al., 1995. Knee joint effusion and proprioception. Arch. Phys. Med. Rehabil. 76, 566–568.

McQuade, K.J., Shelley, I., Cvitkovic, J., 1999. Patterns of stiffness during clinical examination of the glenohumeral joint. Clin. Biomech. 14, 620–627.

Menard, D., 2000. The ageing athlete. In: Harries, M., Williams, C., Stanish, W. et al. (Eds.), Oxford textbook of sports medicine. second ed. Oxford University Press, Oxford, pp. 786–813.

Messner, K., 1999. The innervation of synovial joints. In: Archer, C.W., Caterson, B., Benjamin, M. et al. (Eds.), Biology of the synovial joint. Harwood, Australia, pp. 405–421.

Mooney, V., Robertson, J., 1976. The facet syndrome. Clin. Orthop. Relat. Res. 115, 149–156.

Mow, V.C., Holmes, M.H., Lai, W.M., 1984. Fluid transport and mechanical properties of articular cartilage: a review. J. Biomech. 17 (5), 377–394.

Mow, V.C., Proctor, C.S., Kelly, M.A., 1989. Biomechanics of articular cartilage. In: Nordin, M., Frankel, V.H. (Eds.), Basic biomechanics of the musculoskeletal system. second ed. Lea & Febiger, Philadelphia, pp. 31–58.

Murray, K.J., Woo, P., 2001. Benign joint hypermobility in childhood. Rheumatology 40, 489–491.

Myers, J.B., Lephart, S.M., 2000. The role of the sensorimotor system in the athletic shoulder. J. Athl. Train. 35 (3), 351–363.

Myers, J.B., Wassinger, C.A., Lephart, S.M., 2006. Sensorimotor contribution to shoulder stability: effect of injury and rehabilitation. Man. Ther. 11, 197–201.

Newham, D.J., Hurley, M.V., Jones, D.W., 1989. Ligamentous knee injuries and muscle inhibition. J. Orthop. Rheumatol. 2, 163–173.

Nigg, B.M., 2000. Biomechanics as applied to sport. In: Harries, M., Williams, C., Stanish, W. et al. (Eds.), Oxford textbook of sports medicine. second ed. Oxford University Press, Oxford, pp. 153–171.

Nigg, B.M., Herzog, W., 1999. Biomechanics of the musculo-skeletal system, second ed. John Wiley, Chichester.

Nordin, M., Frankel, V.H., 1989. Basic biomechanics of the musculoskeletal system, second ed. Lea & Febiger, Philadelphia.

Norkin, C.C., Levangie, P.K., 1992. Joint structure and function, a comprehensive analysis, second ed. F A Davis, Philadelphia.

Noyes, F.R., Grood, E.S., 1976. The strength of the anterior cruciate ligament in humans and rhesus monkeys, age-related and species-related changes. J. Bone Joint Surg. 58A (8), 1074–1082.

Noyes, F.R., DeLucas, J.L., Torvik, P.J., 1974. Biomechanics of anterior cruciate ligament failure: an analysis of strain-rate sensitivity and mechanisms of failure in primates. J. Bone Joint Surg. 56A, 236–253.

Noyes, F.R., Butler, D.L., Paulos, L.E., et al., 1983. Intra-articular cruciate reconstruction, 1: perspectives on graft strength, vascularization, and immediate motion after replacement. Clin. Orthop. Relat. Res. 172, 71–77.

O'Hara, B.P., Urban, J.P.G., Maroudas, A., 1990. Influence of cyclic loading on the nutrition of articular cartilage. Ann. Rheum. Dis. 49, 536–539.

Oku, R., Satoh, M., Takagi, H., 1987. Release of substance P from the spinal dorsal horn is enhanced in polyarthritic rats. Neurosci. Lett. 74, 315–319.

Oliver, J., Middleditch, A., 1991. Functional anatomy of the spine. Butterworth-Heinemann, Oxford.

Olsen, K.A., Joder, D., 2001. Diagnosis and treatment of cervical spine instability. J. Orthop. Sports Phys. Ther. 31 (4), 194–206.

Palastanga, N., Field, D., Soames, R., 2002. Anatomy and human movement – structure and function, fourth ed. Butterworth-Heinemann, Oxford.

Palmieri, R.M., Ingersoll, C.D., Cordova, M.L., et al., 2003. The effect of simulated knee joint effusion on postural control in healthy subjects. Arch. Phys. Med. Rehabil. 84, 1076–1079.

Panjabi, M.M., 1992a. The stabilizing system of the spine. Part 1. Function, dysfunction, adaptation, and enhancement. J. Spinal Disord. 5 (4), 383–389.

Panjabi, M.M., 1992b. The stabilizing system of the spine. Part II. Neutral zone and instability hypothesis. J. Spinal Disord. 5 (4), 390–396.

Panjabi, M.M., White, A.A., 2001. Biomechanics in the musculoskeletal system. Churchill Livingstone, New York.

Panjabi, M., Abumi, K., Duranceau, J., et al., 1989. Spinal stability and intersegmental muscle forces: a biomechanical model. Spine 14 (2), 194–200.

Pearcy, M.J., Tibrewal, S.B., 1984. Axial rotation and lateral bending in the normal lumbar spine measured by three-dimensional radiography. Spine 9 (6), 582–587.

Pearcy, M., Portek, I., Shepherd, J., 1984. Three-dimensional X-ray analysis of normal movement in the lumbar spine. Spine 9 (3), 294–297.

Perry, J., Antonelli, D., Ford, W., 1975. Analysis of knee-joint forces during flexed-knee stance. J. Bone Joint Surg. 57A (7), 961–967.

Petty, N.J., 2011. Neuromusculoskeletal examination and assessment: a handbook for therapists, fourth ed. Elsevier, Edinburgh.

Petty, N.J., Maher, C., Latimer, J., et al., 2002. Manual examination of accessory movements – seeking R1. Man. Ther. 7, 39–43.

Phillips, D., Petrie, S., Solomonow, M., et al., 1997. Ligamentomuscular protective reflex in the elbow. J. Hand Surg. [Am.] 22A (3), 473–478.

Pope, M.H., Johnson, R.J., Brown, D.W., et al., 1979. The role of musculature in injuries to the medial collateral ligament. J. Bone Joint Surg. 61A (3), 398–402.

Proske, X.H.E.U., Schaible, H.G., Schmidt, R.F., 1988. Acute inflammation of the knee joint in the cat alters responses of flexor motoneurons to leg movements. J. Neurophysiol. 59 (2), 326–340.

Raja, S.N., Meyer, R.A., Ringkamp, M., et al., 1999. Peripheral neural mechanisms of nociception. In: Wall, P.D., Melzack, R. (Eds.), Textbook of pain, fourth ed. Churchill Livingstone, Edinburgh.

Richie, D.H., 2001. Functional instability fo the ankle and the role of neuromuscular control: a comprehensive review. J. Foot Ankle Surg. 40 (4), 240–251.

Safran, M.R., Borsa, P.A., Lephart, S.M., et al., 2001. Shoulder proprioception in baseball pitchers. J. Shoulder Elbow Surg. 10 (5), 438–444.

Salo, P.T., Theriault, E., 1997. Number, distribution and neuropeptide content of rat knee joint afferents. J. Anat. 190, 515–522.

Salter, R.B., Field, P., 1960. The effects of continuous compression on living articular cartilage: an experimental investigation. J. Bone Joint Surg. 42A (1), 31–49.

Schaible, H.G., Schmidt, R.F., 1983. Responses of fine medial articular nerve afferents to passive movements of knee joint. J. Neurophysiol. 49 (5), 1118–1126.

Schaible, H.G., Schmidt, R.F., 1985. Effects of an experimental arthritis on the sensory properties of fine articular afferent units. J. Neurophysiol. 54 (5), 1109–1122.

Schaible, H.G., Schmidt, R.F., 1988. Excitation and sensitization of fine articular afferents from cat's knee joint by prostaglandin E_2. J. Physiol. 403, 91–104.

Schaible, H.G., Jarrott, B., Hope, P.J., et al., 1990. Acute arthritis in cat's knee joint leads to release of immunoreactive substance P (ir SP) in the spinal cord. Pain (Suppl. 5), S230 (abstract 447).

Schwarzer, A.C., Aprill, C.N., Derby, R., et al., 1994. Clinical features of patients with pain stemming from the lumbar zygapophyseal joints: is the lumbar facet syndrome a clinical entity? Spine 19 (10), 1132–1137.

Seki, K., Taniguchi, Y., Narusawa, M., 2001. Effects of joint immobilization on firing rate modulation of human motor units. J. Physiol. 530 (3), 507–519.

Shakespeare, D.T., Stokes, M., Sherman, K.P., et al., 1985. Reflex inhibition of the quadriceps after meniscectomy: lack of association with pain. Clin. Physiol. 5, 137–144.

Shirley, D., Lee, M., Ellis, E., 1999. The relationship between submaximal activity of the lumbar extensor muscles and lumbar posteroanterior stiffness. Phys. Ther. 79 (3), 278–285.

Shoemaker, S.C., Markolf, K.L., 1982. In vivo rotary knee stability: ligamentous and muscular contributions. J. Bone Joint Surg. 64A (2), 208–216.

Shrive, N.G., Frank, C.B., 1999. Articular cartilage. In: Nigg, B.M., Herzog, W. (Eds.), Biomechanics of the musculo-skeletal system, second ed. John Wiley, Chichester, pp. 86–106.

Simmonds, J.V., Keer, R.J., 2007. Hypermobility and the hypermobility syndrome. Man. Ther. 12, 298–309.

Skoglund, S., 1956. Anatomical and physiological studies of knee-joint innervation in the cat. Acta Physiol. Scand. 36 (Suppl.), 124.

Snyder-Mackler, L., De Luca, P.F., Williams, P.R., et al., 1994. Reflex inhibition of the quadriceps femoris muscle after injury or reconstruction of the anterior cruciate ligament. J. Bone Joint Surg. 76A (4), 555–560.

Solomonow, M., Guzzi, A., Baratta, R., et al., 1986. EMG-force model of the elbows antagonistic muscle pair: the effect of joint position, gravity and recruitment. Am. J. Phys. Med. 65 (5), 223–244.

Solomonow, M., Baratta, R., Zhou, B.H., et al., 1987. The synergistic action of the anterior cruciate ligament and thigh muscles in maintaining joint stability. Am. J. Sports Med. 15 (3), 207–213.

Solomonow, M., Zhou, B.H., Harris, M., et al., 1998. The ligamento-muscular stabilizing system of the spine. Spine 23 (23), 2552–2562.

Stanish, W.D., 2000. Knee ligament sprains – acute and chronic. In: Harries, M., Williams, C., Stanish, W. et al., (Eds.), Oxford textbook of sports medicine, second ed. Oxford University Press, Oxford, pp. 420–440.

Steen, K.H., Issberner, U., Reeh, P.H., 1995. Pain due to experimental acidosis in human skin: evidence for non-adapting nociceptor excitation. Neurosci. Lett. 199, 29–32.

Stener, B., 1969. Reflex inhibition of the quadriceps elicited from a subperiosteal tumour of the femur. Acta Orthop. Scand. 40, 86–91.

Stener, B., Petersen, I., 1963. Excitatory and inhibitory reflex motor effects from the partially ruptured medial collateral ligament of the knee joint. Acta Orthop. Scand. 33, 359.

Stokes, M., Young, A., 1984. The contribution of reflex inhibition to arthrogenous muscle weakness. Clin. Sci. 67, 7–14.

Strasmann, T., Halata, Z., 1988. Applications for 3-D image processing in functional anatomy: reconstruction of the cubital joint region and spatial distribution of mechanoreceptors surrounding this joint in mondelphius domestica, a laboratory marsupial. Eur. J. Cell. Biol. 48 (25 Suppl.), 107–110.

Strasmann, T., van der Wal, J.C., Halata, Z., et al., 1990. Functional topography and ultrastructure of periarticular mechanoreceptors in the lateral elbow region of the rat. Acta Anat. (Basel) 138, 1–14.

Suter, E., Herzog, W., 2000. Muscle inhibition and functional deficiencies associated with knee pathologies. In: Herzog, W. (Ed.), Skeletal muscle mechanics, from mechanisms to function. Wiley, Chichester, ch 21, p. 365.

Suter, E., Herzog, W., Bray, R.C., 1998. Quadriceps inhibition following arthroscopy in patients with anterior knee pain. Clin. Biomech. 13, 314–319.

Threlkeld, A.J., 1992. The effects of manual therapy on connective tissue. Phys. Ther. 72 (12), 893–902.

Tindle, P., 1987. Force/displacement curve of the knee. In: Dalziel, B.A., Snowsill, J.C. (Eds.), Proceedings Manipulative Therapists Association of Australia 5th Biennial Conference, Melbourne, pp. 271–296.

Tipton, C.M., James, S.L., Mergner, W., et al., 1970. Influence of exercise on strength of medial collateral knee ligaments of dogs. Am. J. Physiol. 218 (3), 894–902.

Torry, M.R., Decker, M.J., Viola, R.W., et al., 2000. Intra-articular knee joint effusion induces quadriceps avoidance gait patterns. Clin. Biomech. 15, 147–159.

Tropp, H., Odenrick, P., Gillquist, J., 1985. Stabilometry recordings in functional and mechanical instability of the ankle joint. Int. J. Sports. Med. 6, 180–182.

Urbach, D., Awiszus, F., 2002. Impaired ability of voluntary quadriceps activation bilaterally interferes with function testing after knee injuries. A twitch interpolation study. Int. J. Sports. Med. 23 (4), 231–236.

Vanwanseele, B., Lucchinetti, E., Stussi, E., 2002. The effects of immobilization on the characteristics of articular cartilage: current concepts and future directions. Osteoarthritis Cartilage 10, 408–419.

Vicenzino, B., Souvlis, T., Wright, A., 2002. Musculoskeletal pain. In: Strong, J., Unruh, A.M., Wright, A. et al. (Eds.), Pain: a textbook for therapists. Churchill Livingstone, Edinburgh, pp. 327–349.

Voight, M.L., Hardin, J.A., Blackburn, T.A., 1996. The effects of muscle fatigue on and the relationship of arm dominance to shoulder proprioception. J. Orthop. Sports Phys. Ther. 23, 348–352.

Walla, D.J., Albright, J.P., McAuley, E., et al., 1985. Hamstring control and the unstable anterior cruciate ligament-deficient knee. Am. J. Sports Med. 13 (1), 34–39.

White, A.A., 1969. Analysis of the mechanics of the thoracic spine in man: an experimental study of autopsy specimens. Acta Orthop. Scand. 127 (Suppl.), 1–105.

Wilke, H.J., Wolf, S., Claes, L.E., et al., 1995. Stability increase of the lumbar spine with different muscle groups: a biomechanical in vitro study. Spine 20 (2), 192–198.

Williams, P.L., Bannister, L.H., Berry, M.M., et al., 1995. Gray's anatomy, thirty-eighth ed. Churchill Livingstone, New York.

Woo, S.L.-Y., Akeson, W.H., 1987. Response of tendons and ligaments to joint loading and movements. In: Helminen, H.J., Kiviranta, I., Saamanen, A.M. et al., (Eds.), Joint loading, biology and health of articular structures. Wright, Bristol.

Woo, S.L.-Y., Gomez, M.A., Sites, T.J., et al., 1987. The biomechanical and morphological changes in the medial collateral ligament of the rabbit after immobilization and remobilization. J. Bone Joint Surg. 69A (8), 1200–1211.

Woo, S., Maynard, J., Butler, D., et al., 1988. Ligament, tendon, and joint capsule insertions to bone. In: Woo, S.L.-Y., Buckwalter, J. (Eds.), Injury and repair of the musculoskeletal soft tissues. American Academy of Orthopaedic Surgeons, Park Ridge, Illinois, pp. 133–166.

Wright, V., Johns, R.J., 1961. Quantitative and qualitative analysis of joint stiffness in normal subjects and in patients with connective tissue diseases. Ann. Rheum. Dis. 20, 36–46.

Wyke, B.D., 1970. The neurological basis of thoracic spinal pain. Rheumatol. Phys. Med. 10 (7), 356–367.

Wyke, B.D., Polacek, P., 1975. Articular neurology: the present position. J. Bone Joint Surg. 57B (3), 401.

Yamashita, T., Minaki, Y., Ozaktay, A.C., et al., 1996. A morphological study of the fibrous capsule of the human lumbar facet joint. Spine 21 (5), 538–543.

Young, A., Stokes, M., Iles, J.F., 1987. Effects of joint pathology on muscle. Clin. Orthop. Relat. Res. 219, 21–27.

Zimny, M.L., 1988. Mechanoreceptors in articular tissue. Am. J. Anat. 182, 16–32.

Zimny, M.L., St Onge, M., 1987. Mechanoreceptors in the temporomandibular articular disk. J. Dent. Res. 66, 237.

Principles of joint treatment

3

Karen McCreesh   Anne O'Connor

CHAPTER CONTENTS

There is no pure treatment for joint, that is, treatment cannot be isolated to joint alone; it will always, to a greater or lesser extent, affect muscle and/or nerve tissues. However, some sort of classification system for treatment is needed in order to have meaningful communication between clinicians, and this text follows the traditional classification of joint, muscle and nerve treatment. In this text, a 'joint treatment' is defined as a 'treatment to effect a change in joint'; that is, the intention of the clinician is to produce a change in joint, and therefore it is described as a joint treatment. Similarly, where a technique is used to effect a change in a muscle, it will be referred to as a 'muscle treatment' and where a technique is used to effect a change in nerve, it will be referred to as a 'nerve treatment'. Thus, techniques are classified according to which tissue the clinician is predominantly attempting to affect. This relationship of joint, nerve and muscle treatment is depicted in Figure 3.1.

An example may help to illustrate the impurity of a joint mobilisation technique. A posteroanterior (PA) glide on the head of the fibula will move the superior tibiofibular joint, the lateral collateral ligament of the tibiofemoral joint and also the common peroneal nerve, soleus and biceps femoris. A PA glide to the head of the fibula can therefore be applied to affect any of these structures. It may be used to affect the superior tibiofibular joint, in which case it would be described as a joint treatment, or, for example, it may be used to affect the common peroneal nerve, in which case it is referred to as a nerve treatment. Similarly, physiological joint movements will move local joint, nerve and muscle tissues. The possible desired effects of joint mobilisation on joint, nerve and muscle tissue are summarised in Box 3.1. In the same way, exercise will commonly have an effect on joint, muscle and nerve tissue. For example, active shoulder flexion exercise that moves the glehumeral and scapulothoracic joints will involve muscle contraction of numerous shoulder and scapular muscles while also applying mechanical stress to the nerves of the brachial plexus. Further information on the treatment of muscle and nerve tissue using joint mobilisation and exercise can be found in Chapters 5 and 7. In this chapter it is assumed that joint mobilisation or exercise treatment is being applied to affect joint tissues. The reader is reminded that there are a number of specific precautions and contraindications to joint mobilisation treatment (Petty 2011).

Joint treatment can be used for all of the dysfunctions identified in the previous chapter, including pain, hypomobility, hypermobility and instability, and altered quality of movement (Table 3.1). This

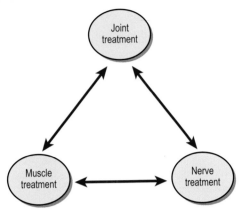

Figure 3.1 • Relationship of treatment techniques one to another: joint, nerve and muscle.

Box 3.1

Desired effect of joint mobilisation

Glide joint surface parallel to plane of joint
Move joint surface to lengthen periarticular tissues
Move joint to rotate joint surfaces
Move joint in such a way as to reproduce the patient's symptoms
Move joint to affect nerve tissue (including pain relief)
Move joint to affect muscle tissue

Joint mobilisations

Types of joint mobilisations

chapter will examine two main types of joint treatments: joint mobilisations and exercise. We will describe them, how they are used, their effects, and the evidence base for their use.

Joint mobilisations are passive joint movements performed in such a way that at all times they are within the control of the patient, and within the

Table 3.1 Joint dysfunction, aims of joint treatment and treatment techniques

Dysfunction	Aims of joint treatment	Treatment techniques
Hypomobility limited by resistance or pain	Increase range of movement and reduce resistance or pain	Accessory movements Physiological movements (active or passive) Accessory with physiological movements (active or passive) Soft-tissue mobilisations Proprioceptive neuromuscular facilitation Electrotherapy Mobilising exercises Hydrotherapy
Hypermobility with pain	Reduce pain	Accessory movements Physiological movements (active or passive) Accessory with physiological movements (active or passive) Soft-tissue mobilisations Proprioceptive neuromuscular facilitation Electrotherapy Proprioceptive exercise
Altered quality of movement	Normalise quality of movement, e.g. instability Increased or decreased resistance to movement	Exercises to enhance motor control (see Chapter 5) Proprioceptive exercise As for hypomobility/hypermobility above
Symptom production with hypomobility, hypermobility or instability	Reduce symptoms	Accessory movements Physiological movements (active or passive) Accessory with physiological movements (active or passive) Soft-tissue mobilisations Electrotherapy Mobilising exercise Proprioceptive exercise Hydrotherapy

physiological range of the joint. This is in contrast to joint manipulation, which involves a sudden movement or thrust at high speed, which cannot be controlled by the patient and often occurs at the end of joint range.

Having identified a dysfunction, treatment aims to restore normal joint function, whether this be restoration of the rotation movement, the translation movement or a combination of the two. This method of treating joints can therefore be broadly divided into physiological movements (which emphasise rotation of the bone) and accessory movements (which emphasise translation of the bone), or a combination of the two (Figure 3.2). The physiological movements can be further subdivided into passive or active physiological movements; accessory movements, by definition, will always be passive. Combinations of accessory and physiological movements are then possible, and include accessory movements with passive or active physiological movements. Details of these accessory and physiological movements are provided in the companion text (Petty 2011).

Accessory movements

Every accessory movement available at a joint can be used as a treatment technique. Having examined and identified a dysfunction of an accessory movement, the clinician can draw a movement diagram and then choose a suitable treatment dose, described in the next section. The accessory movement can be carried out in any part of the physiological range of that joint; for example, an anteroposterior (AP) glide to the tibiofemoral joint can be applied with the knee in flexion, extension or tibial rotation. The chosen position depends on the desired effects of the treatment, discussed later in this chapter.

Figure 3.2 • Classification of joint mobilisations.

Physiological movements

Every physiological movement available at a joint can be converted to a treatment technique and can be carried out actively by the patient or passively by the clinician. Active repetitive movements of the spine have, for example, been advocated by McKenzie (1981, 1983, 1985). Having examined the passive physiological movement, and drawn a movement diagram, the clinician can then choose a suitable treatment dose, described in the next section.

The principles of applying passive physiological movement are:

- The body part is fully supported.
- The movement is fully controlled by the clinician, in terms of: where in the range the movement begins and ends, the amplitude of oscillation, the smoothness of the movement and the speed of the movement.
- The clinician constantly monitors symptoms during the application of the technique.

Passive physiological movement combined with accessory movements

A physiological movement can be applied while also applying an accessory movement. Thus, the physiological movement and the accessory movement can both be oscillated at the same time; the physiological movement can be oscillated while the accessory movement is sustained; or the physiological movement can be sustained while the accessory movement is oscillated. For example, a longitudinal caudad and shoulder abduction can each be oscillated at the same time, the shoulder abduction can be oscillated while the longitudinal caudad is sustained, or the shoulder abduction can be sustained while the longitudinal caudad is oscillated.

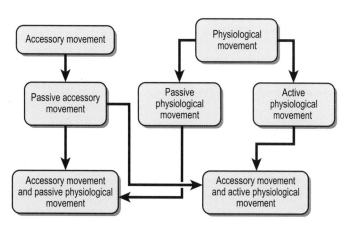

The reader should note that these techniques can be applied in a variety of positions. For example, shoulder abduction with a longitudinal glide can be applied in sitting, lying or standing.

Active physiological movement with accessory movement

As the patient performs an active physiological movement the clinician can apply an accessory movement, often called a mobilisation with movement or MWM (Mulligan 1995). For example, the clinician can apply an AP glide to the talus and ask the patient to dorsiflex the foot actively. For the cervical spine, the clinician can apply a transverse glide to a spinous process and then ask the patient to flex the head laterally. When the physiological movement is performed actively by the patient, as opposed to passively by the clinician, this can sometimes enable the technique to be carried out in a more functional position. For example, it would be extremely difficult, if not impossible, to dorsiflex the foot passively while the patient is weight-bearing. For further information on accessory movement with active physiological movements see Mulligan (1995), or the review by Hing et al. (2008), which proposes an algorithm by which MWMs may be incorporated into patient management.

Manipulation

In a joint manipulation, the joint is moved through its full passive range of motion towards the end of its anatomical range, or to the appropriate movement barrier. A commonly used form of manipulation is a high-velocity, low-amplitude (HVLA) thrust. The purpose of the high-velocity technique is to overcome the patient's protective reflex mechanism which might halt the movement, while the low amplitude may enhance better localisation of the technique and prevent excessive stretch on vulnerable tissues, such as the vertebral artery in the cervical spine. Cavitation of the joint, an audible sound, is thought to be caused by the induced negative joint pressure leading to formation and subsequent collapse of gaseous bubbles in the joint fluid (Unsworth et al. 1971).

Application of joint mobilisations

Dose

The term 'treatment dose' is often used by the medical profession when prescribing the quantity of a drug. The term is used here to describe the nature

Table 3.2 Aspects of treatment dose for joint mobilisation

Factors	Variables
Patient position	e.g. prone, side lie, sitting
Movement	This may be a physiological movement, e.g. flexion, lateral rotation, or an accessory movement or a mixture of the two
Direction of force applied	e.g. anteroposterior, posteroanterior, medial, lateral, caudad, cephalad
Magnitude of force applied	Related to therapist's perception of resistance: grades I–V
Amplitude of oscillation	None: sustained (quasistatic) Small: grades I and IV Large: grades II and III
Speed	Slow or fast
Rhythm	Smooth or staccato
Time	Duration and number of repetitions
Symptom response	Short of symptom production Point of onset or increase in resting symptom Partial reproduction of symptom Full reproduction of symptom

of the movement applied by the clinician or by the patient. The treatment dose incorporates quite a large number of factors, most of which have a number of variables; these variables are outlined in Table 3.2.

An example of treatment dose, which might be used and documented in the patient's notes, is:

> In left side lie with arm back and pelvis rotated, did left rotation grade II in line of femur, slowly and smoothly, for 30 seconds, to partial reproduction of patient's back pain.

This clinical note describes the patient in left side-lying, with the arm resting on the trunk and right hip and the knee flexed so that the knee rests on the couch, in front of the underlying leg. The clinician applied a slow and smooth passive physiological movement (grade II) to the pelvis, in the direction of the line of the femur, for 30 seconds, such that the patient felt only partial reproduction of the back pain.

Patient position

This includes the general position of the patient, such as lying, sitting or standing, and the specific position of the body part; for example, the knee may be flexed or extended during the application of an AP glide on the tibia. The choice of general and specific positioning will depend on a number of factors, including:

- the comfort and support of the patient
- the comfort of the clinician applying the technique
- the desired effect of the treatment
- whether the joints are to be weight-bearing or non-weight-bearing
- to what extent the movement is to be functional
- to what extent symptoms are to be produced.

So, for example, a patient with limitation of knee flexion due to resistance may be positioned in long sitting with the knee flexed to the end of the available range, while the clinician applies an AP glide to the tibia. This technique is comfortable for the patient and the clinician and allows the clinician to apply a strong AP force. An alternative position could be to apply the AP force with the patient in prone, and the knee flexed to the end of available range. The clinician may find this an easier position in which to apply a strong force; however, in this position there may be passive insufficiency of the rectus femoris muscle. The clinician must, therefore, consider carefully the best general, and specific, position of the patient when deciding how to apply a technique.

It should be noted that the resistance to passive accessory movements will depend on the position of the joint; for example, the resistance to a PA force to the humeral head is greatest with the glenohumeral joint in full lateral rotation, while the resistance to an AP force is greatest in medial rotation (McQuade et al. 1999).

Direction of movement

Choice of treatment direction is generally based on the clinician's assessment of passive accessory and physiological motion and symptom response, including knowledge of the normal direction of bone translation (see Chapter 2). Although there is conflicting evidence and opinion regarding the reliability and validity of some of these tests for joint motion (Downey et al. 2003; Harlick et al. 2007; Haxby Abbott et al. 2009), there is evidence to suggest that skilled clinicians can reliably identify symptomatic levels in the lumbar and cervical spine (Jull et al. 1994).

Where a physiological movement is used, a description of the physiological movement and naming the joint will describe this aspect of the treatment dose. For example, knee flexion, hip lateral rotation or lumbar rotation to the left each identifies the

direction of the movement and the joint complex. Where an accessory movement is used, the direction of the force and the joint will describe the movement. Examples include an AP to the tibiofemoral joint, a lateral glide of the glenohumeral joint or an AP to the talocrural joint. Again, each identifies the direction of the force and the joint complex. The general convention would assume that the force was applied to the distal bone of the joint – in the above examples, to the tibia, humerus and talus, respectively. Techniques, of course, can be applied to the proximal bone; when this occurs the bone needs to be identified in the written description. For example, the description may read 'AP to tibiofemoral joint, on femur'.

In the spine, where each spinal level consists of a number of joints, an additional descriptor is added for accessory movements. The point of application of the force needs to be identified. For example, a central PA on L3, a transverse glide to left on T5, a unilateral PA on C5. In these examples, the word 'central' means that the force is applied over the spinous process, 'transverse' to the lateral aspect of the spinous process and 'unilateral' to the articular pillar.

Magnitude of the force

Whenever a clinician passively moves a joint, with either a physiological or accessory movement, the clinician is applying a force. Clearly, this has a certain magnitude and it is commonly described using a grade of movement (Magarey 1985, 1986; Maitland et al. 2001). Grades of movement in this text are defined according to where the movement occurs, within joint resistance. The resistance to movement perceived by the clinician is depicted on a movement diagram (described in Petty 2011). Grades of movement (I to IV+) are then defined according to the resistance curve. The grades of movement defined in this text (Figure 3.3 and Table 3.3) are a modification of Magarey (1985, 1986). The modification allows every possible position in range to be described (Magarey 1985, 1986), and each grade to be distinct from one another (Maitland et al. 2001). A grade V technique is a manipulative thrust.

With most physiological joint movements there is minimal resistance within the range of movement. For example, elbow flexion or knee extension will have little resistance in the early part of the range, and the clinician may mark the onset of resistance (R_1) somewhere towards the end of the movement (Figure 3.3A). Grades of movement available for physiological movements include I, II, III–, IV–, III,

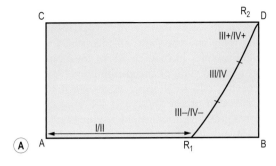

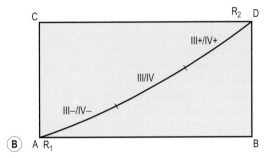

Figure 3.3 • Movement diagram with grades of movement for **A** a typical asymptomatic physiological movement, and **B** a typical asymptomatic accessory movement. The resistance is divided into thirds, so that a large-amplitude movement within the middle third will be a grade III.

Table 3.3 Grades of movement

Grade	Definition
I	Small-amplitude movement short of resistance
II	Large-amplitude movement short of resistance
III−	Large-amplitude movement in the first third of resistance
IV−	Small-amplitude movement in the first third of resistance
III	Large-amplitude movement in the middle third of resistance
IV	Small-amplitude movement in the middle third of resistance
III+	Large-amplitude movement in the last third of resistance
IV+	Small-amplitude movement in the last third of resistance
V	Manipulative thrust

IV, III+, IV+ (Figure 3.3A). With accessory movements, however, resistance occurs at the beginning of range (Petty et al. 2002), that is, R_1 is at A on the movement diagram (Figure 3.3B). Grades of movement available will be limited to grades III−, IV−, III, IV, III+ and IV+ (Figure 3.3B); that is, a grade I and II may not be possible as these grades are defined as movements within a resistance-free range (Table 3.3). The grade of movement is defined according to where the maximum force is applied in resistance, and whether the clinician considers the movement to be large or small.

Amplitude of oscillation

A movement can be a sustained or an oscillatory force. It is impossible for a truly sustained force to be applied – there will always be some variation in the force, albeit very small. For this reason, it is sometimes referred to as a quasistatic force. If the force is deliberately oscillated it is described as having a small or large amplitude. The amplitude is relative to the available range of any particular movement so it will vary quite dramatically between physiological and accessory movements. For example, small-amplitude accessory movements may be a few millimetres of movement, compared with a 40° arc of movement for a physiological movement. The amplitude of oscillatory movement is described within the definition of grades of movement: grades I and IV are small-amplitude movements and grades II and III are large-amplitude movements. Where a clinician applies a sustained force it is suggested that the description would use grades I and IV, with the word 'sustained' written prior to the grade; for example, treatment notes would read 'sustained grade IV'. In this way, the grade is used to describe where in resistance the movement is carried out.

It can be seen that grades of movement describe both the magnitude of force applied and the amplitude of oscillation. The choice of grade of movement is determined by the relationship of pain (or other symptom) and resistance through the range of movement; this is depicted on a movement diagram (Maitland et al. 2001). Where resistance limits the range of movement (Figure 3.4A), and there is minimal pain, a grade III+ or IV+, provoking only a small amount of pain, may be appropriate. Where pain limits the range of movement (Figure 3.4B), and there is minimal resistance, a grade I or II that does not produce any pain may be appropriate. A grade III− or IV− may be chosen if the pain is not severe and not irritable and there is no caution related to the nature of the disorder. Where resistance limits the movement,

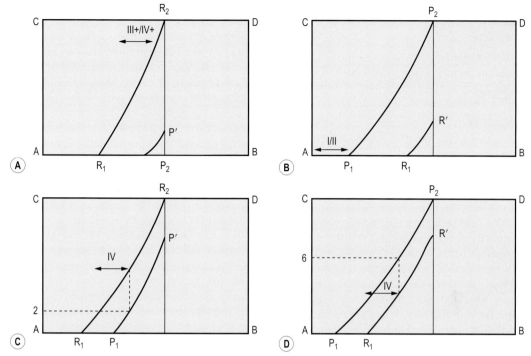

Figure 3.4 • Grades of movement are determined by the relationship of pain and resistance through the range of movement; this is depicted on a movement diagram. **A** Resistance limiting movement. **B** Pain limiting movement. **C** Resistance limiting movement with a significant amount of resistance. **D** Pain limiting movement with a significant amount of pain.

and there is a significant amount of pain, or where pain limits the movement and there is significant resistance, the choice of grade will depend on the degree to which symptoms can be provoked (Figure 3.4C and D). For example, in Figure 3.4C, if a grade IV is chosen at about 50% of resistance, the patient may report an intensity of pain about 2 out of 10 (where A is 0 and C is 10). If a grade IV is chosen for Figure 3.4D, this may provoke about 6 out of 10, which may, or may not, be acceptable to the patient or clinician.

Speed and rhythm of movement
The speed of the movement can be described as slow or fast, and the rhythm as smooth or staccato (jerky); of course, these descriptors will apply only to oscillatory forces. Speed and rhythm go hand in hand; movements will tend to be slow and smooth, fast and smooth or fast and staccato – it would be difficult to apply a slow staccato movement. Using the descriptors of speed as slow or fast, a grade V manipulative thrust may be described as a very fast speed! Grade V techniques to the spine can be referred to as HVLA thrust techniques, shortened to HVLAT (Gibbons & Tehan 2001; Evans 2002).

The tissues around a joint are viscoelastic and, as such, are sensitive to the speed of the applied force. A force applied quickly will produce less movement, provoking a greater stiffness in the tissues; a force applied more slowly, on the other hand, will cause more movement as the stiffness is relatively less (Noyes et al. 1974).

Time
In terms of treatment dose, this relates to the duration for which a movement is carried out in a treatment session, the number of times this is repeated within a treatment session and the frequency of appointments.

Typical clinical practice involves about three repetitions of a treatment technique, each lasting between 30 seconds and 1 minute – most research that has demonstrated the beneficial effects of joint mobilisations has used this time range. The frequency of appointments is decided by the clinician and the patient and will depend on a number of factors. These factors include: the nature of the patient's condition, the severity and irritability of symptoms, the area of the symptoms, the functional limitations of the patient, the stage of the patient's condition, the prognosis, the available time the patient has to attend for treatment and the workload of the clinician.

Symptom response

The clinician decides which symptom, and to what extent each symptom is to be provoked during treatment. Choices include:

- no provocation
- provocation to the point of onset, or increase, in resting symptoms
- partial reproduction
- total reproduction.

The decision as to what extent each symptom is provoked during treatment depends on the severity and irritability of the symptom(s) and the nature of the condition. If the symptoms are severe, that is, the patient is unable to tolerate the symptom being reproduced, the clinician would choose to apply treatment that did not provoke the symptoms. The clinician may also choose not to provoke symptoms if they are irritable, that is, once symptoms are provoked, they take some time to ease. If, however, the symptoms are not severe and not irritable, then the clinician is able to reproduce the patient's symptoms during treatment, and the extent to which the symptoms are provoked will depend on the tolerance of the patient. The nature of the condition may also limit the extent to which symptoms are produced, such as a recent traumatic injury, or acute inflammatory state.

Choice of treatment dose

Where a joint (which includes both intra- and peri-articular tissues) is considered to be the source of the symptoms, the clinician may be able to link the findings of the active and passive physiological movements with the findings of the accessory movements. For example, limited range of wrist extension may be accompanied by limited PA glide of the radiocarpal joint; this would make sense because wrist extension at the radiocarpal joint involves a PA glide of the scaphoid and lunate on the radius. The clinician could choose a physiological wrist extension movement, a PA glide of the proximal carpal bones, or could choose to combine physiological wrist extension with a PA glide to the proximal carpal bones. In the same way, limited dorsiflexion of the ankle may be accompanied by limited AP glide of the talus because these two movements occur together. In this case the clinician could choose to apply a physiological ankle dorsiflexion movement, an AP glide to the talus, or combine physiological ankle dorsiflexion with an AP to the talus. In both examples, the choice would depend on the relative dysfunction of the physiological movement and the accessory movement.

Let us consider treatment to the wrist. If the movements (physiological and accessory) are limited in range by resistance, then the treatment dose will tend to be with the wrist in extension. In this position, the clinician might then apply an end-range sustained or oscillatory grade IV+ PA, to the radiocarpal joint, fast with a staccato rhythm, and continuing for three repetitions of 1 minute each, producing some ache in the wrist. These treatment doses are given in Table 3.4.

At the other end of the spectrum, if the movements are limited in range by pain, then the treatment dose will tend to be applied with the wrist in a painfree position, such as wrist flexion. In this position, the clinician might apply a sustained or oscillatory PA to the radiocarpal joint, grade I or II technique, slowly and smoothly, continuing for three repetitions of 1 minute each, with no production of symptoms. This example highlights how the treatment dose can be varied in terms of grade of movement, speed and rhythm.

Where the clinical presentation is such that there is no clear link between the active/passive physiological movements and the accessory movements, the clinician has to choose a movement(s) to treat.

Table 3.4 Variation in treatment dose depending on whether the joint movement is limited by resistance or by pain

	Resistance limiting movement	Pain limiting movement
Limited radiocarpal extension and limited PA glide of radiocarpal joint	In wrist extension did sustained IV+ PA radiocarpal joint fast and staccato ×3 (1 minute) with some ache	In wrist flexion did II PA radiocarpal joint slowly and smoothly ×3 (1 minute) with no pain provoked

PA, posteroanterior.

The decision will be based on a number of factors, including the:

- number of abnormal joint movement tests
- type and degree of abnormality found
- aim of treatment, in terms of the patient's functional goals
- desired therapeutic effect
- severity and irritability of the symptoms
- nature of the condition.

Modification, progression and regression

The best treatment is the one that improves the patient's signs and symptoms in the shortest period of time. Any physical test that reproduces or eases the patient's symptoms can be converted to a treatment technique by applying components of a treatment dose. Converting positive physical testing procedures to treatment techniques would seem the most logical approach to choosing treatment, as the clinician can be confident that the treatment is, somehow or other, affecting the structure at fault. Reproduction of the patient's symptoms is a vital anchor from which to decide aspects of the treatment dose. Only when symptoms are produced can the clinician be sure that they are affecting, somehow or other, the structure(s) at fault. This may require some careful and time-consuming examination procedures, taking an attitude of the explorer, the researcher or the detective who must explore all possible avenues of investigation. For example, testing elbow flexion overpressure is fully explored only if variations of forearm pronation and supination and variations in direction of flexion medially and laterally are carried out. Similarly, when applying accessory movements, a wide variation in the direction of the force needs to be used before deciding that the accessory movement is not symptomatic.

The choice of treatment dose on second and subsequent treatment occasions needs to be informed by the patient's reponse to the previous treatment (same, better, worse) as well as the level of presenting symptoms and irritability at the time. The decision may be to continue the initial treatment, to modify it in some way, to progress the treatment or to regress the treatment. For instance, if a quick improvement was expected but only some improvement occurred, the clinician may progress treatment. If the patient is worse after treatment the dose may be regressed in some way, and if the treatment made no difference at all then a more

substantial modification may be made. Before discarding a treatment, it is worth making sure that it has been fully utilised as it may be that a much stronger or much weaker treatment dose may be effective.

A treatment is progressed or regressed by altering appropriate aspects of the treatment dose in such a way that more or less treatment is applied to the tissues. The aspects of treatment dose that can be altered are outlined in Table 3.5. It may be important to modify only one or two components of the treatment technique at any one time to avoid excessively irritating symptoms and to be able to identify the treatment components that are having an effect. Treatment with joint mobilisation should continue until the desired treatment goal is reached, or it is no longer having an effect, and ceased if it is having any adverse effect.

Specific examples of how a treatment dose may be progressed and regressed are provided in Table 3.6.

Assessment of outcome

The measurement of outcome is an important part of ensuring that the desired treatment effect is being achieved. In terms of joint mobilisation, the typical outcome is likely to be a change in pain, and/or range of motion, which will be evaluated by reassessment

Table 3.5 Progression and regression of treatment dose

Treatment dose	Progression	Regression
Position	Joint towards end of available range	Joint towards beginning of available range
Direction of force	More provocative	Less provocative
Magnitude of force	Increased	Decreased
Amplitude of oscillation	Decreased	Increased
Rhythm	Staccato	Smoother
Time	Longer	Shorter
Speed	Slower or faster	Slower
Symptom response	Allowing more symptoms to be provoked	Allowing fewer symptoms to be provoked

Table 3.6 Examples of how a treatment dose can be progressed and regressed

Regression	Dose	Progression	Explanation
In cervical extension did central PA C4 IV ×3 (1 minute) slowly and smoothly to partial reproduction of patient's neck pain	In cervical neutral did central PA C4 IV ×3 (1 minute) slowly and smoothly to partial reproduction of patient's neck pain	In cervical flexion did central PA C4 IV ×3 (1 minute) slowly and smoothly to partial reproduction of patient's neck pain	The starting position has been altered. It might be assumed that extension is a position of ease and flexion a more provocative position
In 90° knee flexion did medial glide tibiofemoral joint I ×3 (1 minute) slowly and smoothly short of P1	In 90° knee flexion did medial glide tibiofemoral joint II slowly and smoothly ×3 (1 minute) short of P1	In 90° knee flexion did medial glide tibiofemoral joint III− ×3 (1 minute) slowly and smoothly short of P1	The grade of movement has been altered
Physiological plantarflexion III ×3 (1 minute) slowly and smoothly to full reproduction of ankle pain	Physiological plantarflexion III+ ×3 (1 minute) slowly and smoothly to full reproduction of ankle pain	Physiological plantarflexion III+ ×3 (1 minute) fast and staccato to full reproduction of ankle pain	Grade has been altered as a regression. Speed and rhythm have been altered as a progression

PA, posteroanterior.

of the subjective and physical asterisks; this process is outlined in Figure 3.5. Measuring these variables before, during and after treatment is an appropriate way to assess the ongoing treatment effect. The clinician may choose a relevant joint movement (single plane, or a more functional combination, as relevant) and ask the patient to rate the pain while performing the movement on an 11-point numerical rating scale, an instrument found to be responsive in musculoskeletal pain (Bolton & Wilkinson 1998). This same movement, and question regarding pain intensity, may be used between sets of joint mobilisation to see if the pain level is changing. Equally the range of motion for a relevant movement may be measured using standard goniometry (Soames 2003), or a more functional measure, and this can be repeated at intervals before and after treatment. The importance of patient-based measures such as

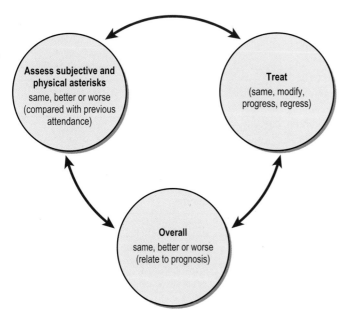

Figure 3.5 • Modification, progression and regression of treatment.

quality-of-life scales, return to work or sport, or satisfaction measures is an important component of measurement of the long-term effect of treatment. See Chapter 9 for further discussion of outcome measures.

Effect of mobilisations

The underlying mechanisms by which joint mobilisations and manipulations can increase range of movement and reduce pain can be broadly divided into mechanical effects and neurophysiological effects.

Mechanical effects

If the cause of hypomobility is shortening of the periarticular tissues, then the underlying mechanism of treatment would aim to elongate these collagenous tissues permanently. This would require the application of a force of sufficient magnitude to produce microtrauma (Threlkeld 1992). The force needs to lie within the plastic zone of the force–displacement curve (Figure 3.6). A force of lesser magnitude, within the elastic zone, will result in only a temporary increase in length owing to creep and hysteresis (Panjabi & White 2001). A rough guide to the amount of force needed to cause a permanent change in length has been estimated to be between 224 and 1136 N (Threlkeld 1992), with microfailure of connective tissue beginning at approximately 3% elongation, and macrofailure at approximately 8% (Noyes et al. 1983). Forces used by clinicians during

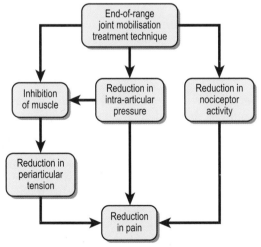

Figure 3.6 • Proposed mechanism for pain relief following end-of-range joint mobilisation treatment (Zusman 1986).

mobilisation of the lumbar spine have been measured up to about 350 N (Harms & Bader 1997), which, in asymptomatic subjects, failed to produce a significant increase in range of movement (Petty 1995, 2000). Whether these forces would produce a mechanical effect on patients with low-back pain, with perhaps some pathological process, has not been determined. It is as yet unknown whether clinically applied forces are able to cause a permanent increase in length. There has been some suggestion that manual forces applied are insufficient to produce microtrauma and that the clinically applied forces lie within the elastic range of the tissues (McQuade et al. 1999).

Repetitive active joint movements (Giovanelli-Blacker et al. 1985) and passive joint movements (Nade & Newbold 1983; Giovanelli-Blacker et al. 1985) have been found to cause a reduction in intra-articular pressure, while another study found a rhythmical increase and decrease in pressure, with active and passive movements (Levick 1979). Intra-articular pressure depends on fluid volume and joint angle (Levick et al. 1999), as well as pressure on the joint capsule by overlying muscles and ligaments (Levick 1979). When synovial fluid volume is greater than normal, in the presence of a joint effusion, for example, the joint angle affects the pressure within the joint (Levick 1979; Levick et al. 1999). In the knee joint, for example, it has been found that flexion increases intra-articular joint pressure (Levick et al. 1999), particularly at end-range (Levick 1979; Nade & Newbold 1983). However, moving a joint to a fully flexed position, and holding this position for a period of time, will cause a reduction in intra-articular pressure at all joint angles. This is thought to be due to absorption of the fluid through the synovial membrane (Levick 1979; Nade & Newbold 1983). This suggests that, where an increased joint pressure is contributing to a patient's symptoms, treatment with positioning and movement may be beneficial.

The mechanical effect of a grade V manipulative thrust technique on the spine is somewhat unclear. The audible 'crack' is due to a mechanism known as cavitation, and is the result of bubbles within the joint being collapsed (Unsworth et al. 1971). The set-up position for a grade V causes the pressure within one part of the joint to be lowered such that carbon dioxide bubbles are formed. Within 0.01 seconds, synovial fluid moves into the area of low pressure and bursts the bubbles, creating the audible sound (Unsworth et al. 1971). The after-effects of cavitation are thought to be therapeutic;

there is an increase in the joint space for approximately 15 minutes (Unsworth et al. 1971), increased range of movement (Surkitt et al. 2000) and muscle inhibition (Brodeur 1995). These immediate effects of manipulation would seem to enhance joint movement, and so active or passive movements may be helpful after carrying out a manipulation. The reader is referred to two useful articles for further information on manipulation, Evans (2002) and Gibbons & Tehan (2001), and to Pickar (2002) for a more specific description of the effects of manipulation.

Neurophysiological effects

A greater knowledge and understanding of the underlying neurophysiological effects of joint mobilisation and manipulation have begun to emerge over the last few years.

Local and spinal mechanisms

It has been proposed that passive joint movement stimulates large-diameter joint afferents which, at the level of the spinal cord, cause inhibition of joint nociceptor activity (Wyke & Polacek 1975), in accordance with the pain gate theory (Melzack & Wall 1965). This is based on the finding that type I mechanoreceptors in joints have been found to have an inhibitory effect, at the spinal cord, on type IV nociceptor afferent activity (Wyke & Polacek 1975). In normal joints, the large-diameter joint afferents are stimulated mainly at the end of joint range (Burgess & Clark 1969; Clark 1975; Grigg 1975; Millar 1975; Grigg & Greenspan 1977; Tracey 1979; Schaible & Schmidt 1983; Guilbaud et al. 1984a). This response is increased with muscle contraction and by movement (Ferrell 1985). This suggests that movements need to be carried out at the end of range to induce pain relief.

However, end-of-range passive movements also cause stimulation of the small-diameter afferents (Clark 1975; Grigg & Greenspan 1977; Schaible & Schmidt 1983; Guilbaud et al. 1984a), and mid-range passive movements of inflamed joints stimulate small-diameter joint nociceptors (Coggeshall et al. 1983; Guilbaud et al. 1984b, 1985; Schaible & Schmidt 1985). This suggests that both mid- and end-range movements would provoke, not relieve, pain.

In addition, experimentally induced joint arthritis in rats has been found to cause a discharge of previously silent small-diameter joint afferents and a reduction in the mechanical threshold of neurones in the dorsal horn of the spinal cord (Menetrey & Besson 1982) and thalamic nuclei (Gautron & Guilbaud 1982; Kayser & Guilbaud 1984). This

has been associated with altered sensorimotor cortex activity (Lamour et al. 1983). In addition, with joint inflammation, static and oscillatory joint movements have been found to cause an increase in activity of the sympathetic nervous system (SNS), with an associated increase in blood pressure and heart rate (Sato et al. 1986).

Another consideration is that passive joint movements will always involve touching the skin, which may affect nociceptor activity. In normal skin, it is known that stimulation of the large-diameter afferents causes inhibition of the skin nociceptors in the spinal cord (Woolf & Wall 1982; Woolf 1983). There is a possibility that, in a painful joint, the increase in skin afferent activity by the clinician may reduce the perception of pain.

Overall, these studies would seem to suggest that the pain gate mechanism does not completely block the transmission of pain from the spinal cord to the brain, and does not fully explain the relief of pain with passive joint movement (Zusman 1986, 1994).

Zusman (1986) proposed a theory for the relief of pain with passive end-range joint movement. It was suggested that end-of-range passive movements reduce pain by inhibiting reflex muscle contraction, reducing intra-articular pressure and reducing the level of joint afferent activity (Figure 3.6). A number of studies have demonstrated that end-of-range passive joint movements cause a reduction in the local and distant reflex muscle contraction (Freeman & Wyke 1967; Baxendale & Ferrell 1981; Taylor et al. 1994) and reduction in muscle tension at the limits of joint movement (Lundberg et al. 1978). This reduction in muscle contraction is thought to reduce ischaemic muscle pain (Freeman & Wyke 1967) and to reduce muscle tension on periarticular and aponeurotic structures, with a subsequent reduction in the peripheral afferent activity (Millar 1973; Grigg 1976). However, activation of joint afferents does not always induce a reduction in muscle activity; stimulation of spinal articular nerves has been found to cause a bilateral increase in electromyogram (EMG) activity in the paraspinal, thigh and abdominal muscles (Nade et al. 1978). It seems reasonably clear, though, that movement of a joint will, somehow or other, alter local and probably distant muscle groups. Exactly what effect, and whether there is a therapeutic effect, remains uncertain.

Active and passive flexion of a joint has been shown initially to increase, and then reduce, intra-articular pressure (Levick 1979; Nade & Newbold 1983). When intra-articular pressure is experimentally induced it is accompanied by an increase in joint afferent activity (Ferrell et al. 1986) owing to the increase in tension in the joint capsule (Wood & Ferrell 1985). Stimulation of joint afferents with joint movement may additionally cause a reduction in the reflex muscle contraction (Spencer et al. 1984). This reduction in reflex muscle contraction may reduce pain, as suggested earlier. After 2 minutes of maintained end-of-range movement there is a decrease in intra-articular pressure (Levick 1979; Nade & Newbold 1983). High intra-articular pressure can be caused by high levels of intra-articular fluid or increased muscle tension on the joint capsule (Levick 1979) and is considered to be partly responsible for the pain and limitation of movement in injured or arthritic joints (Ferrell et al. 1986). If this is so, then end-range passive movement may help to reduce intra-articular pressure, reduce pain and increase range of movement.

The final mechanism put forward by Zusman (1986) to explain the reduction in pain following end-range passive joint movement involves a reduction in the overall joint afferent activity. Oscillatory end-range passive movements have been shown to cause an increase in range of movement (Grigg & Greenspan 1977; Twomey & Taylor 1982; Gibson et al. 1993; McCollam & Benson 1993). When the joint is passively maintained at the end of the range, there is a linear correlation between the stretching of the joint capsule and a reduction in the joint afferent activity (Grigg & Greenspan 1977). If the joint is then moved away from this end-range position, and repositioned, the level of joint afferent activity is substantially reduced or absent (Millar 1975; Grigg & Greenspan 1977), and this can last up to 10 minutes (McCall et al. 1974). This delay is known as hysteresis. McCall et al. (1974) found that this hysteresis effect could be produced with both static and oscillatory passive end-range movements. In arthritic joints, repetitive (Guilbaud et al. 1985) and maintained (Iggo et al. 1984) mechanical stimulation of small-diameter joint afferents produces an increased response, followed by a greater reduced response lasting a few minutes, compared with normal joints. Thus, end-range mobilisations may cause a reduction in joint afferent activity, and hence reduced pain.

Newer methods of investigation, such as transcranial magnetic stimulation (TMS) and functional magnetic resonance imaging (fMRI), have the potential to add important information about the central effects of joint mobilisation and manipulation. One study using TMS found that motor neurone pool excitability appears to be increased by a single L5–S1 manipulation (Dishman et al. 2002), while an MRI study in rats has reported trends toward decreased areas of activation in brain regions associated with pain following physiotherapy joint mobilisation (Malisza et al. 2003).

In summary, then, there is some evidence to support the proposal that end-of-range passive movements reduce pain by inhibiting reflex muscle contraction, reducing intra-articular pressure and reducing the level of joint afferent activity (Zusman 1986).

Supraspinal mechanisms

The periaqueductal grey (PAG) area has been found to be important in the control of nociception. PAG projects to the dorsal horn and has a descending control of nociception (Figure 3.7). It also projects upwards to the medial thalamus, orbital frontal cortex, and so may have an ascending control of nociception (Fields & Basbaum 1999). The PAG has two distinct regions: the dorsolateral PAG (dPAG) and the ventrolateral PAG (vPAG).

The dPAG runs to the dorsolateral pons and ventrolateral medulla, which is involved in autonomic control (Fields & Basbaum 1999). In the rat, stimulation of the dPAG causes analgesia, increased blood pressure, increased heart rate, vasodilation of the hind limb muscles, increased rate and depth of respiration, and coordinated hind limb, jaw and tail movements, suggesting increased activity of the SNS and alpha motor neurones (Lovick 1991). The neurotransmitter from dPAG is noradrenaline (norepinephrine), and the analgesic effect appears to mediate morphine analgesia of mechanical nociceptor stimuli (Kuraishi et al. 1983). At the spinal cord level, dPAG causes inhibition of substance P from peripheral noxious mechanical stimulation (Kuraishi 1990).

The vPAG runs mainly to the nucleus raphe magnus. In the rat, stimulation of vPAG causes analgesia with decreased blood pressure, decreased heart rate, vasodilation of the hind limb muscles and reduced hind limb, jaw and tail movements, suggesting inhibition of the SNS and inhibition of alpha motor neurones (Lovick 1991). The neurotransmitter used in vPAG is serotonin, and the analgesic effect appears to mediate morphine analgesia of thermal nociceptive stimuli (Kuraishi et al. 1983). At the dorsal horn vPAG inhibits the release of somatostatin, produced by peripheral noxious thermal stimulation (Kuraishi 1990). These mechanisms have been linked to the

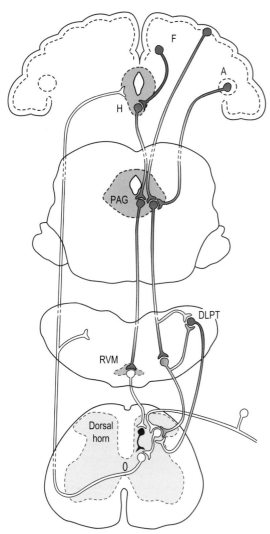

Figure 3.7 • Pain-modulating pathway. Periaqueductal grey (PAG) receives input from the frontal lobe (F), the amygdala (A) and the hypothalamus (H). Afferents from PAG travel to the rostral ventromedial medulla (RVM) and the dorsolateral pontomesencephalic tegmentum (DLPT) and on to the dorsal horn. The RVM has bidirectional control of nociceptive transmission. There are inhibitory (filled) and excitatory (unfilled) interneurones. (From Fields & Basbaum 1999, with permission).

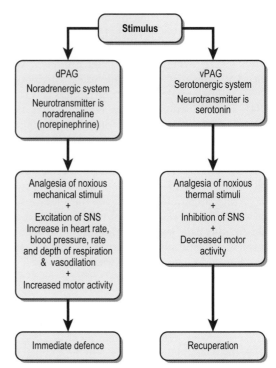

Figure 3.8 • Descending inhibition of mechanical nociception from the dorsolateral periaqueductal grey (dPAG: noradrenergic system), and thermal nociception from the ventrolateral periqueductal grey (vPAG: serotonergic system). SNS, sympathetic nervous system.

behaviour of an animal under threat, which initially acts with a defensive flight-or-fight response, followed by recuperation (Fanselow 1991; Lovick 1991); this is summarised in Figure 3.8.

Noxious stimuli can cause activation of the descending control system (Yaksh & Elde 1981; Fields & Basbaum 1999), which may reduce nociceptive transmission. Noxious stimulation has been found to cause release of enkephalins at the supraspinal and spinal levels (Yaksh & Elde 1981). It has also been found that stimulation of the spinothalamic tract transmitting nociceptive information from one foot can be inhibited by noxious input from the contralateral foot, hand, face or trunk (Gerhart et al. 1981). It has been suggested that this may explain the relief of pain with acupuncture, and pain behaviours such as 'biting your lip and banging your head against a wall' (!) (Melzack 1975). Painful joint mobilisations may also activate the descending control system.

The proposed mechanism by which joint mobilisations relieve pain is outlined in Figure 3.9 (Wright 1995). It is suggested that joint mobilisations almost immediately stimulate the dPAG, to cause hypoalgesia. Using research from acupuncture, it is suggested that vPAG may be stimulated 20–45 minutes later (Takeshige et al. 1992).

A number of research studies that support the proposal by Wright (1995) have investigated the immediate effects of joint mobilisation on noxious

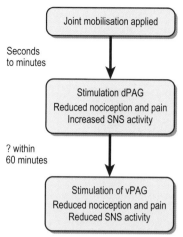

Figure 3.9 • Proposed mechanism by which joint mobilisations may reduce pain (Wright 1995). dPAG, dorsolateral periaqueductal grey; vPAG, ventrolateral periqueductal grey; SNS, sympathetic nervous system.

mechanical and thermal thresholds, and SNS activity. In a number of the studies, noxious mechanical thresholds have been measured using a digital pressure algometer, and noxious thermal thresholds have used a contact thermode system (Wright 1995). Increased activity of the SNS has been measured indirectly by measuring a decrease in skin temperature and an increase in skin conductance (due to a decrease in skin resistance). Skin temperature has been measured using an AT42 skin temperature monitor (Autogenic Advanced Technology, Chicago), and skin conductance has been measured using an AT64 skin conductance monitor (Autogenic Advanced Technology, Chicago).

In a number of studies joint mobilisations have been found to have an immediate hypoalgesic effect on mechanical nociceptor activity and/or to produce increased activity of the SNS. This has been found following a:

- grade III central PA pressure to C5 for three repetitions of 1 minute, on asymptomatic subjects (Petersen et al. 1993)
- grade III central PA pressure to C5 for three repetitions of 1 minute, on asymptomatic subjects (Chiu & Wright 1996). An oscillation frequency of 2 Hz (two cycles per second) caused a greater increase in SNS activity than a slower frequency of 0.5 Hz (one cycle every 2 seconds)
- grade III lateral glide to C5/6 for 30 seconds with the arm in upper-limb tension test positions, on asymptomatic subjects (Vicenzino et al. 1994)

- grade III lateral glide to C5/6 for three repetitions of 30 seconds, on asymptomatic subjects (Vicenzino 1995). This study found an increase in mechanical pain threshold with no increase in noxious thermal threshold
- grade III lateral glide to C5/6 for three repetitions of 30 seconds on patients with chronic lateral epicondylalgia (Vicenzino et al. 1996, 1998)
- grade III unilateral PA pressure to the C5/6 articular pillar for three repetitions of 1 minute (Sterling et al. 2001). This study additionally found that the EMG activity of the superficial neck muscles was reduced during controlled active upper cervical flexion
- grade III unilateral PA pressure on the C5 articular pillar, on asymptomatic subjects (Wright & Vicenzino 1995). This study found an increase in mechanical pain threshold and no increase in noxious thermal threshold
- HVLA upslope manipulation to C5–6 in subjects with lateral epicondylalgia resulted in a significant bilateral increase in mechanical pain threshold in the elbow region with no effect on thermal threshold (Fernández-Carnero et al. 2008).

A correlation between the increased sympathetic activity and the reduction in mechanical pain thresholds has been identified (Vicenzino 1995; Vicenzino et al. 1996, 1998). This supports the hypothesis that joint mobilisations initiate the descending pain inhibitory system because an increase in sympathetic activity and hypoalgesia have been found to occur together (Lovick 1991).

An understanding of the mechanism by which joint mobilisations cause a reduction in a patient's pain is beginning to emerge but is far from complete. Initially, theories that joint mobilisation affected the peripheral painful tissue were put forward and may still partly explain the mechanism of pain relief. More recently, greater emphasis has been placed on the role of the descending inhibitory pathways, with evidence suggesting that joint mobilisation and manipulation activate this system, causing a reduction in nociceptor activity and thus pain perception.

Placebo effect

There is little doubt that the therapeutic relationship between the clinician and patient forms as much a part of the treatment as the manual therapy itself. A number of studies have shown that manual contact alone, without joint mobilisation, can have demonstrable physiological effect (Petersen et al. 1993; Sterling et al. 2001). This evidence makes it difficult to separate out the possibility of some physiological effect due to a placebo response occurring as part of the effect of joint mobilisations. The reader is referred to Chapter 5 of the book by Strong et al. (2002) for a full description of mechanisms of placebo analgesia.

Evidence base for joint mobilisations

As discussed in the section above, there is a large amount of basic science research to support the therapeutic effects of joint mobilisations. However, it is also important to know that these effects translate to an improvement in clinical outcomes for patients. There are numerous randomised controlled trials examining the effectiveness of joint mobilisations in both spinal and peripheral joint dysfunction, enough in fact for researchers to conduct systematic reviews to summarise much of the findings.

Spinal disorders

In spinal joint dysfunction, there is evidence from systematic reviews of moderate benefit for spinal manual therapy in neck disorders (Bronfort et al. 2004; Gross et al. 2004; Sarigiovannis & Hollins 2005), cervicogenic headache (Bronfort et al. 2001) and acute low-back pain (Hettinga et al. 2008). The outcomes in chronic low-back pain have been variable, with some trials finding that manual therapy is an effective treatment (UK BEAM trial 2004) while others have found it not superior to other advocated treatments (Assendelft et al. 2004; Goldby et al. 2006). In trials considering spinal care, the terms manipulation and mobilisation are often used interchangeably, which may affect the outcome of reviews (Kotoulas 2002). In addition, the separation of the manual therapy component from other aspects of physiotherapy care such as exercise and advice is often not achieved. Reflecting this, recent UK clinical guidelines for the management of persistent back pain (National Institute for Health and Clinical Excellence 2009) have recommended that structured exercise, manual therapy and acupuncture all be considered as appropriate treatment options.

As low-back pain is considered not be a homogeneous disorder, many authors support the notion of subclassification of patients with spinal disorders, in order to determine those who may be best managed with specific treatments (Fritz et al. 2007). Using this approach, Flynn et al. (2002) have developed a clinical prediction rule which identifies those patients who respond best to spinal manipulation, i.e. those with recent onset of non-radicular back pain, with low fear avoidance and some local spinal hypomobility. Similar clinical prediction rules have been proposed for the use of cervical (Tseng et al. 2006) and thoracic (Cleland et al. 2007) manipulation.

Peripheral disorders

In the case of peripheral disorders, there is also a moderate level of evidence from systematic reviews for the use of joint mobilisations in lower-limb joint dysfunction (Brantingham et al. 2009), upper-limb joint injury (Michlovitz et al. 2004), lateral epicondylalgia (Herd & Meserve 2008) and ankle sprain (van der Wees et al. 2006) and for the use of MWMs in a variety of peripheral disorders (Hing et al. 2008). Equally, there have been trials that suggest that adding joint mobilisations to a standard physiotherapy programme of exercise and advice does not improve outcomes in peripheral disorders such as radial fractures (Kay et al. 2000), shoulder pain (Chen et al. 2009) and ankle fractures (Lin et al. 2008).

There is widespread concordance that the quality of randomised control trials examining the effect of joint mobilisations needs to be improved, particularly in terms of subject numbers, description of intervention, blinding, inclusion of control groups and length of follow-up (Koes et al. 1996; Bronfort et al. 2004). There is also very limited evidence comparing one type of joint mobilisation with another or indeed comparing dosages. In shoulder capsulitis, Vermeulen et al. (2006) showed that high-grade (more end-range) mobilisations achieved a better outcome than lower-grade. Yang et al. (2007) showed that end-range or MWMs were superior to mid-range mobilisations in improving shoulder kinematics. Undoubtedly this is another area where additional evidence is required in order to provide a sound basis for practice.

Exercise for joint dysfunction

Several types of exercise are utilised in rehabilitation, including strengthening, agility, power training, proprioception and balance exercises, stabilisation, flexibility drills, aerobic exercise and endurance training. Therapeutic exercise has been widely reported to reduce and prevent the incidence of spinal and peripheral pathology as well as influence the rate of healing (Hertling & Kessler 2006a). The benefits of exercise extend to the cardiovascular system, bone and connective tissue. Research supports the theory that exercise can help in improving the strength, integrity and organisation of collagen, an important substance in the healing process (Taunton et al. 1998; Hertling & Kessler 2006a). Furthermore, physical activity can help increase tensile strength in injured tendons and ligaments, and has been shown to be superior to rest in relation to time taken to return to activity (Hertling & Kessler 2006a).

Exercise plays an essential and distinct role in the maintenance of a healthy musculoskeletal system. With regard to joint dysfunction, the aim of exercise is to restore previous function, while remaining cognisant of adequate tissue healing and pain control in the acute stages of healing. In chronic dysfunction the aims of therapeutic exercise will change slightly, although continuing to aim for optimum function. This section will deal with the prescription of, and evidence base for, therapeutic exercise in the acute and chronic stages of joint dysfunction to the point of resisted exercise training, which is dealt with in Chapter 5. The main types of exercise that will be examined are:

- mobilising exercise:
  - passive-of-motion exercise
  - active assisted range-of-motion exercise
  - active exercise
- hydrotherapy
- proprioceptive exercise.

Mobilising exercises

Several types of mobilising exercises exist, and include: passive movements, where the clinician/patient/external device performs the movement without any voluntary muscle activity of the affected limb (Harms & Engstrom 1991); active assisted movement, where the patient takes some part in assisting with movement of the affected limb; and active exercise, where the patient has full control over movement of the limb and may use gravity-assisted or resisted positions in order to increase or decrease the difficulty of the exercise.

Application and effects

In the early stages of mobilisation, passive movement of the joint is often the treatment of choice, as less pain is experienced by the patient. Furthermore, passive movements encourage normal glide and slide of the joint surfaces, enhancing circulation and lubrication of the joint. The benefits of passive movement at this stage of healing are:

- reduction in pain (Frank et al. 1984; Hertling & Kessler 2006b)
- reduced need for analgesia
- promotion of healing through circulatory effects (Frank et al. 1984)
- maintenance of muscle length and tone
- enhanced healing process due to increased protein synthesis
- improved psychological well-being.

Because the patient does not utilise muscle force to move the affected limb, this allows potentially more movement to occur in a painfree range (Hertling & Kessler 2006b).

Active assisted movements are begun when pain has reduced to a level that the patient feels s/he can assist with part of the movement. This is usually judged by the clinician's interpretation of subjective and physical signs as well as any medical protocols that need to be observed. Active assisted movements can be performed with the clinician assisting, or by the patient alone, using the unaffected limb to assist the affected limb; for example, active assisted flexion of the glenohumeral joint, where the patient uses the unaffected upper limb to assist movement of the affected limb. Benefits of active assisted movements are similar to those for passive, although active assisted movements may be hypothesised to have a greater effect on maintaining muscle tone.

Active movement is commenced once the patient can manage to move the limb through an acceptable range of movement, and has an acceptable painfree range of motion available. Active movements can be initiated in gravity-free positions to maximise available movement and then altered to gravity-opposed positions for progression. Once the patient has regained full range of motion or sufficient range for functional movement, the clinician may proceed to resisted exercise. The reader is referred to Chapter 5 for further reading in this area.

Evidence base

It has been proposed that, following injury, immobilisation of a muscle, ligament or joint should be limited to a time period sufficient for adequate repair to have occurred to bear the forces of remobilisation without the threat of reinjury (Jarvinen & Kaariainen 2007). It is widely believed that early movement is crucial from the proliferative stage of ligament injury, owing to the profound effect it has on healing tissue (Taunton et al. 1998). From what is known about the repair and remodelling process, it is clear that there are several important landmarks in the management of injury, not least the fact that the remodelling process of collagen is most effective soon after injury, substantially reducing 2 months postinjury, and is virtually extinct after a year (Taunton et al. 1998). Clearly, this has important implications for rehabilitation, both when considering periods of immobilisation postinjury and initiating remobilisation.

Mobilising exercises, whether passive, active or a combination of both, in these early stages post ligamentous or muscular injury, influence the alignment and orientation of collagen, increase the tensile strength of repair and enhance the proliferative stage of healing as well as the next stage of remodelling (Taunton et al. 1998; Hassenkamp 2005). This emphasises the necessity for early mobilisation of periarticular structures postinjury (Jarvinen & Kaariainen 2007), but mobilisation is also vital for maintenance of healthy intra-articular structures. The effect of joint immobilisation is well documented in animal studies where the environment can be carefully controlled, and the joint immobilised, to identify changes that occur due to immobilisation. These changes include altered proteoglycan synthesis, thinning and softening of articular cartilage tissue (Vanwanseele et al. 2002, 2003; Trudel et al. 2005), reduced motoneuronal firing rate (Kazuhiko & Hiroshi 2007) and increased risk of osteoporosis due to reduced bone mineral density (Jarvinen & Kannus 1998; Uusitalo et al. 2005) and joint stiffness (Harms & Engstrom 1991). The reader is also referred to the section on immobilisation in Chapter 2. Remobilisation following a period of immobilisation of less than 30 days can correct some of these changes. The connective tissue and adhesion formation in the joint space are able to adapt and lengthen with remobilisation (Noyes 1977; Woo et al. 1987), although the atrophy of articular cartilage and subchondral bone remains unchanged (Evans et al. 1960). The length of time taken for recovery is much longer than the period of immobilisation, although functional movement can be restored (Evans et al. 1960).

Hydrotherapy

Hydrotherapy is a therapeutic treatment involving the application of water (Atkinson 2005). Working with the body while immersed in water provides a medium for exercise for clients with orthopaedic, neurological and rheumatological conditions that would otherwise not be possible. This is attributable to the effect of buoyancy, the apparent reduction of one's body weight in water, enabling clients to move freely in this medium.

Application and effects

Buoyancy is used in hydrotherapy to provide support, resistance or assistance, depending on the client's problem (Atkinson 2005). Hydrotherapy may be used for any patient requiring therapy once certain precautions are followed. The reader is referred to further texts for the full scope of the contraindications to hydrotherapy (Atkinson 2005). Several types of hydrotherapy treatments exist, including the Bad Ragaz and Halliwick methods. Increased range of motion can be achieved in water through relaxation methods and slow stretching techniques. Proprioceptive neuromuscular facilitation techniques are often useful for this purpose. The main method of progression of strengthening exercises in water is through the use of resistance, using the effect of water turbulence or by attaching floats to the patient and walking/swimming against the water. The percentage height of the patient above and below the water is also a factor to be considered when addressing range of motion and strengthening exercises.

Evidence base

The effects of hydrotherapy in relation to joint dysfunction include restoration of joint motion after injury (Atkinson 2005; Giaquinto et al. 2010), treatment of joint deformity (Giaquinto et al. 2010) and reduction of pain (Atkinson 2005; Fransen et al. 2007; Giaquinto et al. 2010) and improved function (Giaquinto et al. 2010; Gill et al. 2009). Buoyancy and warmth are hypothesised to contribute to these effects as well as the use of turbulence which can help facilitate increased recovery times postsurgery (Giaquinto et al. 2010). Hydrotherapy is also reported to influence mood (Giaquinto et al. 2010) through a reduction in blood levels of stress hormones such as noradrenaline (Atkinson 2005), which may provide further evidence for its effectiveness in joint-related diseases noted to be affected by stress and anxiety. However, more research is needed in this area to clarify the effectiveness of hydrotherapy and to determine whether it has added benefits over land-based therapies for certain musculo-skeletal disorders.

Pain relief is one of the main effects reported by patients (Atkinson 2005; Giaquinto et al. 2010; Gill et al. 2009). The reason for the decrease in pain experienced is likely to be due to desensitisation of the nerve endings from the warmth of the water. Furthermore the buoyancy effect from immersion can reduce the weight experienced through the joints (Atkinson 2005). Reduction in muscle spasm as a result of the water temperature can provide further pain-relieving effect. High-quality evidence exists to support the effectiveness of hydrotherapy for pain relief in ankylosing spondylitis and rheumatoid arthritis (Hidding et al. 1993; Hall et al. 1996). There is some evidence, of moderate quality, to suggest that hydrotherapy reduces pain experienced in low-back pain (Le Fort & Hannah 1994; McIlveen & Robertson 1998) and osteoarthritis (Fransen et al. 2007; Giaquinto et al. 2010; Green et al. 1993). More randomised controlled trials are required to support hydrotherapy further as a treatment (Geytenbeek 2002). Most of the clinical trials to date have been conducted in the rheumatic, chronic low-back pain and older populations (Geytenbeek 2002), thereby qualifying the perceived benefits for joint-related conditions.

It has been proposed that the warmth of the water and the effect of buoyancy contribute to the increased range of joint motion experienced following hydrotherapy treatment (Atkinson 2005). Some evidence exists to confirm that hydrotherapy increases range of motion (Hidding et al. 1993; Hall et al. 1996; Geytenbeek 2002; Giaquinto et al. 2010). These studies pertain to increased range of joint movement in conditions such as rheumatoid and osteoarthritis and ankylosing spondylitis.

Circulation may be increased following hydrotherapy treatment, although little scientific evidence exists to support this. The reason for the purported effects on circulation is related to physiological principles. Immersion in water causes dilation of the arterioles, reduction in peripheral resistance and increased blood supply to the periphery. This is thought to increase when the temperature of the water is increased (Atkinson 2005).

Proprioceptive exercise

Proprioception is part of the sensorimotor system providing the afferent feedback from joint and soft-tissue mechanoreceptors, present in muscle, ligaments, joint capsule and fascia. Proprioception has three main components: joint position sense, kinaesthesia and sensation of force. Damage to the joint, ligaments, muscle or skin can affect this feedback system and thus cause a loss of proprioception (Blasier et al. 1993; Voight et al. 1996; Hurley 1997; Lysholm et al. 1998; Myers & Lephart 2000; Ageberg 2002; Jackson et al. 2004). However there is a paucity of strong research evidence regarding the value of proprioceptive exercise for improving muscle reaction time, kinaesthetic deficits and postural sway (Hughes & Rochester 2008). Much of this is due to poor methodological quality of the trials conducted.

Hypermobility

Management of hypermobility is challenging owing to the nature of the disorder and is often impeded by setbacks and flare-ups (Simmonds & Keer 2007). Sensitive handling and good interpersonal skills are required to deal with the physical problems as well as potential psychosocial issues that often present in this condition. Prioritisation of main problems is essential in the management of hypermobility, and joint goal-setting between the clinician and the patient can often be the key to treatment success. Advice regarding strengthening and pacing of activities is vital as well as education on management of pain and flare-ups. Although manual therapy can be used for treatment, it is to be applied with extreme caution due to the potential for exacerbating related symptoms of the condition. High-velocity techniques are generally contraindicated except in the most skilful hands, where they may be of benefit in the treatment of a stiff thoracic spine, but careful consideration must be given before pursuing this course of treatment (Simmonds & Keer 2007). A strengthening programme is core to most management programmes for this syndrome. This is based on the principles of overload and specificity in muscle strengthening (American College of Sports Medicine 2009) and has been shown to be effective in providing symptomatic relief (Kerr et al. 2000), although more evidence is required through psychometric testing.

Debate persists as to whether there are consistent proprioceptive deficits in persons with this condition (Hall et al. 1995; Stillman et al. 2002; Mallik et al. 2004), although proprioceptive exercise is strongly advocated in the management of this condition and has been shown to demonstrate improvement ife and proprioceptive acuity (Kerr et al. et al. 2004). However it was shown in Ferrell et al. (2004) that the best improvements occurred in those subjects who demonstrated the poorest initial performance on testing. Reduction in proprioception has been attributed to abnormal output from mechanoreceptors in lax ligaments which may over time predispose to soft-tissue and joint damage (Stillman et al. 2002).

Joint instability

The reader is referred to Chapter 2 for an overview of joint instability. Treatment of joint instability will depend on the degree and underlying cause. Surgical repair may be indicated in some cases: its aim is to repair, augment or realign damaged muscle, ligament, capsule and bony anatomy. It is imperative that the nature of the instability is carefully considered in these cases. Literature reports that less than half of patients with functional ankle instability do not have clinical or radiographic evidence of anatomical abnormalities and thus surgical intervention would be futile (Richie 2001). However, for patients where surgery is indicated it has been shown to restore mechanical stability through re-establishing the mechanical restraints and proprioception, through a possible repopulation of the joint capsule with mechanoreceptors (Lephart et al. 1994, 2002; Cuomo et al. 2005). In contrast to the way that the presence of pain can reduce proprioception (Safran et al. 2001), it is also hypothesised that reduced pain following surgery may contribute to the increased proprioception following surgery (Cuomo et al. 2005).

Treatment of less severe cases of instability, due to a soft-tissue traumatic injury around the joint, will focus on optimising the natural healing process and prevent complications. Initially, pain and inflammation are addressed, followed by a return to normal range of motion, flexibility and strength through manual therapy, advice and rehabilitative exercises. Treatment in these cases will aim to improve muscle activation and muscle control of the joint to improve joint stability and reduce symptoms. Proprioceptive training is necessary from the early stages of rehabilitation to re-establish old, and facilitate new, afferent pathways from the mechanoreceptors to the central nervous system as a substitute for those damaged at the time of injury (Myers & Lephart 2000). Dynamic stabilisation work may be required to restore joint stability. This may incorporate preparatory and reactive muscle activation patterns around the joint as

well as co-activation of muscles known to work in force couples. In patients with spinal instability, such as spondylolysis and spondylolisthesis, for example, specific exercises for the muscles around the lumbar spine have been found to improve the patient's functional status and reduce pain (O'Sullivan et al. 1997). Closed kinetic chain exercise may be a facilitator of muscle co-activation, thus having a potential positive effect on functional stability. As closed chain exercises cause greater joint congruency and increased joint contact, this stimulates joint mechanoreceptors, potentially improving proprioception (Myers et al. 2006). Plyometric training has also been shown to increase proprioception (Swanik et al. 2002), although it is often not included until the latter stages of rehabilitation. Rehabilitation moves from a clinic-based programme to a more functional programme in a controlled manner, using evidence-based outcome measures as a guide for progression.

Degenerative joint disease

As previously mentioned, joint damage, such as in arthritic conditions, may disrupt the afferent feedback loop of the sensorimotor system, causing subsequent loss of muscle activation and/or altered neuromuscular control with subsequent reduction in proprioception (Hurley 1997; Myers & Lephart 2000; Jackson et al. 2004; Cuomo et al. 2005). However, little research has been completed in the area of proprioceptive rehabilitation in degenerative disease and what has been done has involved small sample sizes. It is believed that muscle has an important function in joint proprioception, and muscle strength improvements can cause a concurrent improvement in proprioception (Shakoor & Moisio 2004; Kofotolis & Kellis 2007). The role of ligaments is less clear, with some evidence suggesting that proprioception improves following joint arthroplasty and anterior cruciate ligament reconstruction, and some findings which show no change (Barrett et al. 1991; Ishii et al. 1999; Lee et al. 2009). Owing to the paucity of evidence available on this aspect of rehabilitation, few recommendations can be made regarding the type of exercise that optimises proprioception, although improvements have been shown using quadriceps-strengthening exercises for osteoarthritis of the knee (Kofotolis & Kellis 2007). It is hypothesised that improvements following functional exercise occur due to proprioceptive learning (Chasan 2006). Functional exercises such as closed chain and balance exercises can be progressed by manipulating the environment, either by altering the surface (progressing from hard surface to a foam surface), altering resistance (incorporating resisted rotation using elastic resistance bands) or altering the plane of movement (from single-plane squat to squat with rotation).

Key points and summary

- Joint mobilisations and exercise both form components of evidence-based treatment of joint dysfunction.

- The choice and application of joint mobilisations are dependent on thorough and ongoing assessment of the patient's symptoms and signs, with the need for appropriate modification as required.

- The effect of joint mobilisations is both mechanical and neurophysiological, occurring at local, spinal and supraspinal levels.

- In joint dysfunction, exercise aims to restore function in terms of range and quality of motion and proprioceptive control, while helping to manage pain and enhance tissue healing.

References

Ageberg, E., 2002. Consequences of a ligament injury on neuromuscular function and relevance to rehabilitation using the anterior cruciate ligament-injured knee as model. J. Electromyogr. Kinesiol. 12, 205–212.

American College of Sports Medicine, 2009. ACSM's guidelines for exercise testing and prescription, eighth ed, Lippincott Williams and Wilkins, Philadelphia.

Assendelft, W.J., Morton, S.C., Yu, E.I., et al., 2004. Spinal manipulative therapy for low back pain. Cochrane Database Syst. Rev. (1), CD000447.

Atkinson, K., 2005. Hydrotherapy in orthopaedics. In: Atkinson, K., Coutts, F., Hassenkamp, A. (Eds.), Physiotherapy in orthopaedics, second ed. Elsevier Churchill Livingstone, London.

Barrett, D.S., Cobb, A.G., Bentley, G., 1991. Joint proprioception in normal, osteoarthritic and replaced knees. J. Bone Joint Surg. 73, 53–56.

Baxendale, R.H., Ferrell, W.R., 1981. The effect of knee joint afferent discharge on transmission in flexion reflex pathways in decerebrate cats. J. Physiol. 315, 231–242.

Blasier, R.B., James, E.C., Laura, J.H., 1993. Shoulder proprioception: effect of joint laxity, joint position, direction of motion, and muscle fatigue. Orthop. Rev. 23, 45–50.

Bolton, J.E., Wilkinson, R.C., 1998. Responsiveness of pain scales: a comparison of three pain intensity measures in chiropractic patients. J. Manipulative Physiol. Ther. 21 (1), 1–7.

Brantingham, J.W., Globe, G., Pollard, H., et al., 2009. Manipulative therapy for lower extremity conditions: expansion of literature review. J. Manipulative Physiol. Ther. 32 (1), 53–71.

Brodeur, R., 1995. The audible release associated with joint manipulation. J. Manipulative Physiol. Ther. 18 (3), 155–164.

Bronfort, G., Assendelft, W.J., Evans, R., et al., 2001. Efficacy of spinal manipulation for chronic headache: a systematic review. J. Manipulative Physiol. Ther. 24 (7), 457–466.

Bronfort, G., Haas, M., Evans, R., et al., 2004. Efficacy of spinal manipulation and mobilisation for low back pain and neck pain: a systematic review and best evidence synthesis. Spine J. 4 (3), 335–356.

Burgess, P.R., Clark, F.J., 1969. Characteristics of knee joint receptors in the cat. J. Physiol. 203, 317–335.

Chasan, N., 2006. Functional exercise. In: Hertling, D., Kessler, R.M. (Eds.), Management of common musculoskeletal disorders: physical therapy principles and methods. Lippincott, Williams and Wilkins, Philadelphia, pp. 267–280.

Chen, J.F., Ginn, K.A., Herbert, R.D., 2009. Passive mobilisation of shoulder region joints plus advice and exercise does not reduce pain and disability more than advice and exercise alone: a randomised trial. Aust. J. Physiother. 55 (1), 17–23.

Chiu, T.W., Wright, A., 1996. To compare the effects of different rates of application of a cervical mobilisation technique on sympathetic outflow to the upper limb in normal subjects. Man. Ther. 1 (4), 198–203.

Clark, F.J., 1975. Information signaled by sensory fibers in medial articular nerve. J. Neurophysiol. 38, 1464–1472.

Cleland, J.A., Childs, J.D., Fritz, J.M., et al., 2007. Development of a clinical prediction rule for guiding treatment of a subgroup of patients with neck pain: use of thoracic spine manipulation, exercise, and patient education. Phys. Ther. 87, 9–23.

Coggeshall, R.E., Hong, K.A.H.P., Langford, L.A., et al., 1983. Discharge characteristics of fine medial articular afferents at rest and during passive movements of inflamed knee joints. Brain Res. 272, 185–188.

Cuomo, F., Birdzell, M.G., Zuckerman, J.D., 2005. The effect of degenerative arthritis and prosthetic arthroplasty on shoulder proprioception. J. Shoulder Elbow Surg. 14 (4), 345–348.

Dishman, J.D., Ball, K.A., Burke, J., 2002. Central motor excitability changes after spinal manipulation: a transcranial magnetic stimulation study. J. Manipulative Physiol. Ther. 25 (1), 1–9.

Downey, B., Taylor, N., Niere, K., 2003. Can physiotherapists agree on which lumbar level to treat based on palpation? Physiotherapy 89 (2), 74–81.

Evans, D.W., 2002. Mechanisms and effects of spinal high-velocity, low-amplitude thrust manipulation: previous theories. J. Manipulative Physiol. Ther. 25 (4), 251–262.

Evans, E.B., Eggers, G.W.N., Butler, J.K., 1960. Experimental immobilization on the human knee. J. Bone Joint Surg. 42A, 737.

Fanselow, M.S., 1991. The midbrain periaqueductal gray as a coordinator of action in response to fear and anxiety. In: Depaulis, A., Bandler, R. (Eds.), The midbrain periaqueductal gray matter. Plenum Press, New York, pp. 151–173.

Fernández-Carnero, J., Fernández-de-las-Peñas, C., Cleland, J., 2008. Immediate hypoalgesic and motor effects after a single cervical spine manipulation in subjects with lateral epicondylalgia. J. Manipulative Physiol. Ther. 31 (9), 675–681.

Ferrell, W.R., 1985. The response of slowly adapting mechanoreceptors in the cat knee joint to tetanic contraction of hind limb muscles. Q. J. Exp. Physiol. 70, 337–345.

Ferrell, W.R., Nade, S., Newbold, P.J., 1986. The interrelation of neural discharge, intra-articular pressure, and joint angle in the knee of the dog. J. Physiol. 373, 353–365.

Ferrell, W.R., Tennant, N., Sturrock, R.D., et al., 2004. Amelioration of symptoms by enhancement of proprioception in patients with joint hypermobility syndrome. Arthritis Rheum. 50, 3323–3328.

Fields, H.L., Basbaum, A.I., 1999. Central nervous system mechanisms of pain modulation. In: Wall, P.D., Melzack, R. (Eds.), Textbook of pain, fourth ed. Churchill Livingstone, Edinburgh, pp. 309–329.

Flynn, T., Fritz, J., Whitman, J., 2002. A clinical prediction rule for classifying patients with low back pain who demonstrate short-term improvement with spinal manipulation. Spine 27 (24), 2835–2843.

Frank, C., Akesan, W., Woo, S.L.Y., et al., 1984. Physiology and therapeutic value of passive joint motion. Clin. Orthop. Relat. Res. 185, 113–125.

Fransen, M., Nairn, L., Winstanley, J., et al., 2007. Physical activity for osteoarthritis management. A randomised controlled clinical trial evaluating hydrotherapy or Tai Chi classes. Arthritis Rheum. 57, 407–414.

Freeman, M.A.R., Wyke, B.D., 1967. Articular reflexes at the ankle joint: an electromyographic study of normal and abnormal influences of ankle-joint mechanoreceptors upon reflex activity in the leg muscles. Br. J. Surg. 54 (12), 990–1001.

Fritz, J., Cleland, J., Childs, J.D., 2007. Subgrouping patients with low back pain: evolution of a classification approach to physical therapy. J. Orthop. Sports Phys. Ther. 37 (6), 290–302.

Gautron, M., Guilbaud, G., 1982. Somatic responses of ventrobasal thalamic neurones in polyarthritic rats. Brain Res. 237, 459–471.

Gerhart, K.D., Yezierski, R.P., Giesler, G.J., et al., 1981. Inhibitory receptive fields of primate spinothalamic tract cells. J. Neurophysiol. 46 (6), 1309–1325.

Geytenbeek, J., 2002. Evidence for effective hydrotherapy. Physiotherapy 88, 514–529.

Giaquinto, S., Ciotola, E., Dall'armi, V., et al., 2010. Hydrotherapy after total hip arthroplasty: a follow-up study. Arch. Gerontol. Geriatr. 50, 92–95.

Gibbons, P., Tehan, P., 2001. Patient positioning and spinal locking for lumbar spine rotation manipulation. Man. Ther. 6 (3), 130–138.

Gibson, H., Ross, J., Allen, J., et al., 1993. The effect of mobilization on forward bending range. J. Man. Manip. Ther. 1 (4), 142–147.

Gill, S., McBurney, H., Schulz, D., 2009. Land based versus pool based exercise for people awaiting joint replacement surgery of the hip or knee: results of a randomised controlled trial. Arch. Phys. Med. Rehabil. 90, 388–394.

Giovanelli-Blacker, B., Elvey, R., Thompson, E., 1985. The clinical significance of measured lumbar zygapophyseal intracapsular pressure variation. In: Proceedings Manipulative Therapists Association of Australia 4th Biennial Conference. Brisbane, Queensland, pp. 122–139.

Goldby, L.J., Moore, A.P., Doust, J., et al., 2006. A randomized control trial investigating the efficiency of musculoskeletal physiotherapy on chronic back pain disorder. Spine 31, 1083–1093.

Green, J., McKenna, F., Refern, E., et al., 1993. Home exercises are as effective as outpatient hydrotherapy for osteoarthritis of the hip. Br. J. Rheumatol. 3, 812–815.

Grigg, P., 1975. Mechanical factors influencing response of joint afferent neurons from cat knee. J. Neurophysiol. 38, 1473–1484.

Grigg, P., 1976. Response of joint afferent neurons in cat medial articular nerve to active and passive movements of the knee. Brain Res. 118, 482–485.

Grigg, P., Greenspan, B.J., 1977. Response of primate joint afferent neurons to mechanical stimulation of knee joint. J. Neurophysiol. 40 (1), 1–8.

Gross, A., Hoving, J.L., Haines, T., et al., 2004. Manipulation and mobilisation for mechanical neck disorders. Cochrane Database Syst. Rev. (1), CD004249.

Guilbaud, G., Iggo, A., Tegner, R., 1984a. Sensory receptors in the joints of rats with adjuvant-induced arthritis. J. Physiol. 346, p. 58.

Guilbaud, G., Iggo, A., Tegner, R., 1984b. Sensory changes in joints of arthritic rats. Pain (Suppl. 2), S7(7).

Guilbaud, G., Iggo, A., Tegner, R., 1985. Sensory receptors in ankle joint capsules of normal and arthritic rats. Exp. Brain Res. 58, 29–40.

Hall, M.G., Ferrell, W.R., Sturrock, R.D., et al., 1995. The effect of the hypermobility syndrome on knee joint proprioception. Br. J. Rheumatol. 34, 121–125.

Hall, J., Skevington, S., Maddison, P., et al., 1996. A randomised and controlled trial of hydrotherapy in rheumatoid arthritis. Arthritis Care Res. 9, 206–215.

Harlick, J.C., Milosavljevic, S., Milburn, P.D., 2007. Palpation identification of spinous processes in the lumbar spine. Man. Ther. 12 (1), 56–62.

Harms, M.C., Bader, D.L., 1997. Variability of forces applied by experienced therapists during spinal mobilization. Clin. Biomech. 12 (6), 393–399.

Harms, M., Engstrom, B., 1991. Continuous passive motion as an adjunct to treatment in the physiotherapy management of the total knee arthroplasty patient. Physiotherapy 77, 301–307.

Hassenkamp, A., 2005. Soft tissue injuries. In: Atkinson, K., Coutts, F., Hassenkamp, A. (Eds.), Physiotherapy in orthopaedics, second ed. Elsevier Churchill Livingstone, London.

Haxby Abbott, J., Flynn, T.W., Fritz, J.M., et al., 2009. Manual physical assessment of spinal segmental motion: intent and validity. Man. Ther. 14 (1), 36–44.

Herd, C.R., Meserve, B.B., 2008. Systematic review of the effectiveness of manipulative therapy in treating lateral epicondylalgia. J. Man. Manip. Ther. 16 (4), 225–237.

Hertling, D., Kessler, R., 2006a. Introduction to manual therapy. In: Hertling, D., Kessler, R. (Eds.), Management of common musculoskeletal disorders: physical therapy principles and methods. Lippincott, Williams and Wilkins, Philadelphia.

Hertling, D., Kessler, R.M., 2006b. Shoulder and shoulder girdle. In: Hertling, D., Kessler, R.M. (Eds.), Management of common musculoskeletal disorders: physical therapy principles and methods. Lippincott, Williams and Wilkins, Pennsylvania.

Hettinga, D.M., Hurley, D.A., Jackson, A., et al., 2008. Assessing the effect of sample size, methodological quality and statistical rigour on outcomes of randomised controlled trials on mobilisation, manipulation and massage for low back pain of at least 6 weeks duration. Physiotherapy 94 (2), 97–104.

Hidding, A., Van Der Linden, S., Boers, M.D., et al., 1993. Is group physical therapy superior to individual therapy in ankylosing spondylitis? Arthritis Care Res. 6, 117–125.

Hing, W., Bigelow, R., Bremner, T., 2008. Mulligan's mobilisation with movement: a review of the tenets and prescription of MWMs.

N. Z. J. Physiother. 36 (3), 144–164.

Hughes, T., Rochester, P., 2008. The effects of proprioceptive exercise and taping on proprioception in subjects with functional ankle instability: a review of the literature. Phys. Ther. Sport 9, 136–147.

Hurley, M.V., 1997. The effect of joint damage on muscle function, proprioception and rehabilitation. Man. Ther. 2 (1), 11–17.

Iggo, A., Guilbaud, G., Tegner, R., 1984. Sensory mechanisms in arthritic rat joints. In: Kruger, L., Liebeskind, J.C. (Eds.), Advances in pain research and therapy, vol. 6. Neural mechanisms of pain. Raven, New York, pp. 83–93.

Ishii, Y., Tojo, T., Terajima, K., et al., 1999. Intracapsular components do not change hip proprioception. J. Bone Joint Surg. 81, 345–348.

Jackson, B.D., Wluka, A.E., Teichtahl, A.J., et al., 2004. Reviewing knee osteoarthritis – a biomechanical perspective. J. Sci. Med. Sport 7 (3), 347–357.

Jarvinen, T., Kaariainen, M., 2007. Muscle injuries: optimising recovery. Best Pract. Res. Clin. Rheum. 21, 317–331.

Jarvinen, M., Kannus, P., 1998. Injury of an extremity as a risk factor for the development of osteoporosis. J. Bone Joint Surg. 79-A, 263–276.

Jull, G., Treleaven, J., Versace, G., 1994. Manual examination: is pain provocation a major cue for spinal dysfunction? Aust. J. Physiother. 40 (3), 159–165.

Kay, S., Haensel, N., Stiller, K., 2000. The effect of passive mobilisation following fractures involving the distal radius: a randomised study. Aust. J. Physiother. 46, 93–101.

Kayser, V., Guilbaud, G., 1984. Further evidence for changes in the responsiveness of somatosensory neurons in arthritic rats: a study of the posterior intralaminar region of the thalamus. Brain Res. 323, 144–147.

Kazuhiko, S.K., Hiroshi, Y., 2007. Reduction in maximal firing rate of motoneurons after 1-week immobilization of finger muscle in human subjects. J. Electromyogr. Kinesiol. 17, 113–120.

Kerr, A., Macmillan, C.E., Uttley, W.S., et al., 2000. Physiotherapy for children with hypermobility

syndrome. Physiotherapy 86, 313–317.

Koes, B., Assendelft, W.J., Van der Heijden, G.J.M., et al., 1996. Spinal manipulation for low back pain: an updated systematic review of randomized clinical trials. Spine 21 (24), 2860–2871.

Kofotolis, N.D., Kellis, E., 2007. Cross-training effects of a proprioceptive neuromuscular facilitation exercise programme on knee musculature. Phys. Ther. Sport 8, 109–116.

Kotoulas, M., 2002. The use and misuse of the terms 'manipulation' and 'mobilisation' in the literature establishing their efficacy in the treatment of lumbar spine disorders. Physiother. Can. Winter, 53–61.

Kuraishi, Y., 1990. Neuropeptide-mediated transmission of nociceptive information and its regulation. Novel mechanisms of analgesics. Yakugaku Zasshi 110 (10), 711–772.

Kuraishi, Y., Harada, Y., Aratani, S., et al., 1983. Separate involvement of the spinal noradrenergic and serotonergic systems in morphine analgesia: the differences in mechanical and thermal algesic tests. Brain Res. 273, 245–252.

Lamour, Y., Guilbaud, G., Willer, J.C., 1983. Altered properties and laminar distribution of neuronal responses to peripheral stimulation in the Sml cortex of the arthritic rat. Brain Res. 273, 183–187.

Lee, H.M., Cheng, C.K., Liau, J.J., 2009. Correlation between proprioception, muscle strength, knee laxity, and dynamic standing balance in patients with chronic anterior cruciate ligament deficiency. Knee 16, 387–391.

Le Fort, S., Hannah, E., 1994. Return to work following an aquafitness and muscle strengthening programme for the low back injured. Arch. Phys. Med. Rehabil. 75, 1247–1255.

Lephart, S.M., Warner, J.P., Borsa, P.A., et al., 1994. Proprioception of the shoulder joint in healthy, unstable and surgically repaired shoulders. J. Shoulder Elbow Surg. 3 (6), 371–380.

Lephart, S.M., Myers, J.B., Bradley, J.P., Fu, F.H., 2002. Shoulder proprioception and function following thermal capsulorraphy. Arthroscopy 18 (7), 770–778.

Levick, J.R., 1979. An investigation into the validity of subatmospheric pressure recordings from synovial fluid and their dependence on joint angle. J. Physiol. 289, 55–67.

Levick, J.R., Mason, R.M., Coleman, P.J., et al., 1999. Physiology of synovial fluid and trans-synovial flow. In: Archer, C.W., Caterson, B., Benjamin, M. et al. (Eds.), Biology of the synovial joint. Harwood, Australia, pp. 235–252.

Lin, C.W., Moseley, A.M., Haas, M., et al., 2008. Manual therapy in addition to physiotherapy does not improve clinical or economic outcomes after ankle fracture. J. Rehabil. Med. 40 (6), 433–439.

Lovick, T.A., 1991. Interactions between descending pathways from the dorsal and ventrolateral periaqueductal gray matter in the rat. In: Depaulis, A., Bandler, R. (Eds.), The midbrain periaqueductal gray matter. Plenum Press, New York, pp. 101–120.

Lundberg, A., Malmgren, K., Schomburg, E.D., 1978. Role of joint afferents in motor control exemplified by effects on reflex pathways from 1b afferents. J. Physiol. 284, 327–343.

Lysholm, M., Ledin, T., Odkvist, L.M., et al., 1998. Postural control – a comparison between patients with chronic anterior cruciate ligament insufficiency and healthy individuals. Scand. J. Med. Sci. Sports 8 (6), 432–438.

Magarey, M.E., 1985. Selection of passive treatment techniques. In: Proceedings Manipulative Therapists Association of Australia 4th Biennial Conference. Brisbane, pp. 298–320.

Magarey, M.E., 1986. Examination and assessment in spinal joint dysfunction. In: Grieve, G.P. (Ed.), Modern manual therapy of the vertebral column. Churchill Livingstone, Edinburgh, pp. 481–497.

Maitland, G.D., Banks, K., English, K., et al., 2001. Maitland's vertebral manipulation, sixth ed. Butterworth-Heinemann, Oxford.

Malisza, K., Gregorash, L., Turner, A., et al., 2003. Functional MRI involving painful stimulation of the ankle and the effect of physiotherapy joint mobilization. Magn. Reson. Imaging 21, 489–496.

Mallik, A.K., Ferrell, W.R., McDonald, A.G., et al., 2004. Impaired proprioceptive acuity at the proximal interphalangeal joint in patients with the hypermobility syndrome. Br. J. Rheumatol. 33, 631–637.

McCall, W.D., Farias, M.C., Williams, W.J., et al., 1974. Static and dynamic responses of slowly adapting joint receptors. Brain Res. 70, 221–243.

McCollam, R.L., Benson, C.J., 1993. Effects of postero-anterior mobilization on lumbar extension and flexion. J. Man. Manip. Ther. 1 (4), 134–141.

McIlveen, B., Robertson, V., 1998. A randomised controlled trial of the outcome of hydrotherapy for subjects with low back or back and leg pain. Physiotherapy 84, 17–26.

McKenzie, R., 1981. The lumbar spine, mechanical diagnosis and therapy. Spinal Publications, New Zealand.

McKenzie, R., 1983. Treat your own neck. Spinal Publications, New Zealand.

McKenzie, R., 1985. Treat your own back. Spinal Publications, New Zealand.

McQuade, K.J., Shelley, I., Cvitkovic, J., 1999. Patterns of stiffness during clinical examination of the glenohumeral joint. Clin. Biomech. 14, 620–627.

Melzack, R., 1975. Prolonged relief of pain by brief, intense transcutaneous somatic stimulation. Pain 1, 357–373.

Melzack, R., Wall, P.D., 1965. Pain mechanisms: a new theory. Science 150, 971–979.

Menetrey, D., Besson, J.M., 1982. Electrophysiological characteristics of dorsal horn cells in rats with cutaneous inflammation resulting from chronic arthritis. Pain 13, 343–364.

Michlovitz, S., Harris, B.A., Watkins, M.P., 2004. Therapy interventions for improving joint range of motion: a systematic review. J. Hand Ther. 17, 118–131.

Millar, J., 1973. Joint afferent fibres responding to muscle stretch, vibration and contraction. Brain Res. 63, 380–383.

Millar, J., 1975. Flexion–extension sensitivity of elbow joint afferents in cat. Exp. Brain Res. 24, 209–214.

Mulligan, B.R., 1995. Manual therapy 'nags', 'snags', 'MWMs' etc, third ed. Plane View Series, Wellington.

Myers, J.B., Lephart, S.M., 2000. The role of the sensorimotor system in the athletic shoulder. J. Athl. Train. 35 (3), 351–363.

Myers, J.B., Wassinger, C.A., Lephart, S.M., 2006. Sensorimotor contribution to shoulder stability: effect of injury and rehabilitation. Man. Ther. 11, 197–201.

Nade, S., Newbold, P.J., 1983. Factors determining the level and changes in intra-articular pressure in the knee joint of the dog. J. Physiol. 338, 21–36.

Nade, S., Bell, E., Wyke, B., 1978. Articular neurology of the feline lumbar spine. Abstract. J. Bone Joint Surg. 60B, 292.

National Institute for Health and Clinical Excellence, 2009. Low back pain: early management of persistent non-specific low back pain. NICE guideline 88, London.

Noyes, F.R., 1977. Functional properties of knee ligaments and alterations induced by immobilization: a correlative biomechanical and histological study in primates. Clin. Orthop. 123, 210–242.

Noyes, F.R., DeLucas, J.L., Torvik, P.J., 1974. Biomechanics of anterior cruciate ligament failure: an analysis of strain-rate sensitivity and mechanisms of failure in primates. J. Bone Joint Surg. 56A (2), 236–253.

Noyes, F.R., Butler, D.L., Paulos, L.E., et al., 1983. Intra-articular cruciate reconstruction, 1: perspectives on graft strength, vascularization, and immediate motion after replacement. Clin. Orthop. Relat. Res. 172, 71–77.

O'Sullivan, P.B., Twomey, L.T., Allison, G.T., 1997. Evaluation of specific stabilising exercise in the treatment of chronic low back pain with radiologic diagnosis of spondylolysis and spondylolisthesis. Spine 22 (24), 2959–2967.

Panjabi, M.M., White, A.A., 2001. Biomechanics in the musculoskeletal system. Churchill Livingstone, New York.

Petersen, N., Vicenzino, B., Wright, A., 1993. The effects of a cervical mobilisation technique on sympathetic outflow to the upper limb in normal subjects. Physiother. Theory Pract. 9, 149–156.

Petty, N.J., 1995. The effect of posteroanterior mobilisation on sagittal mobility of the lumbar spine. Man. Ther. 1, 25–29.

Petty, N.J., 2000. Spinal mobilization – the effect of treatment dose on lumbar extension. In: Proceedings International Federation of Orthopaedic Manipulative Therapists Conference, p. 365.

Petty, N.J., 2011. Neuromusculoskeletal examination and assessment: a handbook for therapists, fourth ed. Elsevier, Edinburgh.

Petty, N.J., Maher, C., Latimer, J., Lee, M., 2002. Manual examination of accessory movements: seeking R1. Man. Ther. 7 (1), 39–43.

Pickar, J.G., 2002. Neurophysiological effects of spinal manipulation. Spine J. 2, 357–371.

Richie, D.H., 2001. Functional instability of the ankle and the role of neuromuscular control: a comprehensive review. J. Foot Ankle Surg. 40 (4), 240–251.

Safran, M.R., Borsa, P.A., Lephart, S.M., et al., 2001. Shoulder proprioception in baseball pitchers. J. Shoulder Elbow Surg. 10 (5), 438–444.

Sarigiovannis, P., Hollins, B., 2005. Effectiveness of manual therapy in the treatment of non-specific neck pain: a review. Phys. Ther. Rev. 10 (1), 35–50.

Sato, A., Sato, Y., Schmidt, R.F., 1986. Catecholamine secretion and adrenal nerve activity in response to movements of normal and inflamed knee joints in cats. J. Physiol. 375, 611–624.

Schaible, H.G., Schmidt, R.F., 1983. Responses of fine medial articular nerve afferents to passive movements of knee joint. J. Neurophysiol. 49 (5), 1118–1126.

Schaible, H.G., Schmidt, R.F., 1985. Effects of an experimental arthritis on the sensory properties of fine articular afferent units. J. Neurophysiol. 54 (5), 1109–1122.

Shakoor, N., Moisio, K., 2004. A biomechanical approach to musculoskeletal disease. Best Pract. Res. Clin. Rheum. 18 (2), 173–186.

Simmonds, J.V., Keer, R.J., 2007. Hypermobility and the hypermobility syndrome. Masterclass. Man. Ther. 12 (4), 298–309.

Soames, R., 2003. Joint motion: clinical measurement and evaluation. Churchill Livingstone, Edinburgh.

Spencer, J.D., Hayes, K.C., Alexander, I.J., 1984. Knee joint effusion and quadriceps reflex inhibition in man. Arch. Phys. Med. Rehabil. 65, 171–177.

Sterling, M., Jull, G., Wright, A., 2001. Cervical mobilisation: concurrent effects on pain, sympathetic nervous system activity and motor activity. Man. Ther. 6 (2), 72–81.

Stillman, B., Tully, E., McMeeken, J., 2002. Knee joint mobility and position sense in healthy young adults. Physiotherapy 8 (9), 553–560.

Strong, J., Unruh, A.M., Wright, A., et al., 2002. Pain: a textbook for therapists. Churchill Livingstone, Edinburgh.

Surkitt, D., Gibbons, P., McLaughlin, P., 2000. High velocity low amplitude manipulation of the atlanto-axial joint: effect on atlanto-axial and cervical spine rotation asymmetry in asymptomatic subjects. J. Osteopath. Med. 3 (1), 13–19.

Swanik, K.A., Lephart, S.M., Swanik, C.B., et al., 2002. The effects of shoulder plyometric training on proprioception and selected muscle performance characteristics. J. Shoulder Elbow Surg. 11 (6), 579–586.

Takeshige, C., Sato, T., Mera, T., et al., 1992. Descending pain inhibitory system involved in acupuncture analgesia. Brain Res. Bull. 29, 617–634.

Taunton, J., Robertson Lloyd-Smith, D., Fricker, P., 1998. The ankle. In: Harries, M., Williams, C., Stanish, W. et al., (Eds.), Oxford textbook of sports medicine. second ed. Oxford University Press, Oxford.

Taylor, M., Suvinen, T., Reade, P., 1994. The effect of grade IV distraction mobilisation on patients with temporomandibular pain-dysfunction disorder. Physiother. Theory Pract. 10, 129–136.

Threlkeld, A.J., 1992. The effects of manual therapy on connective tissue. Phys. Ther. 72 (12), 893–902.

Tracey, D.J., 1979. Characteristics of wrist joint receptors in the cat. Exp. Brain Res. 34, 165–176.

Trudel, G., Uhthoff, H., Laneuville, O., 2005. Knee joint immobility induces Mcl-1 gene expression in articular chondrocytes. Biochem. Biophys. Res. Commun. 333, 247–252.

Tseng, Y.L., Wang, W.T.J., Chen, W.Y., et al., 2006. Predictors for the

immediate responders to cervical manipulation in patients with neck pain. Man. Ther. 11, 306–315.

Twomey, L., Taylor, J., 1982. Flexion creep deformation and hysteresis in the lumbar vertebral column. Spine 7 (2), 116–122.

UK BEAM Trial, 2004. United Kingdom Back Pain Exercise and Manipulation (UK BEAM) randomised trial: effectiveness of physical treatments for back pain in primary care. Br. Med. J. doi:10.1136/bmj.38282.669225.AE. Available online at: http://bmj.com (published 29 November 2004).

Unsworth, A., Dowson, D., Wright, V., 1971. 'Cracking joints' a bioengineering study of cavitation in the metacarpophalangeal joint. Ann. Rheum. Dis. 30, 348–358.

Uusitalo, H., Rantakokko, J., Vuorio, E., et al., 2005. Bone defect repair in immobilization-induced osteopenia: a pQCT, biomechanical, and molecular biologic study in the mouse femur. Bone 36, 142–149.

van der Wees, P.J., Lenssen, A.F., Hendriks, E.J.M., et al., 2006. Effectiveness of exercise therapy and manual mobilisation in acute ankle sprain and functional instability: a systematic review. Aust. J. Physiother. 52, 27–37.

Vanwanseele, B., Lucchinetti, E., Stussi, E., 2002. The effects of immobilization on the characteristics of articular cartilage: current concepts and future directions. Osteoarthritis Cartilage 10, 408–419.

Vanwanseele, B., Eckstein, F., Knecht, H., et al., 2003. Longitudinal analysis of cartilage atrophy in the knees of patients with spinal cord injury. Arthritis Rheum. 48, 3377–3381.

Vermeulen, H., Rozing, P.M., Obermann, W.R., et al., 2006. Comparison of high-grade and low-grade mobilization techniques in the management of adhesive capsulitis of the shoulder: randomized controlled trial. Phys. Ther. 86 (3), 355–368.

Vicenzino, B., 1995. An investigation of the effects of spinal manual therapy on forequater pressure and thermal pain thresholds and sympathetic nervous system activity in asymptomatic subjects: a preliminary report. In: Shacklock, M.O. (Ed.), Moving in on pain. Butterworth-Heinemann, Australia, pp. 185–193.

Vicenzino, B., Collins, D., Wright, T., 1994. Sudomotor changes induced by neural mobilization techniques in asymptomatic subjects. J. Man. Manip. Ther. 2 (2), 66–74.

Vicenzino, B., Collins, D., Wright, A., 1996. The initial effects of a cervical spine manipulative physiotherapy treatment on the pain and dysfunction of lateral epicondylalgia. Pain 68, 69–74.

Vicenzino, B., Collins, D., Benson, H., et al., 1998. An investigation of the interrelationship between manipulative therapy-induced hypoalgesia and sympathoexcitation. J. Manipulative Physiol. Ther. 21 (7), 448–453.

Voight, M.L., Hardin, J.A., Blackburn, T.A., 1996. The effects of muscle fatigue on and the relationship of arm dominance to shoulder proprioception. J. Orthop. Sports Phys. Ther. 23, 348–352.

Woo, S.L.-Y., Gomez, M.A., Sites, T.J., et al., 1987. The biomechanical and morphological changes in the medial collateral ligament of the rabbit after immobilization and remobilization. J. Bone Joint Surg. 69A (8), 1200–1211.

Wood, L., Ferrell, W.R., 1985. Fluid compartmentation and articular mechanoreceptor discharge in the cat knee joint. Q. J. Exp. Physiol. 70, 329–335.

Woolf, C.J., 1983. C-primary afferent mediated inhibitions in the dorsal horn of the decerebrate-spinal rat. Exp. Brain Res. 51, 283–290.

Woolf, C.J., Wall, P.D., 1982. Chronic peripheral nerve section diminishes the primary afferent A-fibre mediated inhibition of rat dorsal horn neurones. Brain Res. 242, 77–85.

Wright, A., 1995. Hypoalgesia post-manipulative therapy: a review of a potential neurophysiological mechanism. Man. Ther. 1 (1), 11–16.

Wright, A., Vicenzino, B., 1995. Cervical mobilization techniques, sympathetic nervous system effects and their relationship to analgesia. In: Shacklock, M.O. (Ed.), Moving in on pain. Butterworth-Heinemann, Australia, pp. 164–173.

Wyke, B.D., Polacek, P., 1975. Articular neurology: the present position. J. Joint Bone Surg. 57B (3), 401.

Yaksh, T.L., Elde, R.P., 1981. Factors governing release of methionine enkephalin-like immunoreactivity from mesencephalon and spinal cord of the cat in vivo. J. Neurophysiol. 46 (5), 1056–1075.

Yang, J., Chang, C., Chen, S., et al., 2007. Mobilization techniques in subjects with frozen shoulder syndrome: a randomized multiple-treatment trial. Phys. Ther. 87 (10), 1307–1315.

Zusman, M., 1986. Spinal manipulative therapy: review of some proposed mechanisms, and a new hypothesis. Aust. J. Physiother. 32 (2), 89–99.

Zusman, M., 1994. What does manipulation do? The need for basic research. In: Boyling, J.D., Palastanga, N. (Eds.), Grieve's modern manual therapy, the vertebral column, second ed. Churchill Livingstone, Edinburgh, pp. 651–659.

Function and dysfunction of muscle

4

Laura Finucane

CHAPTER CONTENTS

In this text the word 'muscle' is used to denote both the muscle and its tendinous attachments.

The function of the neuromusculoskeletal system is to produce movement and this is dependent on optimal functioning of each component, that is, muscles, joints and nerves. This interrelationship is depicted in Figure 4.1, which was originally devised to describe the stability of the spine (Panjabi 1992) but is applicable to the function of the whole neuromusculoskeletal system. This interrelationship has been described in relation to the knee as 'a complex systematic sensory–motor synergy, which includes the ligaments, antagonistic muscle pair (flexors and extensors), bones, and sensory mechanoreceptors in the ligaments, joint capsule, and associated muscles' (Solomonow et al. 1987). Once again, this description could equally be applied to the entire neuromusculoskeletal system. Therefore, although this chapter is concerned with the function of muscle, it is important to stress that muscles do not function in isolation but in a highly interdependent way with joints and nerves. For a muscle to function normally there must be normal functioning of the relevant joints and nerves.

Some examples of how muscle, joint and nerve function together may help to highlight this close relationship. Anatomically, muscle often blends with ligaments to form one stability system (Strasmann et al. 1990). For example, the supraspinous ligament and the superficial part of the interspinous ligament is actually the attachment of longissimus thoracis pars thoracis (Adams et al. 2002). In the lumbar spine, multifidus blends with the zygapophyseal joint capsules (Yamashita et al. 1996); in the shoulder, supraspinatus and teres minor blend with the glenohumeral joint capsule; and at the knee joint, biceps femoris fuses with the lateral collateral ligament (Williams et al. 1995). These examples provide evidence that muscle is not an entirely separate tissue – it blends with the periarticular tissue of a joint. As a consequence, there will be a very close functional relationship between these tissues.

There are numerous examples of the close functional relationship between muscle, joint and nerve. When a muscle contracts and produces movement, the movement that occurs will depend on the shape of the articular surface, the ligaments of the joint, other local muscles, intrinsic and extrinsic forces opposing the movement, as well as the cortical

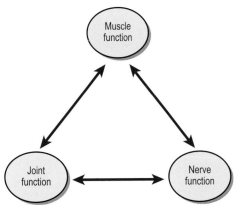

Figure 4.1 • Interdependence of the function of muscle, joint and nerve for normal movement (after Panjabi 1992, with permission). Normal function of the neuromusculoskeletal system requires normal function of muscle, joint and nerve.

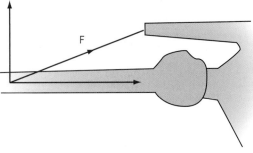

Figure 4.2 • Contribution of deltoid muscle to stability of the glenohumeral joint. The force of contraction F can be resolved into two lines of force: vertically, away from the bone producing the rotation of the humerus, and along the shaft of the humerus to the glenohumeral joint, thus aiding stability. (After Elftman 1966, with permission).

control of movement. Thus, the effect of muscle contraction is dependent on joint and nerve function.

The level of activity of a muscle is dependent on the position of its associated joints. For example, in standing with the knee flexed 15°, the quadriceps force required to support body weight is about 20% of maximum quadriceps strength; when the knee joint angle is increased to 30°, the quadriceps force is increased to about 50% (Perry et al. 1975).

Muscles contribute to the stability of a joint by contributing to joint stiffness. In the cat wrist joint, muscle contributes 41% and tendon 10% to the joint stiffness (Johns & Wright 1962). In the human knee, contraction of the quadriceps and contraction of the hamstring muscles can substantially increase joint stiffness (Louie & Mote 1987; Zhang et al. 1998), with increases of between 200 and 300% for quadriceps and between 100 and 250% for hamstrings (Louie & Mote 1987). Additionally, it has been estimated that co-contraction of the quadriceps and hamstring muscle groups can reduce knee joint laxity by about 70% (Louie & Mote 1987). Contraction of quadriceps and contraction of hamstring muscle groups can each reduce the strain on the anterior cruciate ligament (ACL) (Renstrom et al. 1986). Quadriceps and hamstring contraction thus contributes to joint stiffness and therefore enhances joint stability. At the glenohumeral joint with the arm elevated (Figure 4.2) it can readily be seen that the position and direction of the deltoid muscle produce a force that will compress the humerus against the glenoid cavity, and therefore stabilise the joint (Elftman

1966). It is clear from these studies that muscle contraction directly affects joint stiffness and thus joint stability.

Muscle also enhances joint stability during joint movement (Perry et al. 1975; Pope et al. 1979; Shoemaker & Markolf 1982; Louie et al. 1984; Walla et al. 1985; McGill & Norman 1986; Solomonow et al. 1986, 1987; Louie & Mote 1987; Panjabi et al. 1989; Knatt et al. 1995; Wilke et al. 1995; Phillips et al. 1997; Hortobagyi & DeVita 2000). For example, in the upper limb, isometric contraction of the elbow flexors or extensors at 45, 90 and 135° elbow flexion is coupled with activity in the antagonistic triceps or biceps muscle, which varies with joint angle (Solomonow et al. 1986). The pattern of activity of the antagonistic muscle suggests that it regulates the joint torque, thus enhancing elbow joint stability (Solomonow et al. 1986). In the lumbar spine, during flexion and extension movements, muscles have been shown to affect segmental stability (Panjabi et al. 1989; Wilke et al. 1995). The posterior layer of thoracolumbar fascia is considered to act as an accessory ligament, helping to stabilise the lumbar spine during movement (Bogduk & MacIntosh 1984). It can be concluded that, during movement, muscle directly affects joint stability.

In all of the above examples, where muscle enhances joint stability, a normally functioning nervous system is a prerequisite. A number of studies have identified that muscle activity is directly affected by joint afferent activity. In the cat, for example, stimulation of the articular nerve in the glenohumeral joint produces a reflex activation of the biceps muscle (Knatt et al. 1995). Similarly, the activity of the muscles overlying the medial ligament of the elbow (flexor carpi radialis and ulnaris, flexor digitorum profundus and superficialis, and pronator teres) is increased with stimulation of afferents in the ulnar collateral ligament; this is thought to be a protective reflex to avoid excessive ligamentous tension (Phillips et al. 1997). In the lower limb, in the anaesthetised cat, reflex facilitation of gastrocnemius and inhibition of tibialis anterior is brought about by stimulation of mechanoreceptors in the posterior joint capsule; similarly, facilitation of tibialis anterior and inhibition of gastrocnemius occur with stimulation of mechanoreceptors in the anterior joint capsule (Freeman & Wyke 1967). In the human lumbar spine, reflex contraction of multifidus muscle occurs with stimulation of mechanoreceptors in the supraspinous ligament (Solomonow et al. 1998). In the pig, this also occurs with stimulation of the mechanoreceptors in the facet joint capsule and intervertebral disc (Indahl et al. 1995, 1997) and is thought to be a reflex response for enhancement of spinal stability (Indahl et al. 1995, 1997; Solomonow et al. 1998). Conversely, contraction of muscle around the cat knee joint has been shown to enhance joint mechanoreceptor activity (Ferrell 1985). It has been postulated that the small muscles, such as the intertransversarii and interspinales in the lumbar spine, are thought to be too weak to have a significant role in producing torque; they have been considered to have a sensory feedback role and have thus been regarded primarily as proprioceptive transducers (Bogduk 1997). Afferents in muscle, as well as in joint and skin, are considered to provide the brain with proprioceptive information necessary for movement (Gandevia et al. 1983; McCloskey et al. 1987; Macefield et al. 1990). Collectively, this research clearly links the interdependent relationship of muscle, joint and nerve function during movement.

This section has sought to highlight the complex interrelationship of muscle with joint and nerve. It seems clear from the research findings that normal joint and nerve function are prerequisites for normal muscle function.

Muscle function

This text is limited to the skeletal muscle, as opposed to smooth muscle (in the walls of organs, blood vessels and respiratory passages) and cardiac muscle (in the atria and ventricles of the heart).

The following aspects of joint function will be considered:

- anatomy, biomechanics and physiology of muscle
- nerve supply of muscle
- muscle contraction (strength), power, endurance and motor control and muscle length
- classification of muscle function.

Anatomy, biomechanics and physiology of muscle

Muscle constitutes approximately 40% of the total body weight (Panjabi & White 2001). Muscle is essentially a machine that converts chemical energy into mechanical work, and has been regarded as 'the most efficient and adaptable machine known to man' (Williams et al. 1995). A muscle (that is, muscle and its tendons) can be divided grossly into contractile tissue and non-contractile tissue. The non-contractile tissue includes the connective tissue layers within muscle and the tendons.

Contractile tissue of muscle

The smallest unit of muscle is the myofibril, made up of thin actin and thick myosin filaments, giving a striated appearance under the light microscope (Figure 4.3). The myosin filaments produce the dark A band, and the actin filaments produce the light I band. In addition, elastic titin filaments lie between the myosin filaments (Williams et al. 1995). The titin filaments act like a spring, with increased tension when the sarcomere is lengthened, thus enabling it to return to its resting length when the tension is

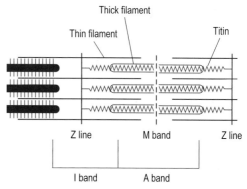

Figure 4.3 • The basic contractile unit of muscle, the sarcomere, formed by the thin actin and thick myosin filaments (from Herzog 1999, with permission).

removed; this is also thought to keep the myosin in the centre of the sarcomere when there is an asymmetrical pull (Horowits et al. 1989). The Z line demarcates the sarcomere, which is the basic contractile unit of muscle.

Individual muscle fibres (or cells) are covered in a membrane called the sarcolemma and by a connective tissue sheath called the endomysium (Figure 4.4). The individual muscle fibres are collected into bundles (or fascicles) by a connective tissue sheath called the perimysium. Numbers of muscle bundles constitute the muscle and are surrounded by a connective tissue sheath called the epimysium and by an outer layer of fascia. These muscle fibres are known as extrafusal fibres, compared with intrafusal fibres, which lie within the muscle spindle (discussed later under nerve supply).

Non-contractile tissue of muscle

Connective tissue is found in layers within the muscle and in the tendons. Connective tissue makes up 30% of muscle mass (Alter 1996) and is vital for normal muscle function. The connective tissue of muscle consists of collagen fibres, and some elastin fibres, held together in a ground substance. The elastin fibres enable muscle to regain its shape, following

shortening with a concentric muscle contraction, or after being in a lengthened position.

Connective tissue forms a sheath around each muscle fibre (endomysium), around bundles of muscle fibres (perimysium) and around the whole muscle (epimysium), as shown in Figure 4.4. The connective tissue, along with the nerves and blood vessels, forms the non-contractile element of the muscle belly. The outer layer of connective tissue enables identification of particular muscles, for example semitendinosus muscle in the thigh, and allows sliding of muscle on adjacent tissues, for example movement of semitendinosus on the biceps femoris and the sciatic nerve. The perimysium around a bundle of muscle fibres provides a channel for blood vessels and nerves. The endomysium, perimysium and epimysium join to form the tendon or aponeurosis that attaches the muscle to bone.

The function of connective tissue in muscle can be summarised as follows:

- It is the architectural structure of the muscle.
- It transmits force and movement from the muscle fibres to the tendinous attachments.
- It resists passive stretching of a muscle.
- It enhances muscle strength by controlling muscle pressure and muscle volume. Cutting the

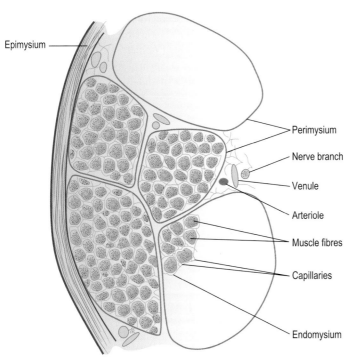

Figure 4.4 • Schematic illustration of the cross-sectional structure of muscle (from McComas 1996, with permission).

Epimysium

Perimysium

Nerve branch

Venule

Arteriole

Muscle fibres

Capillaries

Endomysium

epimysium of a dog hind limb results in a 15% reduction in muscle force and a 50% reduction in intracompartmental pressure (Garfin et al. 1981). In the lumbar spine, the thoracolumbar fascia has been estimated to enhance the strength of the back muscles by 30% (Hukins et al. 1990).

• It provides a channel for blood vessels and nerves.

Connective tissue is also the major constituent of fascia, which is divided into superficial and deep. Superficial fascia lies just below the skin and allows skin movement; it is thick on the plantar aspect of the hands and thin on the dorsum of the hands and feet. Deep fascia acts as retinacula, intermuscular septa, intermuscular aponeurosis and attachment for muscle. In the thoracic and abdominal cavities deep fascia covers and supports the viscera, for example the pleura, pericardium and peritoneum. The flexor and extensor retinacula of the wrist and foot are deep fascia arranged as a transverse thickening to retain tendons deep to it. The intermuscular septa pass between groups of muscles and attach to bone. Muscles can take attachment from the intermuscular septa, which may then be better named intermuscular aponeurosis, for example the rectal sheath. The deep fascia can be a point of attachment for muscle to bone and from muscle to muscle. For example, the tensor fascia lata and gluteus maximus attach to the iliotibial tract (fascia), which then passes down the leg and attaches to the tibia. Deep fascia in the lower leg connects the peroneus longus to the biceps femoris, and, in the upper arm, pectoralis minor to the short head of biceps. Fascial connections around the pelvis have been recognised as important by Vleeming et al. (1997) and have been explored by Myers (2001), who coined the phrase 'myofascial meridians'.

Musculotendinous (or myotendinous) junction

This is the junction between the muscle and the tendon. The contact area is characterised by the muscle cells forming finger-like projections in which the collagen fibres of the tendon insert (Figure 4.5). This arrangement increases the surface area of the contact region and so reduces the tensile force applied to the tissue (Eisenberg & Milton 1984; Kvist et al. 1991). Interestingly, this is reflected in differences in surface area between type I and type II muscle fibres. The area is greater for type II fibres, which are involved in powerful voluntary movements, than for type I fibres, which generate lower forces and are largely involved in postural control (Kvist et al. 1991). There is a high density of glycosaminoglycans, which are thought to increase the adhesive forces between the two regions and thus help to strengthen the region (Jozsa et al. 1992). Despite this arrangement, the region is the weakest part of the tendon–muscle unit and is susceptible to strain injuries (Nikolaou et al. 1987; Garrett et al. 1989; Garrett 1990; Tidball 1991).

Figure 4.5 • Schematic figure of musculotendinous junction (after Jozsa & Kannus 1997, with permission).

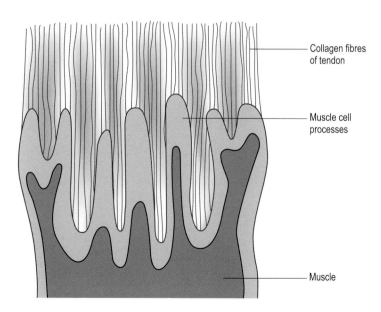

Collagen fibres of tendon

Muscle cell processes

Muscle

Osteotendinous junctions

This is where tendon attaches to bone. Tendons usually attach directly to bone, that is, there is an abrupt well-defined area of attachment with a clear demarcation of tendon and bone; examples include supraspinatus, where it attaches to the superior facet on the greater tuberosity of the humerus, and the medial collateral ligament to the medial condyle of the femur (Woo et al. 1988). Tendons with direct attachments have a superficial layer which blends with periosteum, and a larger deep layer which inserts directly into bone via a thin layer of fibrocartilage (Cooper & Misol 1970; Woo et al. 1988). Sometimes tendons attach rather more indirectly, such that there is a more gradual and less distinct area of attachment (Woo et al. 1988). The superficial layer in this case provides the predominant attachment, blending with the periosteum and bone via Sharpey's fibres (Woo et al. 1988), while the deep layer attaches directly to the bone.

Tendons

Tendons are designed to transmit high tensile force from muscle to bone, and they allow muscles to lengthen and bend around bone. They are therefore flexible, relatively inextensible and able to withstand large tensile forces (Elliott 1965; Jozsa & Kannus 1997). Tendons are made up of approximately 70% of longitudinally arranged collagen tissue, with some elastin tissue, embedded in a proteoglycan–water matrix (Hess et al. 1989). They have a sparse blood supply and so are white in appearance. Between the collagen fibres (the basic unit of tendon) there is loose connective tissue; this provides a channel for vessels and nerve.

Tendons sometimes contain a sesamoid bone (named because of the resemblance to sesame seed) which the ancient Hebrews believed was the resting place of the soul (McBryde & Anderson 1988). Their function is rather more mundane: they increase the mechanical advantage of the muscle and decrease friction between adjacent tissues. They are covered with hyaline cartilage. Examples include the pisiform bone within the flexor carpi ulnaris tendon, the patella within the quadriceps tendon and the sesamoid bone within the flexor hallucis brevis tendon. The existence and shape of sesamoid bones vary between individuals (McBryde & Anderson 1988).

During a muscle contraction, tendon moves on adjacent tissue; the frictional resistance to this movement is minimised by bursae and sheaths which can be classified as fibrous, synovial and paratenon sheaths.

1. A bursa may lie adjacent to tendon to aid gliding movement of the tendon on adjacent tissue; for example, the infrapatellar bursa facilitates gliding movements of the patella.

2. A fibrous sheath may surround a tendon, as in the tendons around the ankle. Bony grooves and notches contain a layer of fibrocartilage, and superficially the tendon is held in place by retinaculum.

3. A synovial sheath may surround a tendon where ease of movement with adjacent tissue is of paramount importance, as in the tendons of the hands and feet. Synovial sheaths are composed of an outer fibrotic sheath and an inner synovial sheath. A thin film of synovial fluid, rich in hyaluronic acid, fills the space between the sheaths and acts as a lubricant reducing frictional resistance (Jozsa & Kannus 1997) and enhancing tendon nutrition (Lundborg 1976; Matthews 1976).

4. A paratenon sheath (or peritendinous sheet) may surround a tendon – for example, the tendocalcaneus tendon. The paratenon is made up of collagen fibres, elastic fibrils and synovial cells, and acts as an elastic sleeve, facilitating movement between the tendon and its surrounding tissues (Hess et al. 1989; Jozsa & Kannus 1997). The paratenon and epitenon are sometimes referred to as the peritendon.

The tendon itself is covered in a fine connective tissue sheath called the epitenon (Figure 4.6) which lies underneath the synovial or paratenon. Most of the fibres that make up the epitenon are arranged at about 60° to the direction of the tendon fibres, but when the tendon is lengthened this angle reduces to about 30°, so that the fibres lie more in line with the direction of stress; this is thought to help protect against overstrain (Jozsa & Kannus 1997).

Underneath the epitenon is the endotenon, which covers tertiary, secondary and primary bundles of collagen fibres together (Elliott 1965; Jozsa & Kannus 1997). These layers of connective tissue enable the fibres to glide on each other, and provide a channel for blood vessels, lymphatics and nerves into the deep portions of the tendon (Elliott 1965; Hess et al. 1989). Collagen fibres are made up of collagen fibrils which are oriented longitudinally, transversely and horizontally to withstand forces from a variety of directions during movement (Jozsa & Kannus

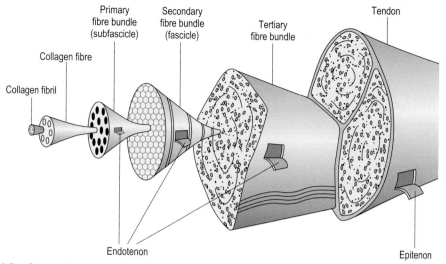

Figure 4.6 • Connective tissue sheaths investing tendon (after Jozsa & Kannus 1997, with permission).

1997). The longitudinal collagen fibrils have a wavy or crimped appearance (Jozsa & Kannus 1997) and cross each other to form spirals and plaits (Figure 4.7) (Elliott 1965; Jozsa et al. 1991); this is thought to increase the tensile strength of tendon (Jozsa & Kannus 1997). The crimped appearance of the collagen fibril varies within and between collagen fibres (Nicholls et al. 1983; Rowe 1985).

Like other tissues in the body, form and function go hand in hand. Tendon tissue is plastic (Brown & Hardman 1987) and so will alter its composition and construction according to the physical demands placed upon it (Elliott 1965). For example, with exercise, there is an increase in tendon thickness (Ingelmark 1948); when a muscle is immobilised in a lengthened position there is an increase in tendon thickness (Elliott 1965), and exercise causes an increase in strength of the tendon at its insertion site (Woo et al. 1988). The stimulus for tendon growth is the tension that is applied and does not appear to be related to the size or strength of the muscle (Elliott 1965).

Tendons have viscoelastic properties; the load–displacement curve for a tendon is shown in Figure 4.8. The toe region is concave and is considered to reflect the straightening of the wavy collagen fibres shown in

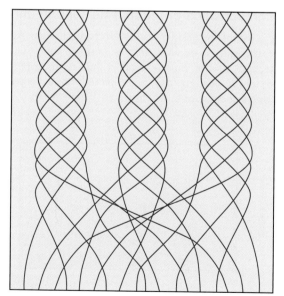

Figure 4.7 • Schematic drawing of the interweaving of tendon bundles near its insertion (from Elliott 1965, with permission).

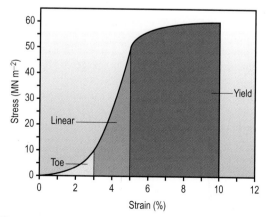

Figure 4.8 • Load–displacement (stress–strain) curve for tendon (from Herzog & Gal 1999, with permission).

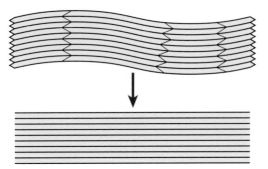

Figure 4.9 • The wavy pattern of a tendon in a relaxed state straightens out when it is stretched (from Jozsa & Kannus 1997, with permission).

Figure 4.9 (Rigby et al. 1959; Hirsch 1974). Little force is required to lengthen the tendon in this region. This region is considered to be responsible for the ability of tendon to absorb shock (Wood T O et al. 1988). With continued lengthening, the wave pattern straightens and the tendon behaves like a stiff spring; this occurs with about 3% elongation (Herzog & Gal 1999). As the force increases, there is an increase in the stiffness of the tendon, producing the linear part of the curve; this occurs at about 4% elongation (Wainwright et al. 1982). Both toe and linear regions are temporary and, on removal of the force, the tendon will return to its resting length. During normal everyday activities, tensile forces on tendon are thought to lie within the toe and linear region and are thought to be less than 4% strain (Fung 1993). If the force continues to elongate beyond this there is a permanent deformation in the yield region of the curve, up to a maximum of approximately 8–15% elongation, where failure occurs (Rigby et al. 1959; Fung 1993). During the yield region, a relatively small increase in force will produce a relatively large increase in displacement. Temperatures of up to 37°C make no difference to the force–displacement curve of tendon; however, by 40°C (104–105°F) displacement of 3–4% will result in breakage of the tendon (Rigby et al. 1959).

The stiffness of tendon is not the same throughout its length. Tendon is stiffest in the middle of its length and least stiff at its insertion. So when a tendon is lengthened there is greatest displacement at the insertion region (Woo et al. 1988).

Blood supply of tendon

Tendons receive their blood supply at the osteotendinous junction, from vessels within bone and periosteum. At the musculotendinous junction it receives blood from vessels within muscle and from the surrounding vessels within the paratenon, mesotenon and synovial sheath (Jozsa & Kannus 1997). The blood supply at the osteotendinous junction is fairly sparse and is limited to where the tendon attaches to bone. Blood vessels are present only in the distal third of the tendon (Jozsa & Kannus 1997). At the musculotendinous junction the blood vessels from within the muscle pass into, and supply, the proximal third of the tendon (Peacock 1959). There is therefore a fairly marked transition between the highly vascular muscle tissue and the relatively poor vascular supply of tendon. The blood vessels around the outer covering of tendons perforate both the epitenon and endotenon, and so supply the superficial and deep portions of the tendon.

Some tendons have an area of poor vascularity; for example, the tendocalcaneus tendon has an avascular area 2–6 cm proximal to its distal attachment (Carr & Norris 1989), the extensor pollicis longus tendon has an area of poor vascularity where it lies underneath the dorsal carpal ligament of the wrist (Jozsa & Kannus 1997), the posterior tibial tendon has an area of poor vascularity posterior and distal to the medial malleolus (Frey et al. 1990), and the supraspinatus tendon has poor vascularity where it inserts onto the humerus (Lohr & Uhthoff 1990; Chansky & Iannotti 1991). Interestingly, the area of poor vascularity in supraspinatus tendon does not increase with age (Lohr & Uhthoff 1990).

Biomechanics of the muscle–tendon unit

It is useful to consider the biomechanical behaviour of the muscle–tendon unit as a single unit. The strength of the muscle–tendon unit with respect to tensile loading can be depicted on a force–displacement curve, as shown in Figure 4.10; this

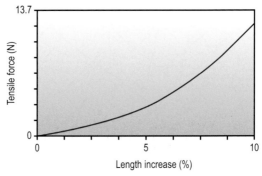

Figure 4.10 • Force–displacement curve of the muscle–tendon unit (after Taylor et al. 1990, with permission).

curve was obtained from the whole tibialis anterior muscle–tendon unit of a rabbit (Taylor et al. 1990). The load or force is plotted against the stretch or deformation. The slope of the curve is the modulus of elasticity, measured in Pa or N/m^2, and is a measure of the 'stiffness' of the muscle–tendon unit (Panjabi & White 2001). It can be seen in Figure 4.10 that only a little force is initially required to deform the muscle–tendon unit, a region referred to as the 'toe' region (Threlkeld 1992) or 'neutral zone' (Panjabi & White 2001). Stiffness then increases, so that greater force is required to deform the muscle–tendon unit; this region is referred to as the elastic zone (Panjabi & White 2001). Forces within the elastic zone will result in no permanent change in length; as soon as the force is released the muscle–tendon unit will return to its preload shape and size (Panjabi & White 2001). The neutral zone and elastic zone fall within the normal physiological range of forces and deformation on the muscle–tendon unit during everyday activities (Nordin & Frankel 1989). Heating muscle beyond $43°C$ causes a 170% increase, and cooling muscle to $+10°C$ causes a 30% decrease in its viscoelastic properties (Talishev & Fedina 1976). Thus, heating muscle will cause it to be less stiff and cooling muscle will cause it to be more stiff.

The strength of a muscle or tendon is measured by stress (force per unit area, measured in Pa or N/m^2) and strain (percentage change in length, from the resting length). The stress–strain properties of muscle and tendon are compared with those of bone, cartilage, ligament and nerve in Table 4.1. The ability of muscle to resist lengthening reduces with age

(Panjabi & White 2001). Failure occurs at 58% elongation in the seventh decade compared with 65% elongation in a teenager (Panjabi & White 2001).

A muscle–tendon unit is viscoelastic, that is, it has time-dependent mechanical properties. These properties affect the behaviour of the muscle–tendon unit to movement and forces and are therefore important principles for clinicians. They can be summarised as:

• elastic nature
• viscous nature
• creep phenomena
• stress relaxation
• loading rate
• hysteresis.

The muscle–tendon unit has elastic properties; it will stretch and return to its original shape like an elastic band.

The muscle–tendon unit has viscous properties; that is, it will gradually elongate over a period of time when a constant force is applied – a phenomenon known as creep.

The muscle–tendon unit undergoes load (or stress) relaxation. In Figure 4.11, the muscle–tendon unit of extensor digitorum longus was lengthened repeatedly 10 times to 78 N. The reduction in tension is indicated by the gradient of the curve. There is a significant ($P < 0.05$) reduction in tension between the first two stretches (Taylor et al. 1990).

The muscle–tendon unit will elongate on loading and is dependent on the rate of loading. When the muscle–tendon unit of tibialis anterior is loaded quickly it will be stiffer and deform less than when it is loaded more slowly (Figure 4.12). This is relevant when applying therapeutic force, as a slower rate will result in less resistance and more movement. An additional effect is that the failure point of the muscle–tendon unit will be higher with a higher loading rate; in other words, it will be stronger and less likely to rupture when the force is applied at a faster rate.

The muscle–tendon unit demonstrates the phenomenon of hysteresis, which is the energy loss during loading and unloading (Figure 4.13). These data are taken from the tibialis anterior muscle–tendon unit of rabbits (Taylor et al. 1990). The unloading curve lies below the loading curve and reflects a greater energy expenditure on loading than the energy regained during unloading. This results in a loss of energy known as hysteresis loss (Panjabi & White 2001). It can also be seen that hysteresis produces an elongation of the muscle–tendon unit.

Table 4.1 Tensile properties of muscle and tendon compared with bone, cartilage, ligament and nerve (Panjabi & White 2001)

Tissue	Stress at failure (MPa)	Strain at failure (%)
Muscle (passive)	0.17	60
Tendon	55	9–10
Cortical bone	100–200	1–3
Cancellous bone	10	5–7
Cartilage	10–15	80–120
Ligament	10–40	30–45
Nerve roots	15	19

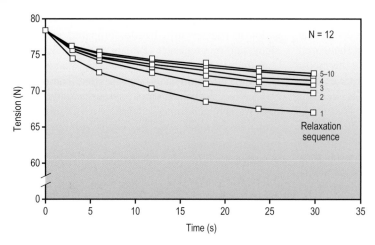

Figure 4.11 • Load relaxation of extensor digitorum longus muscle–tendon unit of the New Zealand white rabbit (from Taylor et al. 1990, with permission). A gradual decrease in tension occurs with the first two repetitions with a force of 78 N.

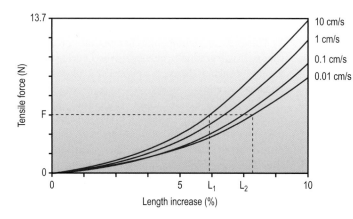

Figure 4.12 • The muscle–tendon unit and rate of loading. When it is loaded quickly it will be stiffer and will sustain a higher force before breaking than when it is loaded more slowly. For example, a given force, if applied at 10 cm/s, it will cause a displacement L_1, but if applied more slowly, at 0.01 cm/s, it will cause a greater displacement to L_2. These data are from the tibialis anterior muscle–tendon unit from New Zealand white rabbits. (After Taylor et al. 1990, with permission).

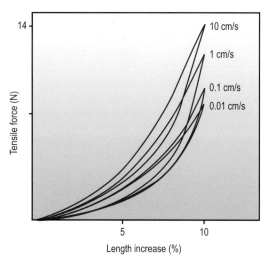

Figure 4.13 • The muscle–tendon unit demonstrates the phenomenon of hysteresis (from Taylor et al. 1990, with permission). The graph was produced from the tibialis anterior muscle–tendon unit of New Zealand white rabbits. The loading rate used was 0.01, 0.1, 1 and 10 cm/s.

The muscle belly is less stiff than the tendon, so when a muscle is passively lengthened most of the length change occurs in the muscle belly and the tendon is minimally affected (Jami 1992). Muscle length refers to the length of the muscle through the available range of joint movement. During normal daily activities muscle lengthens and shortens to allow movement. Muscle length reduces with age (Gajdosik et al. 1996).

Types of muscle fibre

Muscle fibres can be classified in various ways (Table 4.2). Initially, muscle fibres were described according to the speed of shortening and were identified by staining for myoglobin concentration (myoglobin binds oxygen). Muscles were divided into: (1) slow muscles (type I), which stained red owing to a high concentration of myoglobin enabling aerobic energy metabolism, and (2) fast muscles (type II), which stained white owing to a low concentration

Table 4.2 Classification of muscle fibre types (Staron 1997; Scott et al. 2001). The question mark beside fast-twitch oxidative and fast-twitch glycolytic indicates that muscle fibre types IIA and IIB do not always rely on aerobic/oxidative and anaerobic/glycolytic metabolism (McComas 1996)

Myosin ATPase	Myosin ATPase hydrolysis rate	Myosin heavy chain (MHC)	Biochemical identification of metabolic enzymes
I	I	MHCl	Slow-twitch oxidative
	IC	MHCl and MHCIIa	
	IIC	MHCl and MHCIIa	
	IIAC	MHCl and MHCIIa	
IIA	IIA	MHCIIa	? Fast-twitch oxidative
	IIAB	MHCIIa and MHCIIb	
IIB	IIB	MHCIIb	? Fast-twitch glycolytic

of myoglobin enabling anaerobic energy metabolism (Pette & Staron 1990). Fast-twitch fibres (type II) contract more quickly, generate higher forces but fatigue more quickly than slow-twitch (type II) fibres (Table 4.3).

An alternative classification system identified type I and type II myofibrillar actomyosin adenosine triphosphate (ATP) which related to different contractile properties (Pette & Staron 1990). When this classification was combined with the myoglobin classification a metabolic enzyme-based classification was developed (Table 4.2). This classification describes three types of muscle fibre: slow-twitch oxidative (SO), fast-twitch oxidative (FOG) and fast-twitch glycolytic (FG) (Pette & Staron 1990; McComas 1996). Fibres that fall between slow-twitch (type I) and fast-twitch (type IIb) are termed intermediate (type IIa) (Pette et al. 1999). The characteristics of these types of muscle fibre are summarised in Table 4.3.

Although it is convenient to classify muscle fibres into three types, the reality is more of a continuum between fast-twitch and slow-twitch muscles (Pette & Staron 1990; Pette et al. 1999). A third type of fast fibre has since been identified and is known as IID or IIX (Pette et al. 1999).

More recent advances in staining techniques have led to the identification of seven types of muscle

Table 4.3 Characteristics of skeletal muscle and motor neurones (Newham & Ainscough-Potts 2001)

Characteristic	Type I	Type IIa	Type IIb
Muscle fibre type	Slow oxidative (SO)	Fast oxidative glycolytic (FOG)	Fast glycolytic (FG)
Motor unit type	Slow	Fast fatigue-resistant	Fast fatigable
Motor unit size	Small	Medium	Large
Conduction rate of motor neurone	Slow	Fast	Fast
Twitch tension	Low	Moderate	High
Speed of contraction	Slow	Fast	Fast
Resistance to fatigue	High	High	Low
Mitochondrial enzyme activity	High	Medium	Low
Myoglobin content	High	Medium	Low
Capillary density	High	Medium	Low

fibre: I, IC, IIC, IIAC, IIA, IIAB and IIB. The types of muscle fibre can also be classified according to the protein composition of myosin (Staron 1997). Myosin consists of two myosin heavy chains and four myosin light chains (Pette & Staron 1990).

It is worth remembering that these classification systems relate to individual muscle fibres and not to whole muscle. While a few muscles do have a high percentage of type I fibres (80% in adductor pollicis, 86–89% in soleus, 73% in tibialis anterior) or type II fibres (85% in orbicularis oculi, 71% lateral head of rectus femoris), the vast majority of whole muscle contains a range of types of muscle fibre with a large variation between individuals (Johnson et al. 1973). For this reason the classification of individual muscle fibres cannot be applied to whole muscle; that is, generally speaking, whole muscles cannot be classified as fast-twitch or slow-twitch.

For any one motor unit, the characteristic of the muscle fibre type is mirrored by the motor nerve supply (Box 4.1). All muscle fibres that are innervated by the same motor neurone are of the same type; that is, the conduction rate of a motor neurone innervating fast-twitch fibres is faster than that for slow-twitch fibres (Buller et al. 1960). The motor neurone determines the characteristic of a muscle fibre and is described as a phasic or tonic motor neurone. In animals, large, phasic high-threshold motor neurones discharge at the high frequency of 30–60/second compared with small, tonic low-threshold motor neurones with a lower frequency of 10–20/second (Granit et al. 1957). The nerve is so influential on muscle fibre type that, if the motor neurones to fast- and slow-twitch fibres are experimentally switched, the muscle fibre types will also switch characteristics (Buller et al. 1960; Lomo et al. 1980).

The size of the motor unit varies between muscles and within a muscle. There is a tendency for smaller motor units to be composed of slow-twitch fibres and larger motor units to be composed of fast-twitch fibres (Wuerker et al. 1965). The motor neurone of a slow-twitch motor unit innervates 12–180 muscle fibres compared with 300–800 muscle fibres of a fast-twitch motor unit. The fewer number of slow-twitch muscle fibres supplied by a motor neurone enables greater control of muscular contraction. For example, the motor neurone supplies only approximately 12 muscle fibres in the eye (Bors 1926), allowing for the fine control needed. The greater number of fast-twitch muscle fibres supplied by a motor neurone will cause a greater speed and force of contraction of fast-twitch motor units.

The fact that any one muscle contains both small and large motor units providing fine control of muscle contraction, as well as great speed and force of contraction, attests to the multiplicity of muscle functions.

Nerve supply of muscles

Sensory nerve endings in the muscle–tendon units include muscle spindles, Golgi tendon organs and free nerve endings. Large-diameter myelinated group Ia and II fibres supply the muscle spindles, slightly smaller myelinated IIb fibres supply Golgi tendon organs and fine myelinated A δ (or group III fibres) and unmyelinated C (or group IV) fibres supply the free nerve endings.

Muscle spindles

Muscle spindles are proprioceptors acting as stretch receptors controlling the length (or tension) and rate of change in length of muscle. They are sensitive to static and dynamic length changes and are affected by the velocity, acceleration or deceleration of the length change.

Muscle spindles lie within the muscle belly, parallel to extrafusal fibres, and near the musculotendinous junction (Boyd 1976). The muscle spindle consists of intrafusal fibres to distinguish it from the rest of muscle which, in turn, consists of a non-contractile central portion within a capsule with

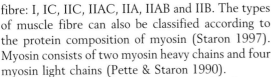

Box 4.1

Characteristics of motor neurone and muscle fibre type (Newham & Ainscough-Potts 2001)

Nerve	Nerve
Large motor neurone	Small motor neurone
Phasic	Tonic
High threshold	Low threshold
High frequency	Low frequency

Muscle fibres	Muscle fibres
Fast-twitch	Slow-twitch
Type Ia – fast oxidative glycolytic	Type I – slow-twitch oxidative
Type IIb – fast glycolytic	
Large motor unit supplies 300–800 muscle fibres	Small motor unit supplies 12–180 muscle fibres

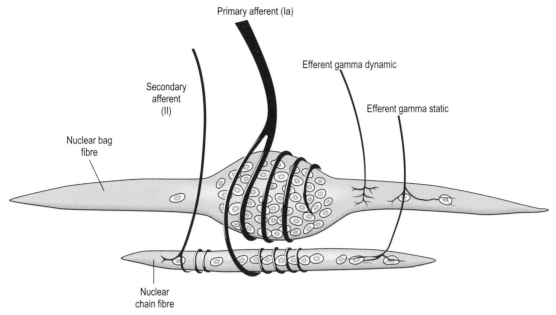

Figure 4.14 • Muscle spindle showing a nuclear bag fibre and a nuclear chain fibre. Group Ia and II afferent fibres supply the muscle spindle. (After Shumway-Cook & Woollacott 1995, with permission.)

contractile ends. The muscle spindle typically consists of one nuclear bag 1 and one nuclear bag 2 (Figure 4.14), distinguished by differences in ATP concentration, and about four or more nuclear chain fibres (Hunt 1990). The nuclear bag fibres extend beyond the fibrous capsule of the muscle spindle while the nuclear chain fibres are contained within the capsule. The nuclear bag fibres are more elastic and less stiff than the nuclear chain fibres.

The group Ia primary afferents terminate in annulo-spiral endings on all of the intrafusal fibres (nuclear bag and nuclear chain) in the spindle (Hunt 1990). The group Ia afferents have a low threshold to stretch, and they respond to both static and dynamic stretches (Shumway-Cook & Woollacott 1995). Even a small change in length will trigger a steep rise in the discharge rate (Hasan & Houk 1975). The group II secondary afferents terminate in 'flower spray' endings on both the nuclear chain fibre and nuclear bag 2 fibres (Hunt 1990). Group II fibres have a higher threshold, responding only to changes in muscle length, and they therefore act as position detectors with little to no dynamic response (Hunt 1990; Shumway-Cook & Woollacott 1995).

The behaviour of muscle spindle to stretch is often identified by stretching a muscle at a constant velocity, then holding it at a new increased length and then releasing the muscle, a procedure known as the ramp-and-hold stretch. When a muscle is stretched at a constant velocity, the primary endings initially have a burst of activity (Hunt 1990). The rate of activity depends on the velocity of the stretch; increased velocity results in an increased rate of activity (Hunt 1990). If the lengthened muscle is then maintained at its new length, there is a reduction in the rate of discharge. The sensitivity of static length is related to muscle length; there is greater sensitivity at greater lengths, although the discharge rate is still relatively small. While the lengthened muscle is maintained at its new length the nuclear bag fibres within the muscle spindle exhibit creep, that is, they lengthen (Boyd 1976). The discharge rate from the secondary group II fibres increases with a maintained position, and so appear to act as position detectors (Hunt 1990). On release from a lengthened position, the discharge rate from the primary endings reduces, and may stop, and then resume at the rate associated with the new length. Because the intrafusal fibres lie parallel to the extrafusal fibres, the discharge from the sensory fibres in the muscle spindle diminishes or ceases when the muscle contracts and increases when the muscle is lengthened (Hunt 1990). In addition to group Ia and II afferent nerve supply, muscle spindles in the cat have been found to receive a sympathetic innervation (Barker & Saito 1981); however, the effect of this is unclear (Hunt 1990).

The nuclear bag and nuclear chain fibres have a motor nerve supply via the gamma motor neurone (or fusimotor) fibres. Nuclear bag 1, sensitive to dynamic lengthening, is supplied by dynamic gamma fibres, whereas nuclear bag 2 and nuclear chain fibres, sensitive to static length, are supplied by static gamma fibres (Hunt 1990; Shumway-Cook & Woollacott 1995). Whenever the alpha motor neurone causes contraction of the extrafusal fibres there is, at the same time, gamma motor neurone activity (static and dynamic gamma activity) causing contraction of the intrafusal fibres. The contraction of the intrafusal fibres causes increased tension of the nuclear bag and nuclear chain fibres and thus maintains the sensitivity of the muscle spindle. If the gamma motor neurone activity did not occur then muscle contraction would shorten the intrafusal fibres and switch off sensory information from the muscle spindle. This enables continuous information of the length of muscle to be relayed to the sensory cortex of the brain. The gamma efferent system is under central nervous system (CNS) control by the cerebellum, basal ganglia and cerebral cortex.

Stretch of the muscle spindle causes excitation of the alpha motor neurones leading to contraction of the extrafusal muscle fibres in which the spindle is situated, and inhibition of the antagonistic muscles. This phenomenon is known as the spindle stretch reflex (Figure 4.15). This phenomenon is used clinically with the reflex hammer to apply a brisk tap to a tendon to produce a reflex contraction of the muscle; for example, a tap to the quadriceps tendon causes a contraction of the quadriceps muscle. Muscle spindles protect and limit the muscle from excessive lengthening by an external force. Clearly, this is a useful protective mechanism to regulate movement and maintain posture (Hunt 1990). Where a muscle becomes shortened, treatment may be directed to lengthen it; slow movements to lengthen a muscle would seem more effective to minimise this protective response.

The density of muscle spindles varies between different muscles. The suboccipital muscles and the muscles of the hand contain a rich density of muscle spindles whereas the large muscles of the arm and leg contain much fewer. The suboccipital muscles, such as the superior oblique and rectus capitus posterior major, have 43 and 30 spindles per gram respectively, the small muscles of the hand such as the lumbricals and opponens pollicis have 16 and 17 spindles per gram respectively, whereas pectoralis major, triceps brachii and latissimus dorsi have only about 1.4 spindles per gram (McComas 1996). The difference in density is probably related to the need for rapid and accurate movements (Armstrong et al. 2008).

Summary of the muscle spindle

Each muscle spindle lying within a muscle belly and the musculotendinous junction is a stretch receptor.

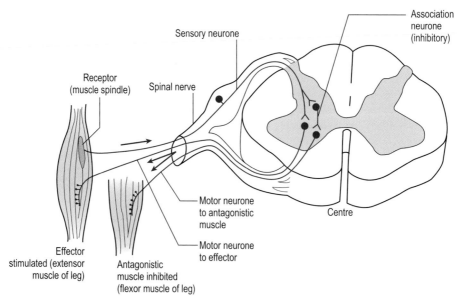

Figure 4.15 • Spindle stretch reflex. Excitation of the muscle spindle causes a reflex contraction of the muscle in which the spindle lies and inhibition of the antagonistic muscle. (From Crow & Haas 2001, with permission.)

A statically maintained muscle length will cause stimulation of group Ia and particularly group II afferents. An increase in muscle length will cause stimulation of group Ia afferents which results in a reflex contraction of the extrafusal fibres of that muscle and inhibition of the antagonist muscle.

Golgi tendon organs

Golgi tendon organs lie in the musculotendinous or musculoaponeurotic junction (Barker 1974); they are not found, as their name implies, in the tendon (Jami 1992). They are encapsulated corpuscles containing collagen fibres, lying in series with 15–20 muscle fibres (Houk & Henneman 1967; Shumway-Cook & Woollacott 1995) (Figure 4.16). Golgi tendon organs are stimulated only by the tension in these muscle fibres in series (Houk & Henneman 1967).

Golgi tendon organs are proprioceptors, particularly sensitive to changes in muscle tension and to the rate of change of this tension produced by active muscle contraction (Houk & Henneman 1967). Golgi tendon organs can be stimulated by passive lengthening of the muscle–tendon unit; however, the threshold for discharge is very high and rarely persists with a maintained muscle stretch (Houk et al. 1971; Jami 1992). Each tendon organ is innervated by a large fast-conducting Ib afferent fibre. The continuous steady state of firing from the Golgi tendon organ is proportional to the muscle tension (Crow & Haas 2001). When the muscle fibres contract there is a lengthening of the musculotendinous junction with approximation of the collagen fibres within the Golgi tendon organ; this compresses the nerve terminals and causes firing of the Ib afferent fibre.

Stimulation of Golgi tendon organs leads to inhibition of the muscle in which they are situated (inhibition of both alpha and gamma motor neurones), a mechanism known as autogenic inhibition, and excitation of the antagonist muscles (Figure 4.17). So, for example, when lifting a weight, such that the muscle contraction and the weight cause excessive force that may damage the musculotendinous junction, the Golgi tendon organs will be stimulated, producing inhibition of the agonist muscles and stimulation of the antagonist. This is a protective mechanism to avoid injury to the musculotendinous junction. However, this mechanism is not seen during competitive sport – for example, wrist wrestling can result in ruptured muscles and tendons. In this case the highly motivated athlete disinhibits the process (Brooks & Fahey 1987).

Summary of the Golgi tendon organ

Golgi tendon organs lie in the musculotendinous junction and help to protect this region from excessive tension brought about by muscle contraction.

Free nerve endings

Free nerve endings have been investigated in the gastrocnemius and soleus muscle of the cat and rat, and it is thought that similar findings are to be found in humans (Stacey 1969; Reinert & Mense 1992). Free nerve endings lie throughout the muscle, in the connective tissue, between intrafusal and extrafusal fibres, in arterioles and venules, in the capsule of muscle spindles and tendon organs, in tendon tissue at the musculotendinous junction and in fat cells (Stacey 1969; Reinert & Mense 1992). This is summarised in Box 4.2. Free nerve endings are supplied

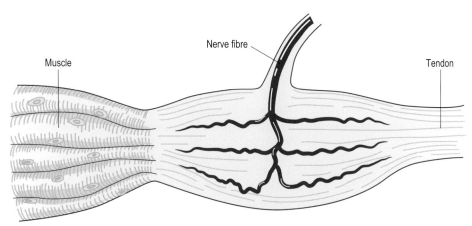

Figure 4.16 • Golgi tendon organ in series with 15–20 muscle fibres (from Shumway-Cook & Woollacott 1995, with permission).

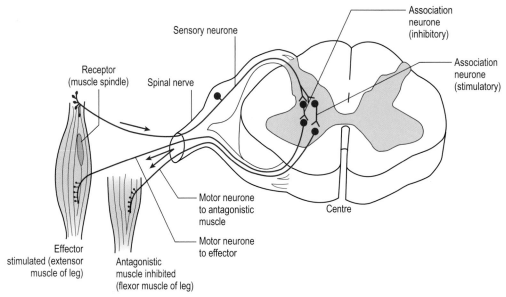

Figure 4.17 • The tendon reflex: stimulation of the Golgi tendon organ causes inhibition of the muscle in which it lies and excitation of the antagonistic muscle (from Crow & Haas 2001, with permission).

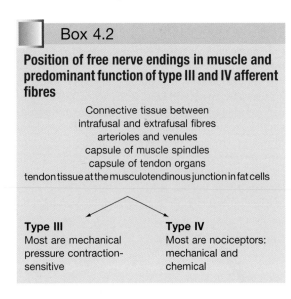

Box 4.2

Position of free nerve endings in muscle and predominant function of type III and IV afferent fibres

Connective tissue between intrafusal and extrafusal fibres
arterioles and venules
capsule of muscle spindles
capsule of tendon organs
tendon tissue at the musculotendinous junction in fat cells

Type III
Most are mechanical pressure contraction-sensitive

Type IV
Most are nociceptors: mechanical and chemical

by myelinated A δ (group III) and unmyelinated C (group IV) fibres.

Type III afferents act as low-threshold mechanical pressure receptors, contraction-sensitive receptors and nociceptors (Mense & Meyer 1985). Most type IV afferents are mainly nociceptors (to both noxious mechanical and chemical stimulation), with a smaller proportion being low-threshold mechanical pressure receptors, contraction-sensitive receptors and thermo-receptors (Kniffki et al. 1978; Mense & Meyer 1985).

Mechanoreceptors

Mechanoreceptors respond to pressure, active muscle contraction and muscle lengthening. The majority of group III fibres respond to local pressure stimulation (Paintal 1960; Iggo 1961; Kaufman et al. 1984a), while very few of the group IV fibres respond to low-threshold innocuous pressure (Franz & Mense 1975).

Group III and IV fibres are activated in a linear fashion to the force of a muscle contraction or the force of a stretch on a muscle (Kaufman et al. 1983; Mense & Stahnke 1983; Mense & Meyer 1985) – the greater the force, the greater the response. Approximately half of the afferents respond to both contraction and lengthening, and half are specific to one or other stimulus (Mense & Meyer 1985).

Afferents responsive to active contraction are often also chemical receptors responsive to bradykinin (Mense & Meyer 1985), a chemical released with inflammation. Group III afferents appear to be stimulated by the mechanical effects of the contraction, whereas group IV receptors seem to be stimulated by the metabolic products produced by the muscle contraction (Kniffki et al. 1978; Kaufman et al. 1982, 1983). Receptors that respond to the metabolic products have been named ergoreceptors (erg is a unit of work or energy) as they are thought to be involved in alterations to the cardiorespiratory system during physical activity (Kao 1963).

Chemical receptors

Some free nerve endings are sensitive to muscle pH, concentrations of extracellular potassium and sodium chloride and changes in oxygen and carbon dioxide. They help to regulate the cardiopulmonary system during exercise or activity (McCloskey & Mitchell 1972; Laughlin & Korthuis 1987). Group IV afferents in muscle are thought to be primarily responsible for producing the reflex changes in cardiorespiratory function with exercise (Kniffki et al. 1978; Kaufman et al. 1982, 1983). Other group IV afferents are activated in the presence of chemicals released with inflammation, such as bradykinin, 5-hydroxytryptamine and potassium ions (Franz & Mense 1975; Kumazawa & Mizumura 1977; Mense 1981; Kaufman et al. 1982). Chemically induced muscle pain in humans is thought to be due to activation of these free nerve endings (Mense 1996).

Thermal receptors

Some group IV receptors respond to small changes of temperature in muscle (Iggo 1961; Kumazawa & Mizumura 1977; Mense 1996). Others have been identified to have a high threshold for thermal stimulation and are thus thermal nociceptors (Iggo 1961; Mense & Meyer 1985). A high proportion of thermoreceptors have also been found to be sensitive to noxious mechanical pressure (Mense & Meyer 1985).

Nociceptors

Muscle nociceptors have a high mechanical threshold and some also have a high thermal threshold. The vast majority of group IV afferents in the cat have been found to be high-threshold mechanoreceptors and thus thought to be nociceptors (Franz & Mense 1975). It is also thought that group III muscle afferents may be capable of acting as nociceptors and thus mediating pain (Paintal 1960). Bradykinin, a chemical released with inflammation, has been found to sensitise muscle and tendon nociceptors (Mense & Meyer 1985). This sensitisation lowers the firing threshold such that an innocuous mechanical stimulus, for example movement or a light touch, causes excitation, a phenomenon known as allodynia (Raja et al. 1999).

Summary of free nerve endings in muscle

The presence of nociceptors indicates that muscle has the potential to be a primary source of symptoms, and this could be brought about by noxious mechanical, chemical or thermal stimulation.

Efferent nerve fibres

Generally, the efferent fibres to muscle consist of the large myelinated alpha motor neurones that supply the extrafusal fibres, and the small myelinated gamma (or fusimotor) fibres that supply the intrafusal fibres within the muscle spindle. Type I muscle fibres are innervated by small, low-threshold, slowly conducting motor nerves while type IIb fibres are innervated by large, higher-threshold, fast-conducting motor nerves.

The efferent fibres enter the muscle around the centre of the muscle belly, a region known as the motor point. Motor nerves divide into small branches to supply each muscle fibre; the presynaptic terminal synapses at the neuromuscular junction, with the motor end-plate (Figure 4.18). When an action potential arrives at the presynaptic terminal, a chain of chemical reactions is initiated which causes diffusion of acetylcholine across the synaptic cleft to the postsynaptic membrane. This chemical causes an increase in the permeability of sodium ions which, if sufficient, will initiate an action potential along the muscle fibre.

Each muscle fibre is supplied by a motor neurone. The motor neurone, and the muscle fibres it

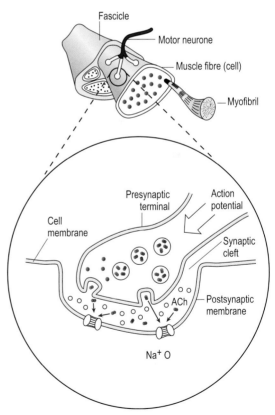

Figure 4.18 • Neuromuscular junction formed by the motor nerve and the motor end-plate (after Herzog 1999, with permission). ACh, acetylcholine.

innervates, is termed a motor unit and is the functional unit of a muscle. Stimulation of the motor neurone initiates and maintains a series of complex events leading to either shortening (concentric contraction) or active lengthening (eccentric contraction) of muscle, and the development of muscle tension. Muscle contraction ceases when the stimulation of the motor nerve stops.

Muscle contraction is thought to be produced by the sliding of myosin and actin filaments so that the length of the sarcomere is shortened; this is termed the sliding filament theory (Figure 4.19). The length of actin and myosin filaments does not change appreciably when a muscle contracts. Myosin contains proteins that extend towards the actin filaments, in the form of a tail and a head. The head contains a binding site for actin (Figure 4.20) and forms the cross-bridge between myosin and actin. The reader is directed to a physiology textbook for a more detailed description of the sliding filament theory.

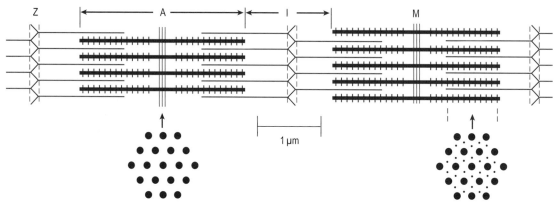

1 μm

Figure 4.19 • The sliding filament model (from Huxley 2000, with permission).

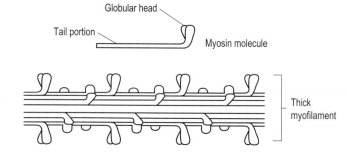

Globular head

Tail portion

Myosin molecule

Thick
myofilament

(A)

Figure 4.20 • A Myosin with tail and head projecting towards the actin filaments (from Herzog 1999, with permission).
B Cross-sectional arrangement of actin and myosin (after Herzog 1999, with permission).

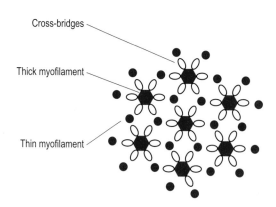

Cross-bridges

Thick myofilament

Thin myofilament

(B)

Muscle and proprioception

Several lines of research support the view that muscle has an important proprioceptive function (Grigg 1994). Isolated movement of a tendon, so as to stretch its muscle, gives a sensation of joint movement (Matthews & Simmonds 1974). In the human hand, it has been found that isolated stimulation of individual spindle afferents is insufficient to cause a perception of joint movement. However, the spatial summation of a number of muscle spindles provides sufficient information for proprioception (Macefield et al. 1990).

In addition, vibration of muscle produces a sensation of joint movement and a sense of joint position (Goodwin et al. 1972). The movement is in the direction that would stretch the muscle being vibrated, so it is the muscle being stretched that provides a sense of joint movement. For example, on elbow extension the elbow flexor muscles will be stretched and give a sense of the extension movement. Because muscle spindles are more sensitive to vibration than Golgi tendon organs it is thought that the illusion of movement is produced by stimulation of the muscle spindles (Goodwin et al. 1972). Further evidence comes from the fact that, if muscle afferent activity is abolished during joint movement, proprioception is less accurate (Gandevia & McClosky 1976; Gandevia et al. 1983) and, conversely, when skin and joint receptor activity is abolished the sense of proprioception remains (Goodwin et al. 1972; Gandevia & McClosky 1976; Clark et al. 1979), albeit poor (Clark et al. 1979; Moberg 1983). Additionally, increased tension in a muscle increases the sensitivity of muscle spindles, and increased muscle tension has been found to enhance proprioception (Goodwin et al. 1972; Gandevia & McClosky 1976; Macefield et al. 1990).

The nerve supply to the skin is also relevant as this will be involved in any movement caused by muscle contraction; details of skin sensation can be found under nerve function in Chapter 6.

Muscle contraction

The strength of a muscle contraction depends on the following factors.

1. The type and number of motor units recruited. The recruitment of muscle fibres is directly related to the size of the motor neurone (Milner-Brown et al. 1973). There is an initial recruitment of small motor neurones and then recruitment of large motor neurones as more force is required (Henneman & Olson 1965; Henneman et al. 1965). This has been referred to as the Henneman's principle, where small motor units (type I) are recruited first and then large motor units (type II). There is a higher predominance of type I muscle fibres in postural muscles, therefore these muscles fire first to provide stability in preparation for movement. The greater the stimulus, the greater the number of muscle fibres stimulated and the greater the strength of contraction. The fact that all muscles contain both type I and II muscle fibres enables graded levels of muscle contraction to occur.

2. The initial length of the muscle. The resting length of a muscle fibre affects its strength of contraction. The optimal length is where there is maximum overlap between actin and myosin. Where a muscle fibre is less or more than the optimal length, fewer cross-bridges between actin and myosin are formed and the tension is lessened. This phenomenon produces a length–tension relationship in muscle which can be depicted on a graph (Figure 4.21). When a single muscle fibre is lengthened there is an uneven lengthening such that the central portion of the muscle fibre lengthens more than the ends of the muscle; so while there is a reduction in the cross-bridges in the central portion there are still cross-bridges at the ends (Huxley 2000).

3. The nature of the neural stimulation of the motor unit. The frequency of the neural stimulation affects the strength of the muscular contraction. A single neural stimulus will result in a muscle twitch. A muscle twitch consists of a brief latent period, then a muscle contraction and then a

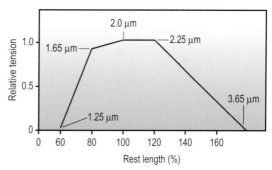

Figure 4.21 • Length–tension relationship in skeletal muscle (from Powers & Howley 1997, with permission).

relaxation period. The total time this takes varies between 10 and 100 ms (Ghez 1991). The strength of the contraction and the total time will depend on the type of muscle fibre, with fast-twitch fibres contracting more quickly, and with more force, than slow-twitch fibres. If a series of neural stimuli are used (1–3 ms apart) (Ghez 1991), the muscle has not had time to relax and so an increase in muscle tension is produced due to the summation of each twitch. If the frequency of the neural stimuli is increased still further, individual contractions are blended together in a single sustained contraction known as fused tetanus (Ghez 1991). This contraction will continue until the neural stimulus is stopped or the muscle fatigues. Muscular contractions that occur during normal body movements are the result of these tetanic contractions.

4. The age of the patient. Age causes a reduction in isokinetic calf strength (Gajdosik et al. 1996) and isometric quadriceps strength (Young et al. 1982a; Grimby 1995; Heyley et al. 1998). Between the fourth and seventh decade there is a 14% reduction in isokinetic quadriceps strength per decade (Hughes et al. 2001).

Muscle strength is proportional to the physiological cross-sectional area of the muscle, reflecting the number of sarcomeres in parallel (Newham 2001). As a muscle contracts, the tension at adjacent sarcomeres is equal and opposite and is therefore not transmitted to the attachments at the end of the muscle. The attachments to bone or fascia are subject to tension from the adjacent sarcomere only. For this reason force is independent of fibre length (Newham 2001). The cross-sectional area of muscle has been found to reduce with age. The quadriceps femoris cross-sectional area for 20-year-olds compared with 70-year-olds has been found to reduce by 27% in both men and women (Trappe et al. 2001) and by 35% in women (Young et al. 1982a). This decrease in cross-sectional area is thought to be mainly responsible for the decrease in muscle strength with age (Akima et al. 2001).

Muscle power

Muscle power is calculated from the force of contraction and the speed of contraction (force multiplied by velocity). Muscle power is determined by the number of sarcomeres in series (muscle length), the angle of pennation of the muscle fibres (the more

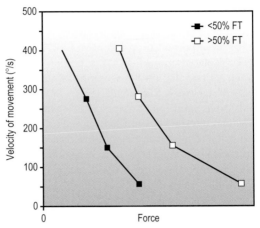

Figure 4.22 • Difference in muscular force and speed of movement between muscles predominantly with fast-twitch (FT) and with slow-twitch muscle fibres (from Powers & Howley 1997, with permission).

parallel to the direction of force, the greater the speed of contraction) as well as the biochemical properties of the muscle (Sacks & Roy 1982). For a given muscular force, the speed of movement is greater in muscles that contain a higher percentage of fast-twitch fibres (Figure 4.22). For both fast- and slow-twitch muscle fibres, the maximum speed of active contraction occurs with the lowest force (Kojima 1991). Fast-twitch fibres are capable of producing greater force at a faster speed than slow-twitch fibres, hence muscles with predominantly fast-twitch fibres have greater power than muscles with predominantly slow-twitch fibres. Speed of contraction is also related to neuromuscular coordination (Kerr 1998). Muscle power reduces with age (Gajdosik et al. 1996).

The relationship of muscle power and velocity is depicted in Figure 4.23. For a given velocity the peak power generated is greater in muscle that contains a high percentage of fast-twitch fibres than in muscle that contains a high percentage of slow-twitch fibres (Powers & Howley 1997). The peak power generated by any muscle increases with increasing speed of movement, up to a movement speed of 200–400°/second.

In vitro muscle studies have demonstrated that the type of muscle contraction affects the force generated by a muscle. The greatest force is produced by an eccentric contraction (Katz 1939), the least force by a concentric contraction; an isometric contraction lies somewhere between the two (Hill 1938; Wilkie 1950). Increased speed of eccentric contraction

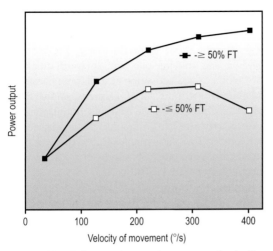

Figure 4.23 • Difference in muscle power and velocity between muscles with predominantly fast-twitch (FT) and slow-twitch muscle fibres (from Powers & Howley 1997, with permission).

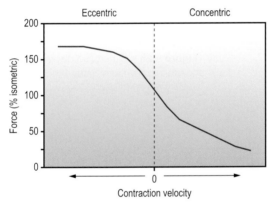

Figure 4.24 • Force–velocity relationship for skeletal muscle (from Newham 1993, with permission).

further increases the force generated (Katz 1939), whereas increased speed of concentric contraction reduces the force generated (Hill 1938). This relationship is depicted in Figure 4.24. In vivo muscle function behaves in a similar, but not identical, fashion (Newham 1993).

Muscle endurance

Muscle endurance is the ability of a muscle to continue an activity over time. It includes all types of muscle contraction and so may include repetitive movement, for example walking, or it may involve holding an isometric contraction over a period of time, for example using the rings in gymnastics. Muscle strength affects the endurance of a muscle. A muscle that is relatively weak, when required to contract during a functional activity, will do so at a proportionally greater level of maximum contraction than a muscle that is relatively strong. Other factors affecting muscle endurance include the energy store and circulation within the muscle (De Vries & Housh 1994).

There is a variety of ways to measure muscle endurance, and they depend on what specific type of muscle contraction is being tested. Measuring muscle endurance involves measuring the resultant muscle fatigue. Holding an isometric contraction at 60% maximum voluntary contraction (MVC) will increase the pressure within the muscle such that there will be no blood flowing into the muscle (Royce 1958). The ability then to continue holding the contraction will depend on the energy store within the muscle. A contraction at less than 60% MVC will enable the contraction to be held for longer, and a contraction at more than 60% MVC will result in the contraction being held for less time. An alternative method for measuring isometric endurance is to measure the increase in electromyogram (EMG) activity that accompanies muscle fatigue (De Vries & Housh 1994).

Measurement of a muscle to repeated isotonic contractions can be obtained by using an ergograph, whereby a constant force is provided through a range of movement and the decrease in endurance is reflected in a reduction in range (De Vries & Housh 1994). Isokinetic endurance can be measured by the strength decrement index, which measures the decline in peak torque during repeated maximal isokinetic contractions. In the clinical situation, muscle endurance may be measured by identifying the length of time a patient can continue to perform a specific activity.

Measurement of more general cardiovascular endurance activity, such as distance running, swimming or cycling, involves measurements of heart rate, volume and composition of expired air to reflect oxygen uptake. An improvement in endurance is reflected, for the same relative amount of work:

• in reduced oxygen uptake and reduced heart rate
• in a reduced sense of effort (Borg 1982)
• in an ability to continue for longer
• in an ability to increase the number of repetitions in the same time period (Newham 2001).

Normal motor control

Normal control of movement occurs as a result of incoming sensory information of position and movement and is integrated at all levels of the nervous system. Automatic and simple reflex movements occur in the spinal cord. Postural and balance reactions occur at the level of the brainstem and basal ganglia. More complicated movements are initiated and controlled at the motor/sensory cortices, and the cerebellum controls and coordinates movement (Crow & Haas 2001). A schematic diagram of these levels of control of voluntary movement is shown in Figure 4.25. Motor control depends 'on the spatial and temporal integration of vestibular, visual, and somatosensory information about the motion of the head and body, and the generation of appropriate responses to that motion' (Speers et al. 2002).

Posture and gait are organised at two levels (Allum et al. 1998). The first level provides direction-specific patterns of movement determining activation, timing and sequencing of muscle. It is formed from hip and trunk proprioceptive input and

vestibular input. The second level allows for particular adaptation for specific tasks, on the basis of the total afferent input from the body. For example, standing and moving one arm forward quickly to 90° flexion causes activation of ipsilateral hamstrings and gluteus maximus. Contralaterally, an increase in activation of tensor fasciae latae and gluteus maximus prior to activation of the shoulder flexors is seen. No such anticipatory activation occurs if the arm movement is produced passively (Bouisset & Zattara 1981; Zattara & Bouisset 1988).

Similar anticipatory muscle activity (Hortobagyi & DeVita 2000) has been found during unsupported rapid elbow flexion where increased activation of gastrocnemius (Cordo & Nashner 1982) and biceps femoris and erector spinae (Friedli et al. 1984) preceded biceps brachii activity. The activation of biceps femoris and erector spinae was reduced if the body was supported (strapped against a wall), reducing the threat to equilibrium (Friedli et al. 1984). Rapid elbow extension causes activation of rectus abdominis, prior to activation of triceps brachii (Friedli et al. 1984). Activation of the rotator cuff muscles and

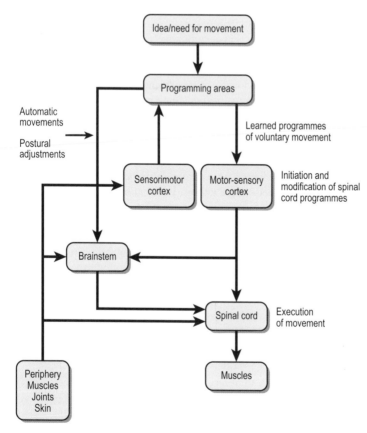

Figure 4.25 • Schematic diagram of the control of movement (after Kidd et al. 1992, with permission).

biceps brachii has been found to occur prior to both concentric and eccentric internal and external rotation of the glenohumeral joint (David et al. 2000). Similarly, activation of the deep abdominal muscles and multifidus has been found to occur prior to rapid leg and arm movements in standing (Hodges & Richardson 1997a–c).

Automatic postural adjustments are constantly being made with functional activities. When a subject stands unsupported, with arms at the side, on a surface that suddenly translates forward, there is increased activity of tibialis anterior to counteract the backward sway, and so maintain equilibrium. If this is repeated with arm support there is very little activity in tibialis anterior but a large increase in activity of biceps brachii (Cordo & Nashner 1982). From this observation, it appears that any muscle may be automatically activated to maintain equilibrium (Cordo & Nashner 1982).

This anticipatory activity is a feedforward mechanism which is thought to enhance balance and reduce postural disturbance (Bouisset & Zattara 1981; Cordo & Nashner 1982; Friedli et al. 1984; Horak et al. 1984; Zattara & Bouisset 1988; Van Vlieta and Heneghan 2006).

Muscle length

Muscle length can be measured by lengthening muscle fully through joint movement and measuring the final joint angle, using a goniometer or by visual estimation. The passive resistance of a muscle to lengthening is more difficult to measure. The clinician can passively lengthen the muscle and estimate the 'feel' of the resistance to movement, or length can be more objectively measured using isokinetic equipment.

Both the non-contractile and contractile components of muscle will contribute to the resistance felt when passively lengthening a muscle. The muscle–tendon unit is viscoelastic, as discussed earlier. Initial lengthening will be achieved with a relatively small force, but as the muscle is stretched out this resistance will increase. The rate at which a muscle is lengthened will affect the resistance felt: increasing the speed will increase the resistance.

Classification of muscle function

There are a number of classification systems of muscle function. Each is useful in understanding muscle, but each has limitations. Classification systems separate out and make distinct that which is often inseparable and indistinct. Enhanced knowledge often tends to produce a blurring of the categories, and a multidimensional continuum is often a more accurate representation. An obvious example is the change in the understanding of pain, which Descartes (1985) described as a signal of tissue damage, and has been developed as having physiological, sensory, affective, cognitive, behavioural, sociocultural and ethnocultural dimensions (Ahles & Martin 1992; McGuire 1995). Each of the systems below is not complete in itself but, taken as a whole, these systems provide insight into muscle function. An overview of the current classification systems is given in Figure 4.26.

Figure 4.26 • Classification systems for muscle.

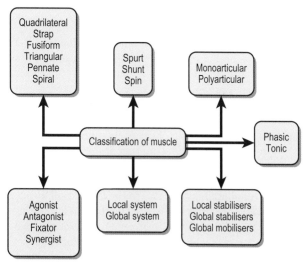

The architecture of a muscle, the monoarticular/ polyarticular and the spurt, shunt and spiral classification systems together cover anatomical and biomechanical aspects of muscle function. The phasic and tonic classification describes an aspect of muscle physiology. The use of agonist, antagonist, fixator and synergist describes the function of a muscle contraction in relation to a specific movement. The final two classification systems of local and global, and local stabiliser, global stabiliser and global mobiliser go one step further and attempt to identify the overall predominant function of a muscle. Each of these classification systems is discussed below.

Muscle architecture

Aspects of architecture include the fibre length, muscle length and pennation angle; each of these aspects will influence the function of the muscle. Each muscle fibre is capable of shortening to approximately half its total length (Norkin & Levangie 1992). Thus, a long muscle is able to shorten over a greater distance than a short muscle, so in terms of joint movement a long muscle will produce more movement of the bone than a short muscle. Long muscles usually lie more superficially than shorter muscles, giving them a greater leverage with which to move bone. Shorter muscles generally lie more deeply and often function to stabilise the joint. The shapes of muscles have been categorised as quadrilateral, strap, fusiform, triangular, pennate and spiral (Figure 4.27).

The direction of the muscle fibres differs with each shape and so affects the direction of force during muscle contraction. A quadrilateral muscle, as the name suggests, is flat and square. The muscle fibres run parallel and extend the length of the muscle. Muscles of this shape, such as pronator quadratus and quadratus lumborum, are well designed to support and stabilise underlying bones and joints.

Strap muscles are long and rectangular in shape, with fibres running the full length of the muscle. They are able to produce movement through a large range, for example sartorius. Rectus abdominis is a strap muscle, but is unusual in that it has three fibrous bands running across it.

Fusiform muscles are in the shape of a spindle with fibres running almost parallel to the line of pull. The two ends of the muscle converge on to a tendon. Biceps brachii consists of two fusiform-shaped muscles, while triceps brachii has three fusiform-shaped muscles.

Triangular muscles have a tendon at one end, and at the other end the muscle attaches to bone via either a flat tendon or an aponeurosis. The shape of the muscle means that some muscle fibres run at quite an oblique angle to the line of pull of the tendon, thus reducing its potential force of contraction. At its flat attachment though, the force of pull is across a broad area. Lower trapezius is an example of a triangular muscle.

Pennate muscles appear like a feather and may be unipennate (fibres attach to only one side of the tendon), bipennate (to both sides of the tendon) or multipennate (a number of bipennate arranged fibres). Examples include flexor pollicis longus (unipennate), rectus femoris (bipennate) and deltoid (multipennate). The oblique direction of the muscle fibres to the line of pull means that the force will be relatively less than if they were parallel; only a component of the force (the cosine of the angle) is available to move the bone. Pennate muscles have shorter and more numerous muscle fibres than do fusiform muscles. The greater number of muscle fibres gives pennate muscles, such as deltoid and gluteus maximus, a greater strength than fusiform muscles.

Spiral muscles twist on themselves, and often untwist on muscle contraction, thus producing a rotation force. Examples include latissimus dorsi twisting 180° through its length to rotate the humerus medially (Lockwood 1998).

These architectural arrangements provide valuable insight into the function of a muscle and have been shown to have more effect on the force-generating capability of a muscle than its fibre-type composition (Bodine et al. 1982; Sacks & Roy 1982; Burkholder et al. 1994).

Monoarticular and polyarticular

Monoarticular muscles cross only one joint whereas polyarticular muscles cross more than one joint. This classification system describes the relationship of muscle to joint, and so provides insight into the movement that will be produced by the muscle. For example, the rectus femoris is a polyarticular muscle crossing the anterior aspect of the hip and knee and therefore causing hip flexion and knee extension on concentric contraction. Muscles crossing more than one joint will be longer, and will produce more movement, than a muscle crossing just one joint. This classification system closely relates to the architecture of muscle and, together, they describe anatomical aspects of muscle.

Figure 4.27 • Shapes of muscles: quadrilateral, strap, fusiform, triangular, pennate and spiral (from Williams et al. 1995).

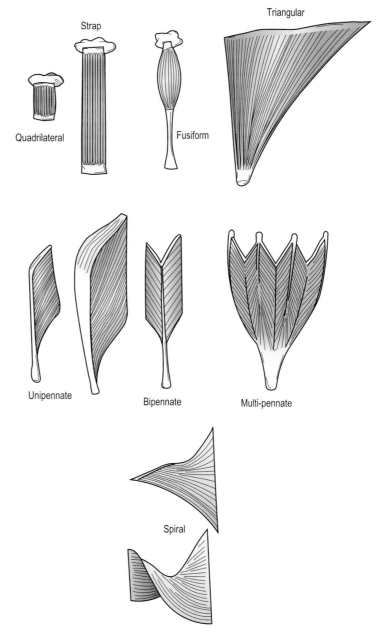

Spurt, shunt and spin

This system describes the biomechanical aspect of muscle function, highlighting the leverage of muscle force on bone. In a spurt muscle the proximal attachment of the muscle lies at a distance from the joint axis, and the distal attachment lies close to the joint axis – for example, the biceps brachii (Figure 4.28). With this arrangement the predominant effect of muscle contraction will be rotation of the bone, i.e. flexion of the elbow, rather than translation of the radius on the humerus.

The direction of the force, however, changes as the bone rotates (Figure 4.29). When the biceps brachii contracts with the elbow at 35° flexion there will be a relatively stronger compression force. At 70° there will be a greater rotational force. At 90° flexion there will be maximum rotational force with no

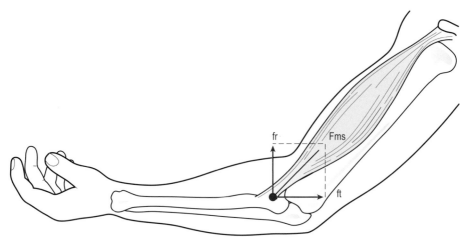

Figure 4.28 • Biceps brachii is acting as a spurt muscle on flexion of the elbow where the force of contraction is Fms; one component of this force (fr) causes a large flexion force, and the other smaller component (ft) causes joint compression (from Norkin & Levangie 1992, with permission).

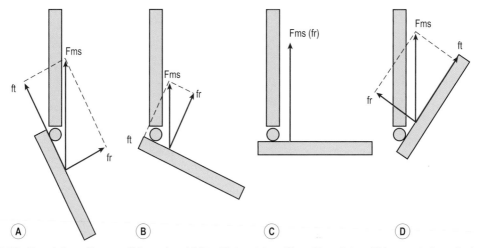

Figure 4.29 • Resolution of forces of biceps brachii (Fms) into rotatory (fr) and translatory (ft) forces at elbow flexion angles of A 35°, B 70°, C 90° and D 145° (from Norkin & Levangie 1992, with permission).

translatory force. Finally, at 145° flexion there will be a relatively greater amount of translatory force that will cause distraction of the joint surfaces. From elbow extension to flexion, then, biceps brachii acts as a shunt (35°), spurt (70 and 90°) and a shunt (145°).

An additional consideration is that, as a muscle contracts, there is a change in the muscle architecture, that is, the muscle fibres change direction relative to the angle of pull (Fukunaga et al. 1997; Kawakami et al. 1998; Maganaris et al. 1998), so this also will alter the angle of pull on the bone.

A shunt muscle is the reverse of this; the proximal attachment is close to the joint axis and the distal attachment lies at a distance from the joint axis – the popliteus at the knee or brachioradialis at the elbow are examples of this arrangement (Figure 4.30). These muscles are positioned in such a way as to apply a predominantly compression force through the joint rather than a rotational force on the bone.

Brachioradialis can be analysed in the same way (Figure 4.31). At all angles, it can be seen that the translatory force is always greater than the rotational force so that the muscle predominantly acts as a shunt muscle (Norkin & Levangie 1992). Maximum rotation force occurs at 90° flexion.

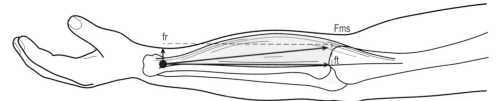

Figure 4.30 • Brachioradialis is acting as a shunt muscle; where the force of contraction is Fms, one component of this force (fr) causes a very small flexion force, and the other larger component (ft) causes joint compression (from Norkin & Levangie 1992, with permission).

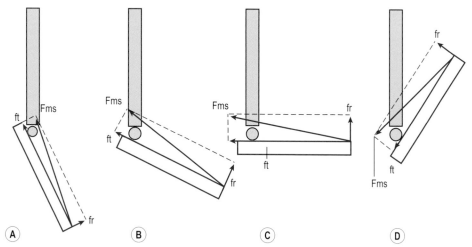

Figure 4.31 • Resolution of forces of brachioradialis (Fms) into rotatory (fr) and translatory (ft) forces at elbow flexion angles of A 35°, B 70°, C 90° and D 145° (from Norkin & Levangie 1992, with permission).

The line of force of a spin muscle is on the tangent of the long axis of the moving bone, so that contraction causes a rotation about its axis. For example, pronator quadratus is positioned to rotate the radius on its longitudinal axis (Figure 4.32).

The classification of a muscle as a spurt, shunt or spin is rather simplistic. The force of a muscle contraction on bone follows simple mechanics and can be resolved into two planes: along the long axis of the bone (F cos θ) and at right angles to the long axis (F sin θ), where θ is the angle between the muscle force and each plane (Figure 4.33). The component of the force along the axis will produce a compression force at the joint; the component of the force at right angles to the long axis will produce rotation of the bone. Hence, for any muscle contraction, there will be both a rotational and compression force applied. The rotational force will produce the spurt function and the compression force will produce the shunt function. Furthermore, if the muscle attaches to one side of the long axis of movement it will produce

spin, such as pronator teres. Some muscles may be described as predominantly spurt or shunt, but with the emphasis on predominant – as most muscles will act as both spurt and shunt. For example, pronator teres combines all three types of muscle action: spurt, shunt and spin. It is positioned such that it weakly flexes the elbow, applies a compression force of the radius on the humerus, and pronates the forearm.

This simplistic classification is further highlighted on analysing a muscle when it reverses its action, that is, when it acts from the distal attachment. In this situation, a muscle that acted as a spurt muscle now acts as a shunt muscle, and vice versa (Norkin & Levangie 1992). For example, when the foot is taken off the ground the hamstring muscle group acts as a spurt muscle to the knee joint and as a shunt extensor muscle to the hip. On returning the foot to the ground, hamstring acts as a shunt flexor muscle to the knee and as a spurt extensor muscle to the hip (Kidd et al. 1992).

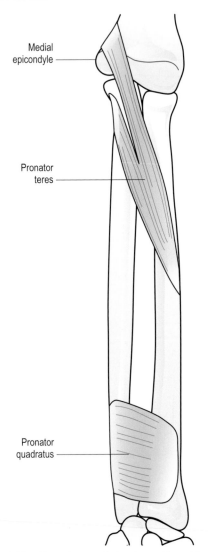

Figure 4.32 • Pronator quadratus is positioned to act predominantly as a spin muscle, while pronator teres combines spurt, shunt and spin functions (from Palastanga et al. 2002, with permission).

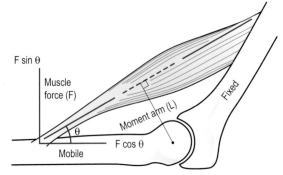

Figure 4.33 • Resolution of force of contraction into a vertical force (F sin θ) and a horizontal force (F cos θ) (after Williams et al. 1995, with permission).

The forces applied by the majority of muscles in the body have a greater translatory force (causing joint compression) than a rotational force, which aids joint stability (Norkin & Levangie 1992).

Phasic and tonic

This classification system attempts to distinguish muscles according to their predominant type of fibre (Norkin & Levangie 1992) or their predominant function (Janda 1985). If a muscle contains a high proportion of type II muscle fibres it is a phasic muscle, and if it contains a high proportion of type I muscle fibres it is a tonic muscle. This system therefore makes the logical assumption that the characteristics of a muscle will reflect the predominant characteristic of its muscle fibre.

There is some overlap between this classification system and that of the spurt, shunt and spin classification system (Norkin & Levangie 1992). Broadly, muscles that are classified as phasic would also be classified as spurt muscles, and muscles that are tonic would also be shunt muscles (Table 4.4).

There are a number of difficulties in attempting to distinguish muscles according to their predominant type of fibre. Orbicularis oculi, sternocleidomastoid and the lateral head of rectus femoris may be considered phasic muscles under this classification system as they each contain a high proportion of type II fibres, and this has been found consistently between individuals (Johnson et al. 1973). Similarly, soleus and tibialis anterior have been found consistently to contain a high proportion of type I fibres (87% and 73% respectively) and can therefore be categorised as having a tonic or postural function. Apart from these few exceptional muscles, the vast majority of muscles contain more or less equal proportions of type I and II fibres (Johnson et al. 1973).

The proportion of type I and II fibres is surprising in some muscles. The erector spinae muscles might be expected to have a predominantly postural role and thus have a higher proportion of type I fibres; however, this has not been found consistently. The percentage of type I fibres in erector spinae between

Table 4.4 Characteristics of phasic (spurt) and tonic (shunt) muscles (Janda 1985; Norkin & Levangie 1992)

	Phasic/spurt	Tonic/shunt
Fibre type	High proportion of type II	High proportion of type I
Fibre arrangement	Strap, fusiform	Pennate
Location	Superficial Cross more than one joint	Deep Cross one joint
Function	Mobility	Stability
Action	Flexion Adduction Medial rotation Tibialis anterior: the vasti glutei rectus abdominis lower stabilisers of the scapular deep neck flexors and extensors of the upper extremity	Extension Abduction Lateral rotation Tibialis posterior Rectus femoris Iliopsoas Tensor fasciae latae Hamstrings Short hip adductors Quadratus lumborum Piriformis Part of paravertebral back muscles Pectoralis major Sternocleidomastoid Upper trapezius Levator scapulae

The situation is further complicated by the fact that, in some individuals, there is a wide variation in the proportion of fibre types within any one muscle; for example, there are more type II fibres in the superficial layer than in the deep layer of deltoid, biceps brachii, adductor magnus, vastus medialis and vastus lateralis, rectus femoris muscles and lateral head of gastrocnemius (Johnson et al. 1973). Additionally, the superficial and deep portions of multifidus have been found to contain 4% and 62.6% respectively of type I fibres at the L4/5 level (Rantanen et al. 1994).

The vast majority of muscles contain more or less equal proportions of type I and type II fibres (Johnson et al. 1973); this is thought to be due to the required variation in muscle activity during functional activities (Saltin et al. 1977; Scott et al. 2001).

There are difficulties in determining the predominant function of a muscle. Muscles can function in a variety of ways. For example, the hamstring group consists of two joint muscles acting over the hip and knee, and will be active during walking or running. In these activities the endurance of the hamstring muscle group is being challenged. However, during the high jump and triple jump it will be strength and power that are required. In gymnastics, on the beam, or in ballet, the hamstring muscle group is required to act with strength, power, control and precision. In the same way, a monoarticular muscle, such as brachialis muscle, is considered to act as a stabiliser. Any suggestion that this muscle functions only to stabilise and fine-tune movement seems rather limited, especially when one considers fast ballistic movements of the upper limb when boxing and weight-lifting.

All muscles contribute to joint stability, including the large polyarticular muscles (Norkin & Levangie 1992). During gait, for example, the hamstring muscle group acts as a shunt extensor muscle to the hip when the foot is taken off the ground, and on returning the foot to the ground the hamstrings act as a shunt flexor muscle to the knee (Kidd et al. 1992). The cross-sectional area of the hamstring muscles is much greater than the small muscles around the hip and knee and therefore the strength of hamstrings is greater. The component of the contraction force of hamstrings compressing the hip and knee joints will therefore be greater than that of the local muscles and may have a significant impact on joint stability.

There are exceptions to this classification system. The internal oblique muscle is considered a global stabiliser, yet it is also thought to act as a local

individuals ranges from 27 to 100% (Johnson et al. 1973) with regional differences such that, in the thoracic spine, there is about 74% type I fibres compared with the lumbar spine, which has about 57% (Sirca & Kostevc 1985). Lumbar multifidus may also be expected to have a postural role and contain a large proportion of type I fibres; however, at L3 they have been found to contain about 63% of type I fibres (Sirca & Kostevc 1985).

Another limitation is that the proportion of types of muscle fibre in any one muscle varies widely between individuals (Johnson et al. 1973) and is considered to be genetically determined (Simoneau et al. 1986), related to gender (Brooke & Engel 1969), and may be related to age and occupation (Johnson et al. 1973). For example, the superficial erector spinae contained 100% type I fibres in one individual but 27% in another individual (Johnson et al. 1973).

stabiliser (Hodges & Richardson 1997a). Serratus anterior is active during forceful shoulder girdle protraction against resistance, in reaching and pushing (Williams et al. 1995), requiring concentric muscle activity. It also contracts isometrically to stabilise the scapula during the early phase of glenohumeral joint abduction. Therefore the suggestion that serratus anterior is a global stabiliser seems too limited.

The scaleni muscles are categorised as global mobilisers yet the position and direction of the muscle fibres would suggest that they will also provide a compression force to the cervical spine and therefore could act as stabilisers. Interestingly, Leonardo da Vinci first suggested this stability function of the cervical spine as early as the 16th century (Gombrich et al. 1989), comparing it to the mast of a ship: 'such a convergence of the muscles of the spine holds it erect as the ropes of a ship supports its mast, and the same ropes, tied to the mast, also support in part the framework of the ships to which they are attached'. He also argued that the muscles will be most effective when they are attached to the ribs further from the axis of the spine, which is, of course, where all the scalene muscles attach. This suggestion – that the neck muscles stabilise the spine in much the same way as ropes attached to a mast of a ship – was also used in a rather more modern review of spinal muscles (Newman 1968).

In conclusion, this classification system seems to be inaccurate and therefore unhelpful in describing the function of muscle.

Prime mover, antagonist, fixator and synergist

This classification system describes the way in which a muscle functions in relation to a specific movement. Any one muscle may act as a prime mover (or agonist), antagonist, fixator or synergist (Williams et al. 1995). The way in which a muscle acts depends on a number of factors which include the start position, the direction and speed of the movement, the phase of the movement and the resistance to movement.

Prime mover and antagonist

When a muscle is active in initiating and maintaining a movement it is acting as a prime mover. A muscle that opposes the prime mover is considered to be the antagonist.

Co-contraction of agonist and antagonist

It might be assumed that when the prime mover is contracting the antagonist is silent. However, there are numerous examples of co-contraction of agonist and antagonist. During maximal voluntary knee extension, the flexors of the knee are also contracting, albeit to a lesser degree (Baratta et al. 1988). When extending the trunk during a lifting task, there is co-contraction of the trunk flexors and extensors (Granata & Marras 1995). When biceps brachii contracts eccentrically, to control extension of the elbow, there is activation of the triceps muscle (Norman & Komi 1979). The antagonistic contraction measured by EMG activity may not be indicative of an opposing torque, as there is a time delay between EMG activity and torque production (Corser 1974; Norman & Komi 1979). With a rapid voluntary movement there is a triphasic pattern of muscle activity, with bursts of activity initially in the agonist, then the antagonist, and then the agonist (Friedli et al. 1984). In alpine skiing, the hip, knee and ankle medial and lateral rotators have been found to co-contract and this is thought to provide postural control during this highly skilled movement (Louie et al. 1984). The effect of co-contraction is to increase stiffness and thus stability of a joint, which is likely to be needed in stressful and complex movements (Figure 4.34). There is therefore activity of the agonist and antagonist muscles during active movements.

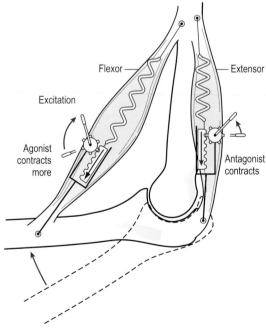

Figure 4.34 • Co-contraction of elbow flexors and extensors to increase joint stiffness and stability (from Ghez 1991, with permission).

Interestingly, the amount of co-contraction can be altered by activity. Athletes who strongly exercised the quadriceps and not the hamstrings had reduced co-contraction of the hamstrings on active knee extension compared with those who exercised both groups of muscles (Baratta et al. 1988). The amount of co-contraction is related to motor control; co-contraction is greater when motor skill is poor and reduces when motor skill is improved (Osu et al. 2002).

The amount of co-contraction increases with age: elderly women compared with young women were found to have over 100% greater activity of hamstring muscles just before and during a step-down movement (Hortobagyi & DeVita 2000) and both men and women were found to have greater co-contraction of biceps femoris during a maximum isometric contraction and one-repetition maximum of quadriceps femoris muscle (Tracy & Enoka 2002).

This increased co-contraction functions to increase joint stiffness and is thought to compensate for the neuromotor impairments associated with the elderly (Hortobagyi & DeVita 2000). The neuromotor impairments include: reduced muscle strength (Hortobagyi et al. 1995), increased time to develop muscle torque (Thelen et al. 1996), reduced proportion and cross-sectional area of type II muscle fibres (Larsson et al. 1979) and poorer proprioception (Skinner et al. 1984; Heyley et al. 1998). It has been found that quadriceps isometric and concentric muscle strength reduces with age much faster than eccentric muscle strength (Hortobagyi et al. 1995).

Fixators

As the name implies, this is when muscles contract to fix a bone. Muscles on either side of a joint sometimes contract together to create a fixed base on which another muscle can contract. For example, the muscles acting around the wrist contract together to fix the wrist when a strong fist is made. The particular wrist muscles in this case are acting as fixators.

Synergists

When a muscle acts over two or more joints, but the required movement is only over one joint, other muscles contract to eliminate the movement. When a muscle acts in this way it is said to act as a synergist (derived from *syn*, together, and *ergon*, work). Contraction of the finger flexors would produce flexion at both the wrist and fingers. The wrist extensors contract to eliminate the wrist flexion during a power grip and thus act as a synergist. Similarly, during elbow flexion with a pronated forearm, the contraction of biceps brachii will produce both elbow flexion

and supination. To maintain the pronated forearm, the pronator quadratus and pronator teres contract and thus act as synergists. In the same way, when muscles around the shoulder contract to produce movement at the glenohumeral joint, muscles around the cervical spine, thoracic spine and scapula must contract to prevent unwanted movement and are therefore acting as synergists.

Any clinician attempting to analyse muscle activity during movement will immediately appreciate the difficulty in doing this. Visual and palpatory cues are simply inadequate to sense whether a particular muscle is active and in what way it is active. The classification system of prime mover, antagonist, fixator or synergist can be used to give a crude and probably inaccurate analysis of muscle activity. A pressure biofeedback unit (PBU, Chattanooga, Australia), ultrasound imaging (Hides et al. 1995) and EMG biofeedback (Richardson et al. 1999) provide information on muscle activity, albeit limited.

Global and local systems

This classification system is very similar to the monoarticular and polyarticular classification systems. It has been used to create a mechanical model of the lumbar spine in order to identify the function of muscle in spinal stability (Bergmark 1989). Muscles were identified as a local system of muscles attaching directly onto the lumbar vertebra and a global system that consists of muscles that attach to the thoracic cage and pelvis (Box 4.3). The global system functions to transfer load between the thoracic cage

Box 4.3

Classification of muscles into local and global muscle systems (Bergmark 1989)

Global system	Local system
Global erector spinae: longissimus thoracis pars thoracis iliocostalis lumborum thoracis	Local erector spinae: longissimus thoracis pars lumborum iliocostalis lumborum pars pars lumborum Multifidus Interspinales Intertransversarii
Quadratus lumborum (lateral fibres) Abdominal muscles: rectus abdominus internal and external obliques	Quadratus lumborum (medial fibres) Abdominal muscles: internal oblique (via thoracolumbar fascia) transversus abdominis

and the thorax and to move one on another. The local system controls the curvature of the lumbar spine and provides sagittal and lateral stiffness to intervertebral segments of the lumbar spine.

The system evaluates muscle specifically in terms of the effect of a muscle on lumbar spine stability and is not attempting to provide a comprehensive description of the function of each of these muscles. For this reason, caution needs to be taken in generalising not only the function of these muscles into global and local systems but in widening this to all muscles in the body. For example, the latissimus dorsi muscle is classified as a global muscle (Bergmark 1989), and this is supported by the movement it produces at the glenohumeral joint, yet it can also act as a stabiliser of the scapula (Williams et al. 1995). Psoas major is categorised as a global muscle, as it actively flexes the hip, yet it also provides a compression-stabilising force to the lumbar spine (Adams et al. 2002). Finally, the internal oblique muscle is considered to be a global muscle, yet it is closely linked anatomically with transversus abdominis, which is considered part of the local system; it might be expected that where there is a close anatomical relationship there would be a close functional relationship. Some evidence supports a local function of internal oblique, which has been found to be activated along with transversus abdominis in a feedforward manner prior to hip movements, suggesting a possible stabilising role (Hodges & Richardson 1997a). These examples further highlight the difficulty in categorising muscle according to function.

Local stabilisers, global stabilisers and global mobilisers

The two classification systems, the monoarticular system and polyarticular system, and the local and global system, have been combined by Comerford & Mottram (2001a, b). Muscle function, in this system, is divided into local stabilisers, global stabilisers and global mobilisers.

Local stabilisers
Local stabilisers function to control the underlying joint movement. These muscles are sometimes referred to as postural or tonic muscles. Transversus abdominis has been described as a local stabiliser, and this has been supported by a number of research studies. Transversus abdominis has been found, using needle EMG, to contract a few milliseconds prior to rectus femoris, tensor fasciae latae and gluteus maximus during rapid hip flexion, abduction and

extension respectively (Hodges & Richardson 1997a). This pre-emptive contraction has been demonstrated prior to deltoid muscle activity during rapid arm flexion, extension and abduction (Hodges & Richardson 1997b, c). Transversus abdominis has also been found to be the major abdominal muscle responsible for increasing intra-abdominal pressure (Cresswell et al. 1992; Cresswell 1993; Cresswell & Thorstensson 1994). The anticipatory activity of transversus abdominis, and its ability to raise intra-abdominal pressure, provides evidence to suggest that it functions as a local stabilising muscle for the trunk (Cresswell et al. 1992; Cresswell 1993; Cresswell & Thorstensson 1994; Hodges & Richardson 1997a–c). This is supported by the observation that low-back pain patients have been found to have a delayed activation of transversus abdominis (Hodges & Richardson 1996).

In the lower limbs vastus medialis oblique and vastus lateralis may also act to stabilise the knee. In prone-lying the EMG activity of vastus medialis oblique and vastus lateralis did not alter with active knee flexion and extension movements, nor with increasing speeds of movement – unlike rectus femoris and hamstring muscle groups, which were activated according to the cycle of the movement and with increase in activity with increasing speed (Richardson & Bullock 1986). Vastus medialis oblique and vastus lateralis appeared therefore to be continually contracting and not in relation to the knee movement, suggesting a possible stabilising function.

Throughout the body, small muscles often contract alongside much larger muscles to fine-tune the gross movement produced by the larger muscles (Peck et al. 1984). Examples include supination produced by the larger biceps brachii and the smaller supinator; extension of the spinal column with the larger erector spinae and multifidus and the smaller occipital muscles, interspinales and intertransversarii. In all cases, the smaller muscles contain appreciably more muscle spindles than longer muscles (Cooper & Daniel 1963; Abrahams 1977, 1981; Peck et al. 1984) and are thus thought to provide proprioceptive input (Peck et al. 1984; Bastide et al. 1989; Adams et al. 2002).

Global stabilisers
The global stabilisers are considered to generate force to control movement through eccentric control, particularly of the inner and outer range of joint movement (Comerford & Mottram 2001a, b). They are thought to provide rotational control during functional movements. Stabiliser muscles have been

referred to as monoarticular muscles (Comerford & Mottram 2001b). Eccentric muscle contraction is considered to provide shock absorption by decelerating the body during activities such as walking and running (Stauber 1989). Examples of muscles in this category are the internal and external oblique muscles, spinalis, gluteus medius, serratus anterior and longus colli (M Comerford, personal communication, 2000).

Global mobilisers

The global mobilisers are considered to generate force to produce movement through concentric contraction, particularly in the sagittal plane (Comerford & Mottram 2001a, b). These muscles are often long superficial muscles, strap or fusiform in shape, and could also be categorised as spurt, phasic or polyarticular muscles designed for power and speed (Mitchell 1993). Examples could include rectus abdominis, iliocostalis, hamstrings, latissimus dorsi, levator scapulae and the scaleni.

This classification system attempts to identify the overall predominant function of a muscle, with the suggestion that global (polyarticular) muscles control movement and alignment while local (monoarticular) muscles provide stability (Comerford & Mottram 2001b). The limitations of this system are similar to that of the phasic and tonic classification: there are major difficulties in suggesting that a muscle has a predominant function.

Summary of classification of muscle function

Each of the classification systems provides insight into muscle function. The theory of motor control provides a valuable context in which to consider these functions. Muscle contraction is not an isolated event in the body; it is controlled by various levels of the CNS. The motor cortex that initiates muscle contraction does not function in relation to individual muscles; rather, it controls the coordinated contraction of a large number of muscles to control movement. The CNS is thus concerned with movement, and it can be argued that analysis should focus more on gross movement than on individual muscle activity. This is reinforced by the fact that muscle is in a constant state of change; muscle activity per se is highly unstable and is being constantly altered by the CNS to maintain balance and coordinate movements.

Because almost all muscles contain similar proportions of type I and type II muscle fibres, it can be presumed that the characteristics of whole muscles reflect both characteristics. That is, all muscles can contract slowly and gently for a long period of time, exhibiting endurance. All muscles can contract quickly and strongly, exhibiting strength and power; the actual amount will depend on factors such as the cross-sectional area of the muscle, leverage and architecture. It seems reasonable to suggest that all muscles will have a role in posture and balance, and all muscles will have a role in movement. The CNS will activate type I fibres in all types of muscle in order to provide the necessary posture and balance and will activate the type II fibres in all types of muscle in order to provide strength and power. The relative amounts of activation, and in which muscles, will depend on the specific position and the movement that is being carried out.

Muscle dysfunction

Just as the function of muscles depends on the function of joints and nerves, so dysfunction of muscles can lead to dysfunction of joints and nerves. They

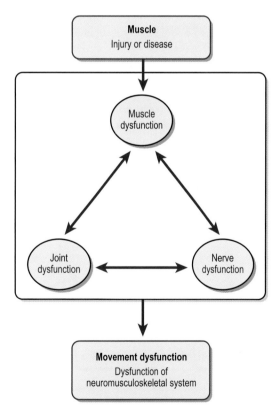

Figure 4.35 • Dysfunction of muscle can produce joint and/or nerve dysfunction, and can lead to movement dysfunction.

are dependent on each other in both normal and abnormal conditions; this is depicted in Figure 4.35. The following examples may help to highlight how muscle dysfunction will often be accompanied by joint and/or nerve dysfunction.

Dysfunction in muscle and joint often occur together. For example, abnormality of the eccentric muscle force of the quadriceps muscle may be a contributing factor in anterior knee pain (Hughston et al. 1984; Bennett & Stauber 1986) and lateral epicondylitis is associated with tears of the lateral collateral ligament of the elbow (Bredella et al. 1999). This evidence highlights the close relationship of muscle and joint dysfunction.

There is overwhelming evidence that weakness of a muscle occurs with joint pathology and dysfunction. This has been demonstrated in the knee in the presence of a variety of pathologies: rheumatoid arthritis (deAndrade et al. 1965), osteoarthritis (deAndrade et al. 1965; Hurley & Newham 1993), ligamentous knee injuries (Kennedy et al. 1982; Newham et al. 1989; Hurley et al. 1992, 1994; Snyder-Mackler et al. 1994; DeVita et al. 1997; Urbach & Awiszus 2002) and following meniscectomy (Stokes & Young 1984; Shakespeare et al. 1985; Hurley et al. 1994; Suter et al. 1998a); in the elbow in the presence of rheumatoid arthritis (Hurley et al. 1991) and in the glenohumeral joint in the presence of anterior dislocation (Keating & Crossan 1992). The inhibition of muscle is thought to be due to inhibitory input (Iles et al. 1990; Suter & Herzog 2000; Torry et al. 2000) or abnormal input (Hurley et al. 1991; Hurley & Newham 1993) from joint afferents. Thus, joint pathology leads to altered neural activity, which alters muscle activity. A muscle that is inhibited will, over time, weaken and this may make the joint vulnerable to further injury (Young et al. 1982b; Stokes & Young 1984). For example, it is thought that weakness

of the posterior rotator cuff muscles may make the glenohumeral joint vulnerable to recurrent anterior dislocation (Keating & Crossan 1992). This sequence of events is outlined in Figure 4.36.

Another example of the close relationship between joint, nerve and muscle is the effect of joint immobilisation. Following 3 weeks of finger and thumb immobilisation there is reduced maximal voluntary contraction of the muscles around the joint and a decrease in the maximal firing rate of motor neurones supplying the muscles (Seki et al. 2001).

Muscle activity around a joint is altered in the presence of ligament insufficiency and joint instability. During throwing, EMG activity of the elbow muscles is altered with ligament insufficiency of the elbow (Glousman et al. 1992). Similarly, during throwing, the EMG activity around the shoulder region is altered with shoulder instability (Glousman et al. 1988). In the lower limb, the EMG activity of quadriceps and hamstring muscle groups is altered with ACL deficiency during knee movement (Solomonow et al. 1987) and during gait and functional activities (Berchuck et al. 1990; Ciccotti et al. 1994). Figure 4.37 identifies a proposed cycle of events of progressive knee instability following an initial ligament injury (Kennedy et al. 1982).

Muscle activity is directly affected by joint nociceptor activity. Pain around the knee causes a nociceptive flexor withdrawal response: hip and knee flexion and ankle dorsiflexion. There is increased alpha motor neurone excitability of the muscles to produce this movement (Stener & Peterson 1963) and reciprocal inhibition of the knee extensors (Stener & Peterson 1963; Stener 1969; Young et al. 1987). For example, pressure or tension on a partially ruptured medial collateral ligament results in an increased activity of sartorius and semimembranosus (knee flexors) with inhibition of the vastus medialis (extensor) (Stener

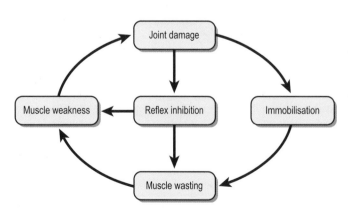

Figure 4.36 • Effect of joint damage and/or immobilisation on muscle and nerve tissues (Reproduced with permission, from Stokes M, Young A 1984, Clinical Science 67:7–14. © The Biochemical Society and the Medical Research Society. (http://www.clinsci.org)).

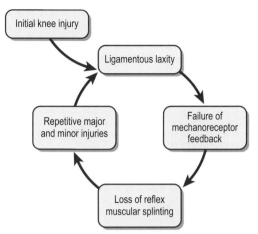

Figure 4.37 • A proposed cycle of progressive knee instability following an initial ligament injury (from Kennedy et al. 1982, with permission).

and Peterson 1963). Pain over the lateral femoral epicondyle leads to inhibition of the vastus medialis and lateralis, both knee extensors (Stener 1969). In the lumbar spine, pain from the zygapophyseal joint causes increased activity of the hamstring muscle group (Mooney & Robertson 1976).

Interestingly, activation of type I, II and IV receptors in the zygapophyseal joints of the cervical spine have more widespread effects than just on the muscles around the neck: they also influence the muscles around the eye and mandible (Wyke & Polacek 1975). This research clearly indicates that nociceptor activity increases the activation of some muscles and decreases the activation of others.

Nociceptor activity is thought to influence muscle activity via the alpha motor neurone (Wyke & Polacek 1975). Nociceptor activity is thought to have a greater inhibitory effect upon the low-threshold motor units supplying type I muscle fibres than on the high-threshold motor units supplying type II fibres (Gydikov 1976). If this is true, it might be speculated that a muscle containing a relatively higher proportion of type I fibres, such as soleus and tibialis anterior, may be more affected by nociceptor activity than a muscle that has a more equal proportion of type I and II fibres.

The functions of a muscle are essentially to produce and allow movement to occur. That is, it will contract with strength, power and endurance, it will lengthen and shorten with movement and, under the control of the CNS (motor control), it will produce coordinated movement. The signs and symptoms of muscle dysfunction are related to these functions, that is,

Box 4.4

Signs and symptoms of muscle dysfunction

Reduced muscle strength
Reduced muscle power
Reduced muscle endurance
Altered motor control
Reduced muscle length
Production of symptoms

there may be one or more of the following: reduced muscle strength, reduced muscle power, reduced muscle endurance, altered motor control, reduced muscle length or production of symptoms. Box 4.4 highlights these characteristics of muscle function and dysfunction. A particular mix of these signs and symptoms occurs with a muscle or tendon injury, and these are discussed at the end of the chapter.

Reduced muscle strength

Reduced muscle strength can occur as a result of disuse such as immobility (Berg et al. 1997), immobilisation (Sargeant et al. 1977; Vaughan 1989; Labarque et al. 2002), trauma (Newham et al. 1989; Hurley et al. 1992; Snyder-Mackler et al. 1994; DeVita et al. 1997; Urbach & Awiszus 2002), weightlessness (Edgerton et al. 1995; Fitts et al. 2000, 2001) and pathology (Sirca & Kostevc 1985; Zhao et al. 2000; Yoshihara et al. 2001). As will be seen later, a reduction in muscle strength will produce a reduction in muscle power and a reduction in endurance.

A body of knowledge is emerging on the effects of space flight on the musculoskeletal system in anticipation of a manned mission to Mars (Fitts et al. 2000, 2001). While the reader is unlikely to be managing patients recovering from the effects of space flight, the effects on muscle are of interest in furthering our understanding of the plastic nature of the muscle. Space flight causes a reduction in muscle strength and power (Edgerton et al. 1995; Fitts et al. 2000, 2001). Initially, space flight causes greater atrophy and weakness of the leg extensors, but after 110 days there is a similar 30% loss in dorsiflexion and plantarflexion strength (Greenleaf et al. 1989). It is thought that the rate of muscle atrophy plateaus such that little further atrophy will occur beyond this period of time (Antonutto et al. 1999; Fitts et al. 2000).

With microgravity, atrophy of human soleus muscle is greater than the atrophy of gastrocnemius

(Fitts et al. 2001; Widrick et al. 2001). This might be expected as microgravity will affect type I fibres more than type II fibres; moreover, as soleus has such a high proportion of type I fibres, this muscle may be affected more than gastrocnemius with a lower percentage of type I fibres (H Fiddler, personal communication, 2004). Within the human soleus muscle, two studies (Edgerton et al. 1995; Widrick et al. 2001) have found greater atrophy of type II than type I fibres, while one study found similar degrees of atrophy for both types of fibre (Fitts et al. 2001). The results of these studies are not conclusive as the number of subjects was small and there was a large variation between individuals. Microgravity has also been found to cause a 50% reduction in muscle power (Antonutto et al. 1999), which is thought to be caused by an alteration in the recruitment of motor units (Antonutto et al. 1999; Fitts et al. 2000).

Muscle atrophy has been found to occur with pathology. For example, in patients who underwent surgery for a chronic lumbar disc herniation there was atrophy of the multifidus and longissimus muscles (Sirca & Kostevc 1985). In another similar study a biopsy of multifidus at L4/5 and L5/S1 levels also revealed muscle atrophy on the side of herniation, with smaller type I and type II fibres (Zhao et al. 2000). Patients with an L4/5 disc herniation and L5 nerve root compression (identified at surgery) were found to have atrophy of multifidus with a 6.4% reduction in cross-section area of type I fibres and a 9.8% reduction in type II fibres at the level of the herniation; interestingly, no atrophy was found at the L4 level (Yoshihara et al. 2001).

It should be remembered that there are normal age-related changes in muscle strength. For instance, there is a reduction in isokinetic calf strength (Gajdosik et al. 1996) and isometric quadriceps strength (Young et al. 1982a; Grimby 1995; Heyley et al. 1998). Between the fourth and seventh decade there is a 14% reduction in isokinetic quadriceps strength per decade (Hughes et al. 2001).

Muscle strength is profoundly affected by immobilisation. Immobilisation also affects the non-contractile portion of muscle, the musculotendinous junction and the tendon, and these are discussed below.

Immobilisation

Immobilisation affects the contractile portion of muscle, the non-contractile portion of muscle, the musculotendinous junction and the tendon. The reduced strength resulting from immobilisation is thought to be due to muscle atrophy, that is, reduced fibre area and diameter (Sargeant et al. 1977; Young et al. 1982b; Berg et al. 1997) and reduced neural input to the muscle (Berg et al. 1997). The effects of immobilisation on muscle depend on the length of time, the position of the muscle when immobilised and the predominant muscle fibre type within the muscle.

Time of immobilisation

If a muscle does not contract at all muscle strength will decrease by approximately 5% a day, but one contraction at half maximum contraction (0.5 repetition maximum) is considered sufficient to prevent this reduction (Muller 1970). Normally, some degree of muscle contraction may occur while a muscle is immobilised, giving a more realistic estimate of 2–3% reduction in muscle strength per day (Muller 1970; Appell 1990); bed rest is estimated to cause a 1–1.5% reduction per day (Muller 1970).

Following 2 weeks of elbow immobilisation, subjects developed a significant decrease ($P < 0.01$) in elbow flexion strength; interestingly, there was no significant decrease in extensor strength (Vaughan 1989). It appears that if the elbow is immobilised for a longer period of time, 5–6 weeks, reduction of extensor strength occurs and decreases by 41% (MacDougall et al. 1980). With knee immobilisation there is uniform atrophy of all the heads of quadriceps (Lieb & Perry 1968). It is sometimes suggested that there is selective wasting of muscle groups; however, there is no research evidence to support this.

Position of the muscle

The effects of immobilisation on muscle depend on the position in which the muscle is held, whether it is in a shortened or lengthened position.

The effects of immobilisation in a shortened position are summarised in Box 4.5. The changes in muscle demonstrate the plastic nature of muscle, which changes its structure as a consequence of a change in function. The decrease in the number of sarcomeres and increase in length of each sarcomere ensure that the muscle is able to contract maximally in the shortened immobilised position. The connective tissue loss, due to immobilisation, occurs at a lower rate than the loss of contractile tissue, resulting in a relative increase in connective tissue (Goldspink & Williams 1979); this can occur as early as 2 days after immobilisation (Williams & Goldspink 1984). In addition, the connective tissue remodels during immobilisation to produce a thicker perimysium and endomysium (Goldspink & Williams 1979).

Box 4.5

Effects of immobilisation on muscle in a shortened position

Decrease in muscle weight and fibre size	Williams & Goldspink 1978 Witzmann 1988
Decrease in the number of sarcomeres	Goldspink 1976 Tabary et al. 1972 Williams & Goldspink 1973 Williams & Goldspink 1978
Increase in the sarcomere length	Williams & Goldspink 1978, 1984
Increase in amount of perimysium	Williams & Goldspink 1984
Increase in ratio of collagen concentration	Goldspink & Williams 1979 Williams & Goldspink 1984
Increase in ratio of connective tissue to muscle fibre tissue	Goldspink & Williams 1979 Williams & Goldspink 1984
Reduction in the cross-sectional area of the intrafusal fibres of the muscle spindle	Jozsa et al. 1988
Increase in the thickness of the capsule surrounding the muscle spindle	Jozsa et al. 1988

These changes produce an increased stiffness to passive lengthening, which is thought to occur to prevent the muscle from being overstretched (Tabary et al. 1972; Goldspink & Williams 1979).

The increase in connective tissue associated with immobilisation in a shortened position can be prevented by 15 minutes of passive stretch on alternate days (Williams 1988). This intermittent stretching regime, however, does not influence the reduction in muscle fibre length and subsequent reduction in range of movement (Williams 1988).

The muscle spindle is also affected by immobilisation. Three weeks of immobilisation of rat calf muscle caused a 40% reduction in the cross-sectional area of the intrafusal fibres of the muscle spindle, and a marked increase in the thickness of the capsule surrounding the muscle spindle (Jozsa et al. 1988). The effect of these changes on muscle function is unclear.

When the immobilisation ceases the muscle will be weak and shortened and will have an increased resistance to passive lengthening. The plastic nature of muscle is further demonstrated by the fact that the changes to immobilised muscle (in cat and mouse) revert to normal with removal of the immobilisation (Tabary et al. 1972; Williams & Goldspink 1973). It has been demonstrated that the new sarcomeres on remobilisation are added at the ends of the muscle fibres (Williams & Goldspink 1973).

Two weeks' immobilisation of the human knee held in almost full extension (shortened position for knee extensors and relative lengthened position for knee flexors) resulted in a 27% reduction in knee extensor torque and an 11% reduction in knee flexor torque (Labarque et al. 2002). The reduction in knee extensor torque agrees with the estimate of 2–3% reduction per day in muscle strength (Muller 1970; Appell 1990).

The effects of immobilisation of muscle in a lengthened position are summarised in Box 4.6. There is an increase in the number of sarcomeres that lie in series, thus lengthening the muscle (Tabary et al. 1972; Williams & Goldspink 1973, 1976, 1978; Goldspink 1976). The length of the sarcomeres is reduced (Tabary et al. 1972; Williams & Goldspink 1978, 1984). There is hypertrophy, which may then be followed by atrophy (Williams & Goldspink 1984). Functionally the muscle has a greater capacity to generate tension. There is no change in the muscle stiffness to passive lengthening (Tabary et al. 1972; Williams & Goldspink 1978).

Predominant type of muscle fibre within the muscle

There is some suggestion that the effect of immobilisation on a muscle is affected by its proportion of type I and type II muscle fibres. The effect of immobilisation in near-resting length of a guinea pig soleus (predominantly type I muscle fibres)

Box 4.6

Effects of immobilisation on muscle in a lengthened position

Increase in the number of sarcomeres in series	Goldspink 1976 Tabary et al. 1972 Williams & Goldspink 1973, 1976, 1978
Decrease in the length of sarcomeres	Tabary et al. 1972 Williams & Goldspink 1978, 1984
Muscle hypertrophy that may be followed by atrophy	Williams & Goldspink 1984

has been compared with immobilisation of gastrocnemius (predominantly type II muscle fibres) (Maier et al. 1976). In both muscles type I fibre atrophied to a greater extent than type II fibres, and interestingly this was greater in soleus than in gastrocnemius (Maier et al. 1976). The capacity of gastrocnemius to create tension was significantly ($P <0.05$) reduced, whereas in soleus there was no significant reduction (Maier et al. 1976). In contrast, another study found that type II fibres atrophied more than type I fibres (MacDougall et al. 1980). Following 5–6 weeks of elbow immobilisation there was a 30% reduction in cross-sectional area of type II fibres and a 25% reduction in type I fibres (MacDougall et al. 1980).

Effect of immobilisation on the musculotendinous junction and the tendon

Immobilisation has widespread effects on the musculotendinous junction and the tendon (Box 4.7). At the musculotendinous junction, 3 weeks of immobilisation of the rat gastrocnemius–soleus–tendon unit in a shortened position resulted in over 40%

reduction in the contact area between the muscle and the tendon (Kannus et al. 1992). Other changes included an increase in scar tissue in the area, reduced glycosaminoglycans, and an increase in weaker type III collagen fibres (Kannus et al. 1992).

Collectively, these changes will reduce the tensile strength of the musculotendinous junction. An experimental muscle strain and 2 days of immobilisation resulted in a significant ($P <0.001$) reduction in tensile strength and stiffness at the musculotendinous junction (Almekinders & Gilbert 1986). In addition, a 30% reduction in blood vessels in the musculotendinous junction has been observed following immobilisation (Kvist et al. 1995). Three weeks of immobilisation of rat calf muscle caused a marked increase in the thickness of the capsule surrounding the Golgi tendon organ (Jozsa et al. 1988); the effect of this on muscle function is unclear.

In tendons it has been found that 5 weeks of disuse of rat Achilles tendon resulted in a reduction in the number of collagen fibres, causing a reduction in tensile strength (Nakagawa et al. 1989). There is also reduced energy supply, oxygen consumption and enzyme activity within the tendon following a period of immobilisation (Jozsa & Kannus 1997).

The effect of remobilisation of tendon following a period of immobilisation is still largely unclear. The 30% loss of vascularity at the musculotendinous junction can be restored following remobilisation (Kvist et al. 1995). There is acceleration of collagen synthesis and enzyme activity (Karpakka et al. 1990). However, the collagen content and orientation of remobilised tendon may continue to be inferior despite remobilisation (Jozsa & Kannus 1997).

Box 4.7

Effects of immobilisation on the musculotendinous junction and tendon

Musculotendinous junction

Reduction in the contact area between muscle and tendon	Kannus et al. 1992
Increase in scar tissue	Kannus et al. 1992
Reduced glycosaminoglycans	Kannus et al. 1992
Increase in the weaker type III collagen fibres	Kannus et al. 1992
Reduced tensile strength	Almekinders & Gilbert 1986
	Kannus et al. 1992
Reduced stiffness	Almekinders & Gilbert 1986
Reduction in blood vessels	Kvist et al. 1995
Increase in the thickness of the capsule of the Golgi tendon organ	Jozsa et al. 1988
Tendon	
Reduced collagen fibres	Nakagawa et al. 1989
Reduced energy supply, oxygen consumption and enzyme activity	Jozsa & Kannus 1997

Measurement of muscle strength

Muscle strength is often clinically assessed using manual muscle testing with a scale from 0 (no contraction) to 5 (normal strength). The value of this is severely limited as the accuracy and sensitivity are very poor (Newham 2001). In one study a muscle which was only 8% of normal strength was rated as grade 4, clearly underestimating true muscle strength (Agre & Rodriquez 1989).

Quadriceps muscle wasting has been measured clinically by using a tape measure around the circumference of the thigh. There are difficulties with this measure as it includes the subcutaneous fat and hamstring muscle group, which can conceal the quadriceps muscle wasting (Young et al. 1982b). The measurement has been found to underestimate the extent of the quadriceps muscle atrophy (Sargeant et al. 1977; Young et al. 1980, 1982b, 1983; Arangio et al. 1997) and is of questionable value in the clinical environment (Arangio et al. 1997).

Muscle strength can be more objectively tested by measuring muscle cross-sectional area, or by measuring muscle force or pressure during active contraction. Physiological cross-sectional area can be measured by ultrasound, computed axial tomography and magnetic resonance imaging. The physiological cross-sectional area, however, underestimates muscle strength; Young et al. (1983) found a 15% increase in isometric strength of the quadriceps following a training period, but only a 6% increase in physiological cross-sectional area. Force or pressure can be measured using devices such as the handheld dynamometer for grip strength and the large isotonic or isokinetic dynamometers for larger muscle groups (Watkins et al. 1984). Where strength is measured by an active contraction, muscle length and the motivation and effort by an individual will affect the force measurement. Muscle strength testing is further complicated by the fact that asymptomatic subjects have been found to vary the maximal voluntary contraction over different days of testing (Allen et al. 1995; Suter & Herzog 1997).

Reduced muscle power

Muscle power is a function of force and velocity and if either is reduced there will be a subsequent reduction in power. Where there is a reduction in muscle strength, there will be, by definition, a reduction in muscle power. Velocity is a function of force and distance and therefore any reduction in muscle length or any reduction in the speed of contraction will result in a reduction in muscle power. It has already been identified that immobilisation in a shortened position causes a reduction in strength and a reduction in length; both of these changes will cause a reduction in muscle power.

The velocity of a contraction is determined, in part, by the proportion of fibre types within the muscle – the greater the proportion of type II fibres, the greater the power (Newham 2001). Any reduction in type II fibres within a muscle would potentially reduce its power.

No difference in atrophy of type I and type II fibres in vastus lateralis was found in healthy volunteers confined to 6 weeks' bed rest (Berg et al. 1997). Any reduction in muscle power would not be as a result of a reduction in type II fibres; however, all subjects had an 18% reduction in cross-sectional area of the muscle and this would reduce muscle strength, and hence power.

A number of studies have investigated the effect of knee immobilisation on the proportion of type I and type II fibres in vastus lateralis (Sargeant et al. 1977; MacDougall et al. 1980; Haggmark et al. 1981; MacDougall 1986; Hortobagyi et al. 2000). Three weeks of knee immobilisation resulted in a 13% reduction in type I fibres and a 10% reduction in type II fibres (Hortobagyi et al. 2000). Following a lower-limb fracture and knee immobilisation for up to 7 weeks there was a 46% reduction in type I fibres and a 37% reduction in type II fibres (Sargeant et al. 1977). Following knee surgery and 5 weeks of knee immobilisation there was a reduction only in the cross-sectional area of type I fibres with no alteration in type II fibres (Haggmark et al. 1981). The studies suggest that knee immobilisation causes a greater atrophy of type I fibres than of type II fibres in vastus lateralis.

The effect of immobilisation on the atrophy of type I and type II fibres has also been investigated in triceps muscle (MacDougall et al. 1980; MacDougall 1986). Two studies have investigated type I and II atrophy following elbow immobilisation and found greater reduction in type II fibres (MacDougall et al. 1980; MacDougall 1986). Following 6 weeks of elbow immobilisation there was a 38% reduction in cross-sectional area of type II fibres and a 31% reduction in type I fibres (MacDougall 1986). In a similar study, 5–6 weeks of elbow immobilisation resulted in a 33% reduction in type II fibres and a 25% reduction in type I fibres (MacDougall et al. 1980). In the triceps muscles it appears that immobilisation causes greater atrophy in type II fibres than in type I fibres.

From the above studies on vastus lateralis and triceps muscles it appears that muscle fibre types in different muscles respond slightly differently to immobilisation. While the proportional atrophy of type I fibres and II fibres differs in vastus lateralis and triceps, the magnitude of the difference is, in all cases, less than 9%, which seems quite a small difference.

Reduced muscle endurance

Reduced muscle endurance may be manifested by a reduced ability to repeat a contraction, or a reduced ability to hold an isometric contraction over a period of time (McArdle et al. 2000). In order to avoid testing muscle strength it is suggested that the resistance is sufficiently low to allow 15–20 repetitions.

More general cardiovascular endurance training such as distance running, swimming or cycling involves measurements of volume and composition of expired air to reflect oxygen uptake and heart rate. An improvement in endurance is reflected, for the same relative amount of work, in:

• reduced oxygen uptake and reduced heart rate
• a reduced sense of effort (Borg 1982)
• an ability to continue for longer
• an ability to increase the number of repetitions in the same time period (Newham 2001).

Altered motor control

Aspects of altered motor control include:

• muscle inhibition
• timing of onset
• increased muscle activation
• altered activation of agonist and antagonist.

Muscle inhibition

Muscle inhibition may be identified by the clinician by visual and/or palpatory cues. While these methods are clearly practical in the clinical setting and require no special equipment, they may have questionable reliability. Some muscles are superficial and may be relatively easy to identify – for example sternocleidomastoid; the vast majority of muscles overlap with other muscles or lie deep underneath a whole muscle, so that identification of these muscles is extremely difficult, if not impossible. This has led to the development of instrumentation to help the clinician identify muscle inhibition; it includes ultrasound imaging (Hides et al. 1995) and EMG biofeedback (Richardson et al. 1999). In research, voluntary muscle activity can be measured using the interpolated twitch technique (ITT) and involuntary muscle activity by a reduction in the Hoffman (H)-reflex.

The ITT involves applying a single electrical twitch to a nerve during a maximal isometric contraction and indicates the motor unit activity (Rutherford et al. 1986; Hales & Gandevia 1988; Gandevia et al. 1998), although a high-frequency train of stimuli is considered to be a more sensitive measure than the single twitch (Kent-Braun & Le Blanc 1996).

A dynamometer measures muscle torque during the active contraction, and if there is full motor unit activity then the addition of nerve stimulation will not produce any increase in torque. Any increase in torque (referred to as 'interpolated twitch torque': Suter & Herzog 2000) indicates muscle inhibition due to incomplete activation.

In asymptomatic subjects, the ITT will produce, on average, a 4% increase in isometric quadriceps muscle torque at 90° flexion (Suter et al. 1996). It should be noted that the extent of muscle inhibition measured by the ITT is dependent on the joint angle; at 60°, knee flexion muscle inhibition is three times greater than with the knee in extension (Suter & Herzog 1997).

Involuntary muscle activity is measured by a reduction in the H-reflex, indicating an inhibition of the alpha motor neurone pool (Spencer et al. 1984; Iles et al. 1990). The H-reflex is a small muscle contraction (via alpha motor neurones) in response to low-intensity stimulation of a mixed nerve (via stimulation of group Ia fibres from muscle spindles). This reflex inhibition continues to be present during active contraction of the muscle (Iles et al. 1990).

Both acute and chronic joint pathology, effusion, pain and immobilisation have been found to lead to inhibition of the overlying muscle, a response sometimes referred to as arthrogenous muscle inhibition (Stokes & Young 1984). All of the research studies identified in Box 4.8 have been carried out on the knee, apart from those on rheumatoid arthritis of the elbow joint. The muscle inhibition of an active voluntary contraction seems to be related to the extent of the joint damage: the greater the injury, the greater the inhibition of muscle (Newham et al. 1989; Urbach & Awiszus 2002).

The presence of pain can cause muscle inhibition (Arvidsson et al. 1986; Rutherford et al. 1986), although the mechanism is not fully understood. It has been suggested that muscle inhibition can be due to inhibitory input (Shakespeare et al. 1985; Iles et al. 1990; Snyder-Mackler et al. 1994; Suter & Herzog 2000; Torry et al. 2000) or abnormal input (Hurley & Newham 1993) from joint afferents, which reduces the motor drive to muscles acting over the joint.

The presence of effusion can cause muscle inhibition. This inhibition has been found by measuring a voluntary active contraction (deAndrade et al. 1965; Wood L et al. 1988), using the H-reflex (Spencer et al. 1984; Iles et al. 1990), measuring EMG activity

Box 4.8

Possible causes of arthrogenic muscle inhibition

Causes	Reference
Rheumatoid arthritis of knee	deAndrade et al. 1965
Rheumatoid arthritis of the elbow	Hurley et al. 1991
Osteoarthritis (knee joint) with no pain or effusion	deAndrade et al. 1965 Hurley & Newham 1993
Articular cartilage Degeneration of the patellar or tibial plateau	Suter et al. 1998a
Subperiosteal tumour of the femur	Stener 1969
Anterior knee pain	Suter et al. 1998 a, b
Muscle pain	Rutherford et al. 1986
Ligamentous knee injuries without pain or effusion	DeVita et al. 1997 Hurley et al. 1992 Newham et al. 1989 Hurley et al. 1994; Snyder-Mackler et al. 1994 Urbach & Awiszus 2002
Postmeniscectomy (knee joint)	Hurley et al. 1994 Shakespeare et al. 1985 Stokes & Young 1984 Suter et al. 1998 a
Presence of pain	Arvidsson et al. 1986 Rutherford et al. 1986
Effusion of the knee joint	deAndrade et al. 1965 Fahrer et al. 1988 Kennedy et al. 1982 Jones et al. 1987 Iles et al. 1990 Spencer et al. 1984 Stratford 1981 Wood L et al. 1988
Anterior cruciate ligament Deficiency of the knee joint	Newham et al. 1989 Hurley et al. 1994 Snyder-Mackler et al. 1994 Suter et al. 1998 a, b
Immobilisation	Vaughan 1989

(Torry et al. 2000) and by using the interpolated twitch technique (Fahrer et al. 1988). One study found that a knee effusion had no effect on quadriceps strength or power (McNair et al. 1994).

The effect of knee joint effusion and muscle inhibition has a marked effect on gait (Berchuck et al. 1990; Torry et al. 2000). This inhibition is thought to be due to increased intra-articular pressure causing an increase in tension in the joint capsule that stimulates mechanoreceptors in the intracapsular receptors and causes a reflex inhibition of the alpha motor neurone pool (Spencer et al. 1984; Iles et al. 1990; Torry et al. 2000). The inhibition is thought to affect both voluntary and involuntary muscle activity.

In experimentally produced effusion there is a linear relationship between the volume of the effusion and the reduction in the H-reflex amplitude, that is, the greater the effusion the greater the muscle inhibition (Spencer et al. 1984; Iles et al. 1990). In chronic effusions, associated with arthritis, the degree of effusion is not related to the amount of inhibition (Jones et al. 1987). In one study an effusion immediately caused inhibition of rectus femoris (Iles et al. 1990), while 50–60 ml was needed in another study to inhibit rectus femoris and vastus lateralis and between 20 and 30 ml to inhibit vastus medialis (Spencer et al. 1984).

With experimentally induced knee joint effusion, aspiration reduces the muscle inhibition (Spencer et al. 1984), whereas in chronic or recurrent knee joint effusions muscle inhibition remains the same post aspiration (Jones et al. 1987). The amount of inhibition of the muscle is related to the angle of the joint, with greater inhibition occurring with the knee in extension than in flexion (Krebs et al. 1983; Shakespeare et al. 1983; Stokes & Young 1984; Jones et al. 1987). This is thought to be due to the difference in intra-articular pressure, which is greater in full extension than in a few degrees of flexion (Levick 1983).

There has been some suggestion that the heads of a muscle are inhibited separately, that is, there is selective inhibition. One study found greater inhibition of vastus medialis than vastus lateralis or rectus femoris following effusion of the knee joint, although only 10 subjects were investigated (Kennedy et al. 1982). Another study found all heads of the quadriceps inhibited following knee joint effusion (Spencer et al. 1984).

Interestingly, a number of studies have found that muscle inhibition is not just restricted to the local muscles but also occurs in the contralateral limb (Newham et al. 1989; Hurley & Newham 1993; Hurley et al. 1994; Suter et al. 1998a, b; Urbach & Awiszus 2002). The clinician needs to be aware of this when comparing muscle function on the side of injury with the unaffected side as the degree of inhibition may be underestimated. The reason for the change on the unaffected side is unclear: it has been suggested to be due to altered movement patterns (Berchuck et al. 1990; Frank et al. 1994).

Another explanation may be the connection of nerve pathways in the spinal cord.

In rats, experimental injury to one paw produces hyperalgesia and swelling on the opposite side (Levine et al. 1985a), a response known as reflex neurogenic inflammation (Levine et al. 1985b). It should be noted that research in this area has been restricted to rats, and the effects have not yet been demonstrated in humans.

Timing of onset

The timing of onset of muscle activation during movement and functional activities has been identified in patients. Patients with chronic low-back pain have exhibited delayed activation of transversus abdominis muscle when asked to perform rapid arm movements (Hodges & Richardson 1996). There was also a significant (P <0.05) delayed activation found in the internal oblique, external oblique and rectus abdominis muscles during rapid shoulder flexion (Hodges & Richardson 1996).

Altered timing of the vastus medialis oblique relative to the vastus lateralis has been identified in patients with anterior knee pain (Voight & Wieder 1991; Cowan et al. 2002). It was found that, in normal subjects, the reflex response of vastus medialis preceded the vastus lateralis but in the patient group this was reversed: vastus lateralis was activated before vastus medialis oblique (Voight & Wieder 1991; Witvrouw et al. 1996).

It should be noted that there are normal age-related changes in the activation of muscles. For example, with age there is increased coactivation of quadriceps and hamstring muscle groups during a step-down movement (Hortobagyi & DeVita 2000). In addition, older subjects have been found to have a delay in muscle activation in the lower limb when stepping to regain balance during a fall (Thelen et al. 2000).

Increased muscle activation

Increased muscle activation is brought about by an increase in the activation of the alpha motor neurone pool supplying the muscle. The alpha motor neurone pool can be activated by the CNS, as part of motor control, or by peripheral input from muscle spindles, skin, joint, nerve and muscle afferents, including nociceptors. The underlying causes are therefore wide-ranging, and could include the perception of pain, as well as joint, nerve or muscle dysfunction.

Baseball players with known elbow medial collateral ligament insufficiency have been found to have increased EMG activity of extensor carpi radialis longus and brevis and reduced EMG activity of triceps, flexor carpi radialis and pronator teres compared with a control group (Glousman et al. 1992). Flexor carpi radialis and pronator teres might have been expected to demonstrate increased activity to compensate for the ligamentous insufficiency, but this was not the case.

Baseball players with known anterior shoulder instability have been found to have reduced EMG activity of pectoralis major, subscapularis, latissimus dorsi and serratus anterior and increased activity of biceps and supraspinatus compared with a control group (Glousman et al. 1988). The authors postulate that the reduced muscle activity exacerbates the anterior shoulder instability while the increased activity of biceps and supraspinatus compensates for the anterior instability.

This compensation or protective mechanism has also been suggested in another study that found increased EMG activity of biceps femoris, vastus lateralis and tibialis anterior in patients with an ACL-deficient knee (Ciccotti et al. 1994).

Experiments on the rabbit, cat and rat have identified that sympathetic efferent activity causes an increase in muscle tone (Passatore et al. 1985). There was an increase in activity, and decrease in position sensitivity, of the muscle spindle. This suggests that the increase in muscle tone was due to contraction of the intrafusal fibres of the muscle spindle and some extrafusal fibres.

Altered activation of agonist and antagonist

This alteration in the relative activation of agonist and antagonist can result from the above consequences of increased or decreased muscle activation. In addition to these dysfunctions, there is also evidence of a specific alteration in the agonist and antagonist activation patterns.

Pain around the knee causes a nociceptive flexor withdrawal response: hip and knee flexion and ankle dorsiflexion. To produce this movement there is increased alpha motor neurone excitability of the hip and knee flexors and ankle dorsiflexors (Stener & Peterson 1963) and reciprocal inhibition of the knee extensors (Stener & Peterson 1963; Stener 1969; Young et al. 1987). Stener & Peterson (1963) observed that pressure or tension on a partially ruptured medial collateral ligament resulted in increased muscle activity of sartorius and semi-membranosus (knee flexors) with inhibition of vastus medialis (knee extensor). Stener (1969) found that pain over the lateral femoral epicondyle caused inhibition of the vastus medialis and lateralis.

Patients with more chronic ACL deficiency (16 months–21 years) have been found to have less quadriceps and gastrocnemius activity and greater hamstring activity during the stance phase, and increased hamstring activity during the swing phase of gait (Branch et al. 1989). In another study of patients with chronic ACL deficiency (2–3 years), horizontal walking failed to show any difference in EMG activity of quadriceps and hamstrings but on walking uphill the hamstring muscle was activated much earlier than in control subjects (Kalund et al. 1990). Patients with an ACL-deficient knee following 6 months' rehabilitation continued to have increased EMG activity of vastus lateralis, biceps femoris and tibialis anterior muscles during functional movements, compared with a control group (Ciccotti et al. 1994).

A number of studies have demonstrated that chronic ACL deficiency and post-ACL reconstruction cause an alteration of the motor control around the knee (Branch et al. 1989; Berchuck et al. 1990; Kalund et al. 1990; Ciccotti et al. 1994; Beard et al. 1996; DeVita et al. 1997). Patients who have had an ACL reconstruction were found to have an altered gait pattern such that, compared with control subjects, the knee was in more flexion at heel contact and mid-stance, and a greater range of extensor torque was present during the stance phase (DeVita et al. 1997). Patients with chronic ACL deficiency, longer than 6 months without repair, were found to walk with the knee in more flexion at heel contact and mid-stance and this correlated with an increased duration of hamstring activity (Beard et al. 1996).

A clinical observation of the reaction of muscle to pain has been described (Janda 1985). It has been suggested that postural (or tonic) muscles become hypertonic and short, while phasic muscles are thought to become hypotonic and weak. Muscle shortness describes a muscle which, when inactive, has a length less than normal and limits the full range of joint movement (Schmid & Spring 1985). Janda (1985), however, uses the classification system that a muscle is either postural or phasic (Box 4.9), which is difficult because it is a rather flawed classification system. The vast majority of muscles contain equal proportions of type I and type II muscle fibres and

Box 4.9

The reaction of postural and phasic muscles to pain (Janda 1985)

Postural muscles which become tight, short or hypertonic	Phasic muscles which become inhibited, weak and hypotonic
Soleus	Tibialis anterior
Gastrocnemius	The vasti
Tibialis posterior	Glutei
Rectus femoris	Rectus abdominis
Iliopsoas	Lower stabilisers of the scapula
Tensor fasciae latae	Deep neck flexors
Hamstrings	Extensors of the upper extremity
Short hip adductors	
Quadratus lumborum	
Piriformis	
Part of paravertebral back muscles	
Pectoralis major	
Sternocleidomastoid	
Upper trapezius	
Levator scapulae	

therefore cannot easily be divided into these two categories.

There is, nevertheless, some evidence to support the muscle reaction proposed by Janda (1985). For example, pain around the knee has been found to cause increased activation of the hip flexors, which might be assumed to include rectus femoris and iliopsoas (Stener & Peterson 1963), and increased activation of the knee flexors (Stener & Peterson 1963), which would mean the hamstring group, and inhibition of the knee extensors (Stener & Peterson 1963; Stener 1969; Young et al. 1987), which can be assumed to include the vasti. This research therefore supports the contention that rectus femoris, iliopsoas and hamstrings tend to react to pain by becoming hypertonic and the vasti react by being hypotonic.

Research supports the observation that the deep neck flexor muscles become hypotonic and weak (Janda 1985). Patients with recurrent headaches were found to have reduced isometric strength and endurance of the deep neck flexors, compared with a control group (Watson 1994).

Finally, arm pain produced by an upper-limb tension test (ULTT2a; Butler 2000) in asymptomatic subjects was found to be associated with an increase in EMG activity of the upper fibres of trapezius (van der Heide et al. 2001). This provides further support to the observation of Janda (1985) that the upper trapezius muscle reacts to pain by becoming hypertonic.

Altered muscle length

The most obvious reduction in muscle length is seen following immobilisation of a joint, with the muscle held in a shortened position. In this situation the muscle will be shortened and will have an increased resistance to passive lengthening (Tabary et al. 1972; Goldspink 1976; Goldspink & Williams 1979). Upon removal of the immobilisation, in the cat soleus muscle, the muscle returns to its original length within 4 weeks (Tabary et al. 1972; Goldspink 1976).

When muscle is immobilised in a lengthened position it increases the number of sarcomeres and thus becomes longer; there is no change in resistance to passive lengthening. Again, on removal of the immobilisation, in the cat and mouse, the muscle quickly returns to its original length (Tabary et al. 1972; Williams & Goldspink 1976).

Muscle length can be measured by lengthening muscle fully and measuring the final joint angle using a goniometer, or by visual estimation. The passive resistance of muscle to lengthening is more difficult to measure. The clinician can passively lengthen the muscle and estimate the 'feel' of the resistance to movement or the muscle can be more objectively measured using isokinetic equipment.

Production of symptoms

Symptoms from muscle dysfunction are commonly a pain or an ache. Symptoms may be felt when the muscle is at rest, when it is lengthened or when it contracts. The clinician attempts to obtain an accurate assessment of the behaviour of symptoms with each of these tests (palpation, length and contraction) so that they can be used as a sensitive measure on reassessment of the patient. If symptoms are produced when a muscle is lengthened, the detailed behaviour of when the symptom is first produced during the movement P_1, and what happens to its intensity with any continued movement P_2 or P', can be depicted on a movement diagram (Petty 2011). The symptom may be sufficiently intense to be the cause of the limitation in range, depicted as P_2 on a movement diagram (Figure 4.38A), or may reach a particular intensity at the limit of range P', spoken as 'p prime' (Figure 4.38B). Symptoms may be produced in muscle with a 'normal' or hypomobile range of movement, with or without altered quality of movement.

Pain limiting movement

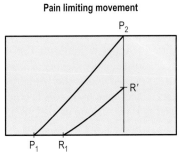

Pain is first felt at ¼ range and increases to limit range (P_2) to ¾ range (L). Resistance is first felt at ½ range and increases to about 5/10 at limit of range

Figure 4.38 • Movement diagram of hamstring length in supine depicting A P_2 with some resistance and normal range, and B P' and resistance limiting movement.

Resistance limiting movement

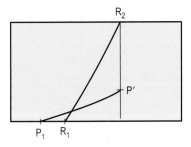

Resistance is first felt at 1/2 range and increases to limit range (R_2) to ¾ range (L). Pain is first felt at ¼ range and increases to about 3/10 at limit of range (where 0 is no pain and 10 is maximum pain ever felt by patient)

Free nerve endings supplied by group III and IV afferents can be found throughout muscle. They lie in the connective tissue, in between the intrafusal and extrafusal fibres, in arterioles and venules, in the capsule of muscle spindles and tendon organs, in tendon tissue at the musculotendinous junction and in fat cells (Stacey 1969; Reinert & Mense 1992). Muscle can therefore be a primary source of pain. Both A δ and C fibres can be activated by noxious thermal, mechanical and chemical stimuli (Kumazawa & Mizumura 1977; Kaufman et al. 1982; Mense 1996). The last two, noxious mechanical and chemical forms of irritation, are the probable causes in patients with muscle pain seen in the musculoskeletal field. The pain from muscle can therefore be classified as mechanical or chemical nociceptive pain (Gifford 1998).

Mechanical pain occurs when certain movements stress injured tissue, increasing the mechanical deformation and activation of nociceptors; other movements may reduce the stress on injured tissue, reducing the mechanical deformation and activation of nociceptors. Thus, with mechanical pain, there are particular movements which aggravate and ease the pain, sometimes referred to as 'on/off' pain. The magnitude of the mechanical deformation may be directly related to the magnitude of nociceptor activity; this has been found in the skin of the cat where greater forces cause greater nociceptor activity (Garell et al. 1996).

Chemical nociceptive pain can be produced by the chemicals released as a result of inflammation, ischaemia or sympathetic nervous system activity (Gifford 1998).

Experimentally induced inflammation of muscle in the cat and rat has been shown to cause an increased irregular resting discharge in both group III and IV afferents in muscle (Berberich et al. 1988; Diehl et al. 1988). This increased resting discharge or sensitisation produces primary hyperalgesia (Raja et al. 1999). In addition, inflammation was found to lower the mechanical threshold of group IV afferents and is the probable cause of muscle tenderness on palpation (Berberich et al. 1988; Diehl et al. 1988), a response known as allodynia (Raja et al. 1999). An increase in the levels of substance P from muscle afferent fibres has been found to initiate background activity of muscle nociceptors (Reinert et al. 1992); thus, with muscle injury, substance P may, in part, be responsible for muscle pain (Reinert et al. 1992; Mense 1996).

Clinical features of inflammatory pain are redness, oedema and heat, acute pain and tissue damage,

a close relationship of stimulus response and pain, a diurnal pattern with pain and stiffness worst at night and in the morning, signs of neurogenic inflammation (redness, swelling or symptoms in the neural zone) and a beneficial effect of anti-inflammatory medication (Butler 2000).

Ischaemic nociceptive pain in muscle is not yet fully understood (Mense 1996). It may be related to chemical irritation (Moore et al. 1934), build-up of potassium ions (Harpuder & Stein 1943), lack of oxidation of metabolic products (Pickering & Wayne 1933–1934) or the presence of bradykinin (Nakahara 1971). Experimentally induced ischaemia of muscle activated only 10% of muscle nociceptors. However, when a muscle contracts under ischaemic conditions there is much stronger activation of group IV nociceptors (Mense & Stahnke 1983; Kaufman et al. 1984b). With muscle hypoxia there is an increase in group III and IV mechanoreceptor and nociceptor afferent activity (Kieschke et al. 1988). The underlying mechanism of ischaemic contraction causing nociceptor activity appears to be related to chemical sensitisation of muscle nociceptors (Mense 1996).

Clinical features of ischaemic pain are thought to be symptoms produced after prolonged or unusual activities, rapid ease of symptoms after a change in posture, symptoms towards the end of the day or after the accumulation of activity, a poor response to anti-inflammatory medication and sometimes absence of trauma (Butler 2000).

The sympathetic nervous system can cause pain. Increased concentrations of adrenaline (epinephrine) in muscle cause an increased discharge frequency of muscle nociceptors, and this response is enhanced with the addition of noxious mechanical stimulation (Kieschke et al. 1988). In the presence of tissue injury or inflammation, sympathetic nervous system activity can maintain the perception of pain or enhance nociception in inflamed tissue (Raja et al. 1999). Sympathetically maintained pain can occur with complex regional pain syndromes and may play a part in chronic arthritis and soft-tissue trauma (Raja et al. 1999). Thus, it appears that the sympathetic nervous system can cause muscle pain.

The effect of nociceptor activity by a mechanical or chemical stimulus alters the physiology of the nociceptor itself; in this way the nociceptor is plastic: it alters according to its environment. Nociceptor activity causes an increased sensitivity of the nociceptors so there is a lower threshold for response, an increased response to suprathreshold stimuli and spontaneous activity (Raja et al. 1999). For example, 5-hydroxytryptamine and prostaglandin E_2 cause sensitisation of group IV afferents that are sensitive to these substances (Mense 1981). This increased sensitivity of nociceptors leads to a decreased pain threshold, an increased pain to suprathreshold stimuli and spontaneous pain – changes collectively referred to as primary hyperalgesia. If a stimulus is applied which would normally not provoke pain, such as movement or a light touch, and pain is provoked, then this is termed allodynia (Raja et al. 1999). In addition, mechanoreceptors in adjacent uninjured tissue develop the ability to evoke pain, a phenomenon known as secondary hyperalgesia (Raja et al. 1999). It is thought to be due to an increase in the responsiveness of second-order nociceptor neurones in the spinal cord that become activated by mechanoreceptor activity, a response known as central sensitisation (Raja et al. 1999).

Constant experimentally induced muscle pain in humans has been found to cause an increase in the stretch reflex of the relaxed muscle, suggesting that muscle pain increases the sensitivity of the muscle spindle to stretch (Matre et al. 1998). In the same study, muscle pain did not alter the H-reflex, suggesting that muscle pain does not directly alter the sensitivity of alpha motor neurone activity, although it may have an indirect effect by causing a reduction in descending inhibition on the alpha motor neurone activity and thus cause an increase in the stretch reflex (Matre et al. 1999). Inducing muscle pain also increases the stretch reflex of the antagonist muscle group; pain in tibialis anterior increases the stretch reflex of soleus (Matre et al. 1998). The increased stretch reflex induced by muscle pain is present only when the muscle is relaxed – there is no change in stretch reflex during an isometric muscle contraction or during walking (Matre et al. 1999).

Muscle pain is thought to have a greater inhibitory effect upon low-threshold motor units supplying type I fibres than high-threshold motor units supplying type II muscle fibres (Gydikov 1976). If this is correct then it can be speculated that pain over the soleus muscle, for example, which has a high proportion of type I fibres, would have a greater effect than pain in a muscle that has a more even distribution of fibre types.

It should be noted that the information given here has focused on pain from muscle tissue only. Clearly, pain may be felt from a number of tissues, including the skin, joint and nerve overlying the joint. Joint pain

is discussed in Chapter 2, pain from skin and nerve is discussed in Chapter 6, and Chapter 8 provides a broad overview of pain.

Referral of pain from muscle

In the upper and lower limbs, muscle pain is often felt over the joint that the muscle moves, provided that the joint has the same segmental innervation as the muscle (Kellgren 1939). Some generalisations can be made about the pattern of pain referral from muscle. The segmental distribution of muscle is given in Figure 4.39.

An early investigation of referred pain from muscle was made by Kellgren in 1938. Observations of pain referral were made following noxious injection of saline into muscle in three asymptomatic co-workers. The chart of pain referral for various muscles is shown in Figure 4.40. The study investigated differences in the quality of pain from muscle, from tendon and from fascia. Fascia and tendon tended to produce sharp localised pain, while muscle tended to produce some localised pain and a diffuse referred pain with tenderness of structures deep to the skin.

The limb muscles are generally innervated by more than one spinal segment; for example, infraspinatus is supplied by C5 and C6 and this produces a more widespread area of referral than the dermatome areas for skin (Kellgren 1938). Pain from muscle appears to be referred to regions corresponding to the spinal segments from which it obtains its motor supply; this is clearer in the upper limb than in the lower limb (Kellgren 1938).

Pain from muscle may be poorly localised to muscle; for example, pain from flexor digitorum profundus may refer to the metacarpophalangeal joint, and when this joint is injected the pain is considered to be very similar to that from the muscle (Kellgren 1938). In the same way, pain from the lumbar erector spine muscle produces pain similar to that caused by injection of the gluteal fascia. Some muscles, such as rectus abdominis and muscles in the hand, are much more sensitive and produce more severe pain than biceps brachii and glutei muscles. Metabolic muscle disease, in contrast, typically causes pain that the patient is able to locate as 'in the muscle'; it is not vague and does not refer (Petty 2003).

Referred pain from muscle has also been investigated by another group of researchers (Feinstein et al. 1954). Injection of saline (6%) into the paravertebral muscles (immediately on either side of the

Figure 4.39 • Myotomes of **A** upper limb, anterior view, **B** upper limb, posterior view, **C** lower limb, anterior view, and **D** lower limb, posterior view (Reproduced with permission, from Kellgren J H 1938 Clinical Science 3:175–190. © The Biochemical Society and the Medical Research Society (http://www.clinsci.org)).

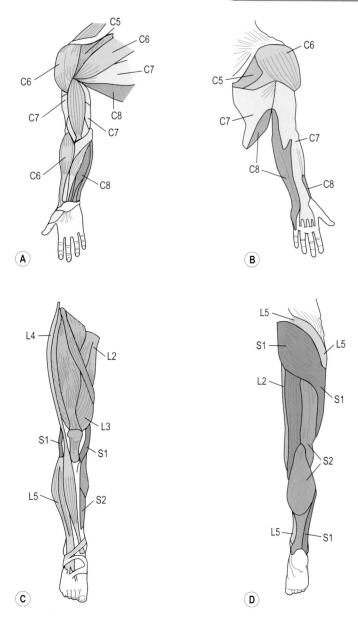

midline) at each segmental level of the spine resulted in referral maps obtained from five subjects (Figure 4.41). The pain was described as a deep ache that was 'boring', 'heavy', 'crampy' or 'lumpy'. The intensity of pain was related to the amount of saline that was injected – greater amounts caused more pain. Injection of the thoracic paravertebral muscles was also accompanied by autonomic symptoms of pallor and sweating, and sometimes bradycardia, reduced blood pressure, faintness and nausea.

Injection of saline (6%) into peripheral muscles was also carried out on three or four subjects (Figure 4.42). The muscles injected were serratus anterior, infraspinatus, pectoralis major, brachialis, flexor carpi ulnaris and extensor digitorum. The area of pain spread variable distances from the injection site. In most cases of spinal and peripheral injection the pain was accompanied by deep tenderness and skin hypoalgesia (diminished pinprick sensation) and in some cases by muscle spasm.

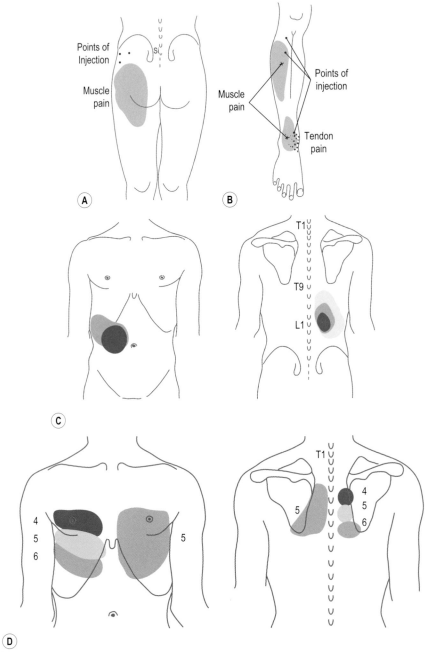

Figure 4.40 • Referred pain from muscle (reproduced, with permission, from Kellgren 1938. © The Biochemical Society and the Medical Research Society). A Gluteus medius. B Tibialis anterior; stippling is tendon pain. C Horizontal hatching from multifidus, vertical hatching from intercostals and stippling from rectus abdominis. D From 4th, 5th and 6th intercostal muscles.

(*Continued*)

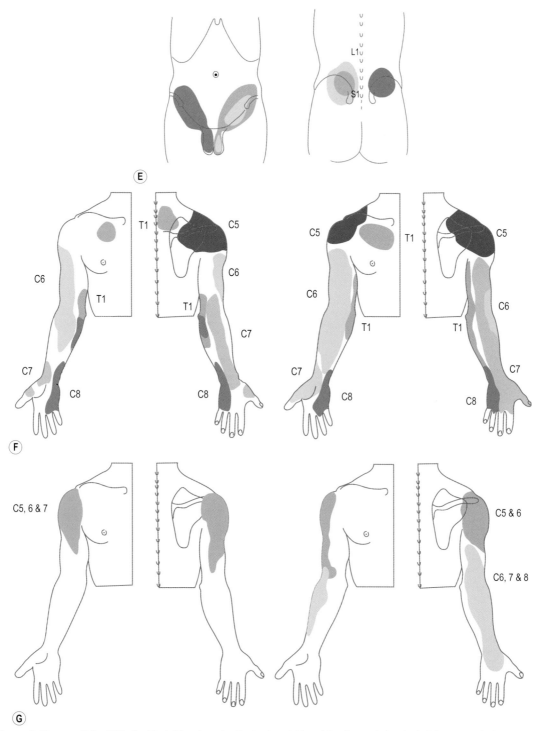

Figure 4.40—cont'd • E Vertical hatching from testis, horizontal hatching from abdominal obliques and stippling from multifidus. F Crosses from rhomboids, oblique hatching from flexor carpi radialis, stippling from abductor pollicis longus, vertical hatching from third dorsal interosseous, horizontal hatching from first intercostal space. G Vertical hatching from serratus anterior, oblique hatching from infraspinatus and stippling from latissimus dorsi.

(Continued)

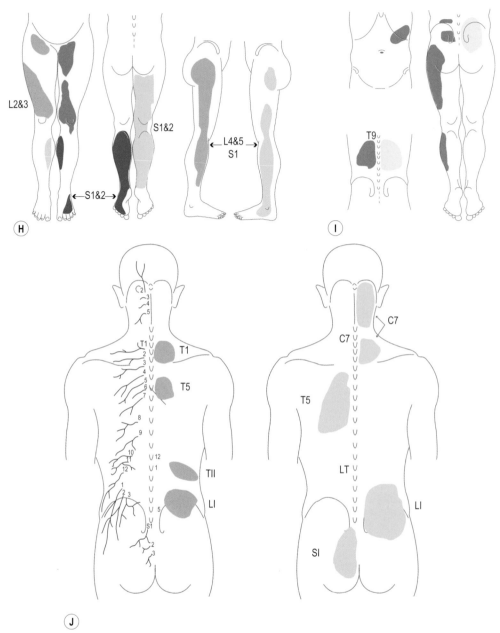

Figure 4.40—cont'd • H Left leg with oblique hatching from adductor longus, right leg with oblique hatching from sartorius, vertical hatching from gastrocnemius, horizontal hatching from first interosseous, crosses from tensor fasciae latae and stippling from peroneus longus. I Vertical hatching from erector spinae and horizontal hatching from multifidus stimulated opposite T9 and L5. J Left figure represents anterior aspect of erector spinae and right figure posterior aspect of erector spinae at the spinal level indicated.

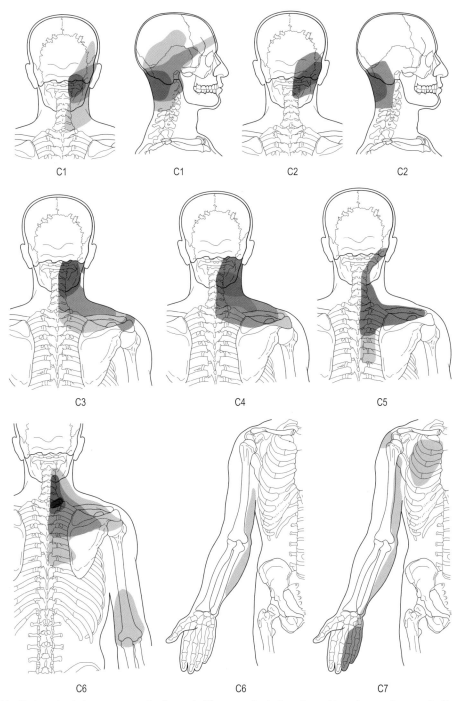

Figure 4.41 • Referred pain from paravertebral muscle. The area of pain from five subjects is superimposed. (From Feinstein et al. 1954. © The Journal of Bone and Joint Surgery, Inc.)

(Continued)

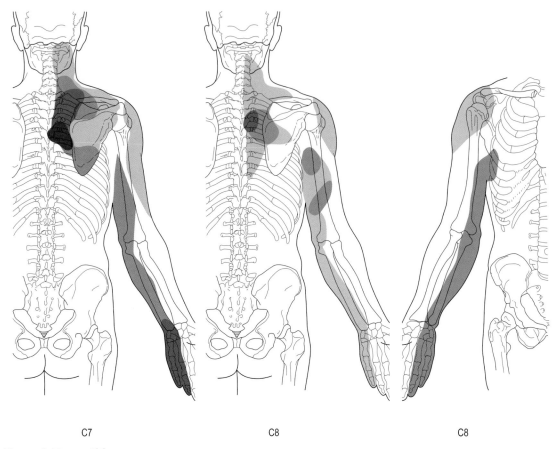

C7 C8 C8

Figure 4.41—cont'd

(Continued)

Referred pain from muscle has been more recently investigated by stimulating the median nerve fascicles innervating muscles in the forearm and hand (Torebjork et al. 1984). Intraneural stimulation of the median nerve at the elbow gave rise to an aching cramp-like pain deep in the forearm and thumb, and in 50% of cases (13 of 26) superficial pain over the hand. In some subjects there was also referred pain, that is, pain felt outside the innervation area of the median nerve, with deep cramp-like pain felt in the upper arm, axilla or mammillary region (Torebjork et al. 1984). The results of this study support the existence of myotomes (Inman & Saunders 1944). This study also provided the interesting observation that dysfunction of the median nerve at the elbow may refer pain proximally to the upper arm, axilla and mammillary region.

In a similar study, stimulation of muscle nociceptors of the common peroneal nerve also produced a deep cramp-like pain (Simone et al. 1994). Stimulation of tendon nociceptors produced a sharp and localised pain (Simone et al. 1994).

The mechanism of referred pain is thought to be due to the convergence of afferents in the periphery and in the dorsal horn (Torebjork et al. 1984). This is depicted in Figure 4.43. In the periphery, proximal to the spinal cord, sensory neurones from skin and muscle converge (Wells et al. 1994). In the dorsal horn, there is convergence of skin afferents and group III and IV muscle afferents on to wide dynamic range cells (Foreman et al. 1979). In both cases, activation of nociceptors from the muscle, for example, is perceived by the brain to come from the skin; the brain thus misinterprets the information.

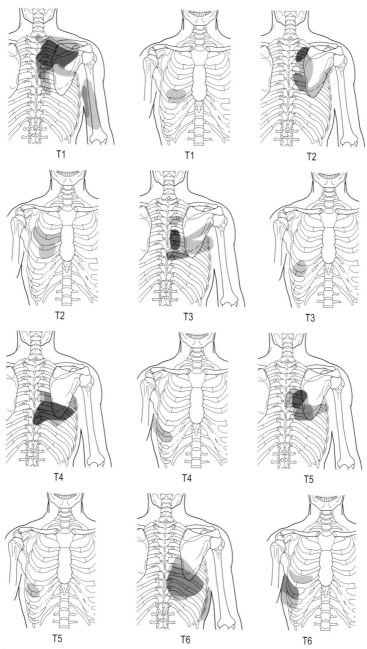

T1   T1   T2

T2   T3   T3

T4   T4   T5

T5   T6   T6

Figure 4.41—cont'd

(Continued)

Summary of symptom production

The commonest symptom from a muscle is pain. The perception of pain occurs in the CMS and is multidimensional, i.e. it includes sensory, physiological, affective, cognitive, behavioural and sociocultural factors. Nociceptors are found throughout muscle, so that muscle can be a potential source of pain. Muscle nociceptors are sensitive to mechanical deformation and chemical irritation and thus can produce mechanical or chemical nociceptive pain. Chemical

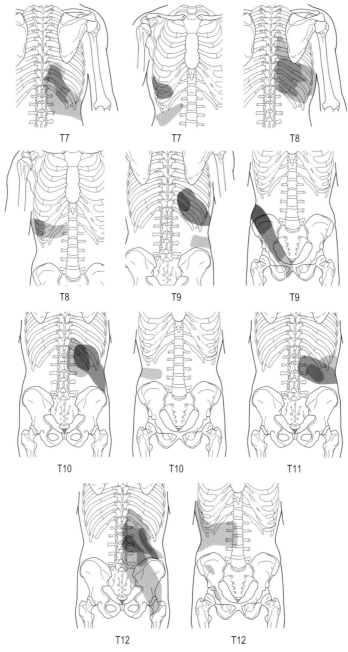

T7   T7   T8

T8   T9   T9

T10   T10   T11

T12   T12

Figure 4.41—cont'd

(Continued)

irritation may be due to inflammation, ischaemia or sympathetic nervous system activity. Pain from muscle tends to be deep and localised over the muscle with some diffuse referred pain and tenderness to touch some distance away, possibly over the underlying joint, and may follow a segmental distribution.

Tendon injury and repair

Tendons can tear in the middle region, by avulsion of bone, and more rarely at the insertion site (Woo et al. 1988). Repetitive strain of a tendon can produce micro- and macrotrauma of the tendon. The amount

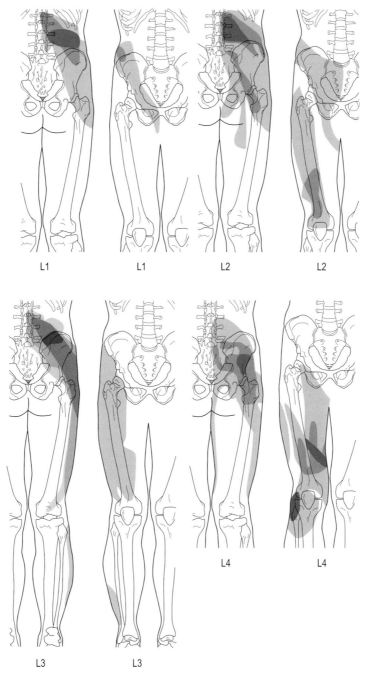

L1   L1   L2   L2

L3   L3   L4   L4

Figure 4.41—cont'd

(Continued)

of strain needed to cause micro- and macrotrauma is given in Figure 4.44. Repetitive strain may alter the collagenous structure of tendon with resultant inflammation, oedema and pain (Jozsa & Kannus 1997). Overuse injury occurs where this repetitive strain, causing tissue damage, is greater than the natural repair and healing process and this may lead, with further strain, to partial or complete rupture of the tendon (Archambault et al. 1995; Jozsa & Kannus 1997). Terms such as tendinitis, peritendinitis and

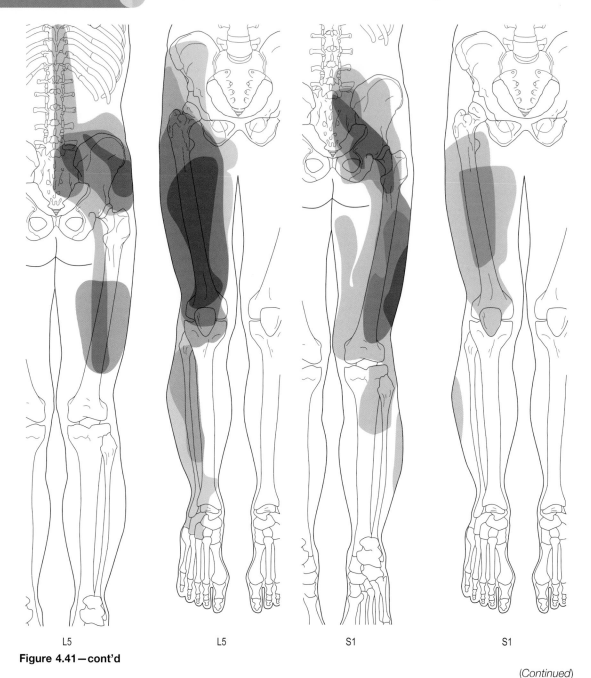

L5   L5   S1   S1

Figure 4.41—cont'd

(Continued)

tenosynovitis have traditionally been used to describe conditions affecting the tendon; however, the preferred term is tendinopathy as evidence suggests that very little inflammation exists within the tendon (Rees et al. 2006; Woodley et al. 2007). Often, these overuse injuries are seen in the upper extremity in occupations that require repetitive movement of the hands and forearms, and in the lower extremities in sport-related injuries.

The aetiology of sports-related lower-limb tendon injuries is thought to include vascularity of the tendon, malalignments, leg length discrepancy, age and

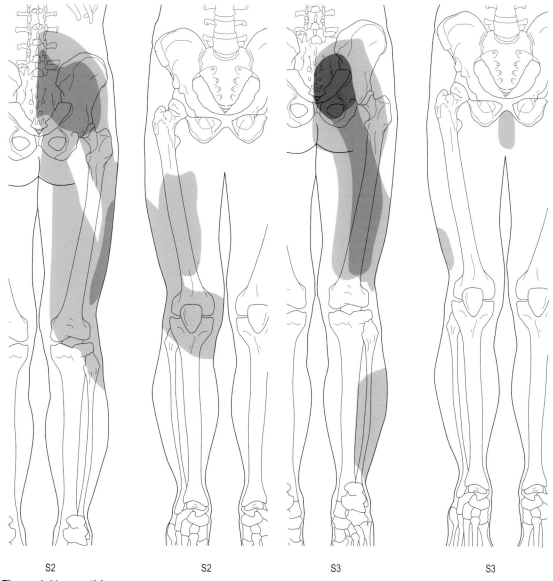

S2   S2   S3   S3

Figure 4.41—cont'd

weight (Clement et al. 1984; Jozsa et al. 1989b; Jozsa & Kannus 1997), as well as extrinsic factors such as type of sport, training errors, environmental conditions, equipment and ineffective rules (Clement et al. 1984; Jozsa & Kannus 1997).

Vascularity is thought to be an important aetiological factor because tendon injuries often occur where there is a relatively poor blood supply (Clement et al. 1984; Carr & Norris 1989; Frey et al. 1990; Reynolds & Worrell 1991; Archambault et al. 1995). For example, the tendocalcaneus tendon has an

avascular area 2–6 cm proximal to its distal attachment (Carr & Norris 1989), and it is in this region where the most severe tendon degeneration and spontaneous ruptures occur (Jozsa et al. 1989b; Jozsa & Kannus 1997). The posterior tibial tendon has an area of poor vascularity posterior and distal to the medial malleolus, and it is in this region that it frequently ruptures (Frey et al. 1990). The supraspinatus tendon has poor vascularity where it inserts on to the humerus (Lohr & Uhthoff 1990; Chansky & Iannotti 1991), and, again, it is in this region where

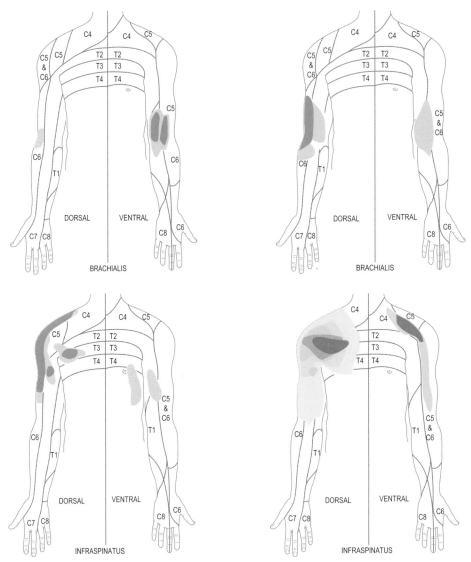

Figure 4.42 • Referred pain from peripheral muscle. The area of pain from three or four subjects is superimposed. Cross-hatching represents deep pain, and vertical hatching cutaneous hypoalgesia. (From Feinstein et al. 1954. © The Journal of Bone and Joint Surgery, Inc.)

(Continued)

the tendon ruptures (Jozsa & Kannus 1997). Age-related degenerative changes within the tendon can cause narrowing or obliteration of blood vessels, further reducing the vascularity of the tendon (Kannus & Jozsa 1991).

In work-related upper-limb tendon injuries the strain placed on tendon may not be excessive, but the repetitive nature of the task may be sufficient to cause change in the tissue. It is proposed that, initially, in the first 5 days, there is ischaemia, metabolic disturbance and cell membrane damage leading to inflammation (Jozsa & Kannus 1997). The increase in tissue pressure further impairs the circulation and enhances the ischaemic changes. In the proliferation phase (5–21 days) there is fibrin clotting and proliferation of fibroblasts, synovial cells and capillaries. This is followed by the maturation phase (<21 days) in which adhesions and thickening of the tenosynovium and paratenon occur (Kvist & Kvist 1980; Jozsa & Kannus 1997).

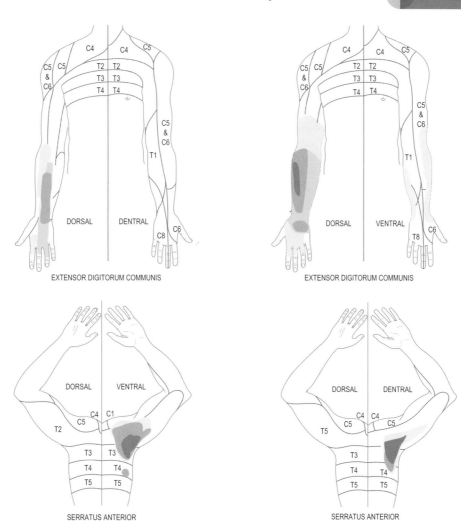

Figure 4.42—cont'd

(Continued)

Spontaneous tendon rupture is associated with degenerative changes (Jozsa et al. 1989b). The diameter of collagen fibres decreases in degenerative tendon, suggesting an increase in weaker type III collagen fibres (Jozsa et al. 1989a). Degenerative changes were found in 97% of ruptured tendons, which included the Achilles tendon, biceps brachii and extensor pollicis longus from nearly 900, compared with 35% in a control group (Kannus & Jozsa 1991).

Tendon repair

Healing of tendon is similar to that of other soft tissues and consists of three phases: lag or inflammation phase (1–7 days), regeneration or proliferation phase (7–21 days) and remodelling or maturation phase (21 days to 1 year) (Jozsa & Kannus 1997). Initially type III collagen is laid down; this is replaced by type I collagen tissue during the late proliferation stage and maturation phase (Coombs et al. 1980).

Muscle injury and repair

Muscle strain injury can occur with eccentric exercise, producing delayed muscle soreness (Friden et al. 1983; Jones et al. 1986). Pain, weakness and muscle stiffness are felt after unaccustomed eccentric exercise. There is disruption of the Z band, predominantly of type II fibres, with repair largely

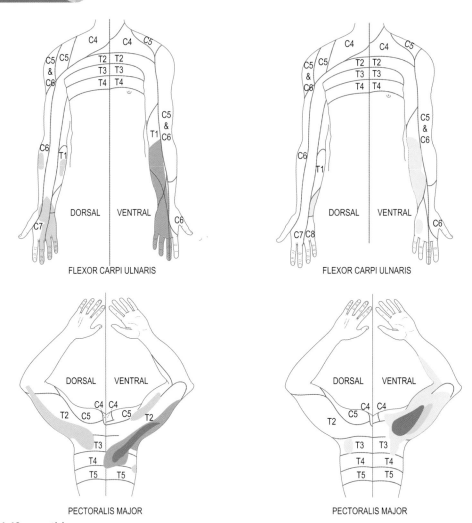

Figure 4.42—cont'd

completed by 6 days (Friden et al. 1983; Jones et al. 1986). The reason for the delayed muscle soreness following eccentric contraction may be that eccentric contraction produces more force within the muscle than other types of muscle contraction (Katz 1939). The myotendinous region is the weakest part of the tendon–muscle unit and is the region most susceptible to strain injuries (Nikolaou et al. 1987; Garrett et al. 1989; Garrett 1990; Tidball 1991).

Muscle repair

Repair of muscle injury follows the typical healing process of all soft tissues: the lag phase, regeneration and remodelling.

There is initially the development of a necrotic zone at the site of damage and the adjacent uninjured myofibrils retract and begin the repair process, with activation of satellite cells (McComas 1996). The satellite cells migrate into the necrotic area and differentiate into myotubes, which begin to bridge the gap between the retracted uninjured myofibrils.

An experimental crush injury of the semitendinosus muscle of the rat reveals necrosis in the first 2 days, with new myotubes within the damaged area at 5 days and regeneration of muscle fibres bridging the necrotic area by 10 days, with full regeneration at 30 days (Stuart et al. 1981). A controlled strain injury of the musculotendinous junction of tibialis anterior muscle was carried out on New Zealand white rabbits

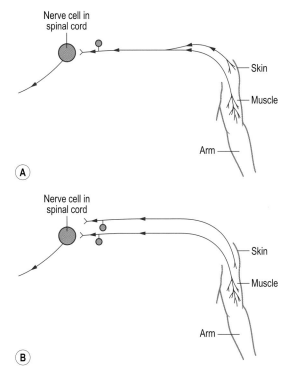

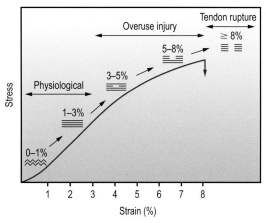

Figure 4.44 • Stress–strain curve of tendon depicting the amount of stress involved in microtrauma (3–8%) and macrotrauma (<8%) (from Jozsa & Kannus 1997).

A

B

Figure 4.43 • Referred pain due to convergence of afferents **A** in the periphery and **B** in the spinal cord (after Wells et al. 1994, with permission).

(Nikolaou et al. 1987). Necrosis and infiltration of inflammatory cells, oedema and haemorrhage occurred after 1 day. After 2 days the damaged fibres had been broken down with proliferation of inflammatory cells, macrophages and fibroblasts. After

7 days inflammation was reduced and fibrocytes were evident (Nikolaou et al. 1987). Clear evidence of muscle regeneration was evident after 4 days following an experimental strain injury of a rat tendon (Almekinders & Gilbert 1986).

Summary of muscle dysfunction

Common muscle dysfunctions seen clinically are reduced muscle strength, power and endurance, altered motor control, reduced muscle length and the production of symptoms. Muscle dysfunction does not exist in isolation; joint and nerve will also to some extent be involved. The next chapter discusses treatment of muscle dysfunction.

References

Abrahams, V.C., 1977. The physiology of neck muscles; their role in head movement and maintenance of posture. Can. J. Physiol. Pharmacol. 55, 332–338.

Abrahams, V.C., 1981. Sensory and motor specialization in some muscles of the neck. Trends Neurosci. 4, 24–27.

Adams, M.A., Bogduk, N., Burton, K., et al., 2002. The biomechanics of back pain. Churchill Livingstone, Edinburgh.

Agre, J.C., Rodriquez, A.A., 1989. Validity of manual muscle testing in post-polio subjects with good or normal strength. Arch. Phys. Med. Rehabil. 70 (Suppl.), A17–A18.

Ahles, T.A., Martin, J.B., 1992. Cancer pain: a multidimensional perspective. In: Turk, D.C., Feldman, C.S. (Eds.), Noninvasive approaches to pain management in the terminally ill. Haworth, New York, pp. 25–48.

Akima, H., Kano, Y., Enomoto, Y., et al., 2001. Muscle function in 164 men and women aged 20–84 yr. Med. Sci. Sports Exerc. 33 (2), 220–226.

Allen, G.M., Gandevia, S.C., McKenzie, D.K., 1995. Reliability of measurements of muscle strength and voluntary activation using twitch interpolation. Muscle Nerve 18, 593–600.

Allum, J.H.J., Bloem, B.R., Carpenter, M.G., et al., 1998. Proprioceptive control of posture: a review of new concepts. Gait Posture 8, 214–242.

Almekinders, L.C., Gilbert, J.A., 1986. Healing of experimental muscle strains and the effects of nonsteroidal antiinflammatory medication. Am. J. Sports Med. 14 (4), 303–308.

Alter, M.J., 1996. Science of flexibility, second ed. Human Kinetics, Illinois.

Antonutto, G., Capelli, C., Girardis, M., et al., 1999. Effects of microgravity on maximal power of lower limbs during very short efforts in humans. J. Appl. Physiol. 86, 85–92.

Appell, H.J., 1990. Muscular atrophy following immobilisation, a review. Sports Med. 10 (1), 42–58.

Arangio, G.A., Chen, C., Kalady, M., et al., 1997. Thigh muscle size and strength after anterior cruciate ligament reconstruction and rehabilitation. J. Orthop. Sports Phys. Ther. 26 (5), 238–243.

Archambault, J.M., Wiley, J.P., Bray, R.C., 1995. Exercise loading of tendons and the development of overuse injuries, a review of current literature. Sports Med. 20 (2), 77–89.

Armstrong, B., McNair, P., Taylor, D., 2008. Head and neck position sense. Sports Med. 38 (2), 101–117.

Arvidsson, I., Eriksson, E., Knutsson, E., et al., 1986. Reduction of pain inhibition on voluntary muscle activation by epidural analgesia. Orthopaedics 9 (10), 1415–1419.

Baratta, R., Solomonow, M., Zhou, B.H., et al., 1988. Muscular coactivation. The role of the antagonist musculature in maintaining knee stability. Am. J. Sports Med. 16 (2), 113–122.

Barker, D., 1974. The morphology of muscle receptors. In: Hunt, C.C. (Ed.), Handbook of sensory physiology. Muscle receptors 3. Springer-Verlag, Berlin, p. 124 part 2.

Barker, D., Saito, M., 1981. Autonomic innervation of receptors and muscle fibres in cat skeletal muscle. Proc. R. Soc. Lond. B Biol. Sci. 212, 317–332.

Bastide, G., Zadeh, J., Lefebvre, D., 1989. Are the 'little muscles' what we think they are? Surg. Radiol. Anat. 11, 255–256.

Beard, D.J., Soundarapandian, R.S., O'Connor, J.J., et al., 1996. Gait and electromyographic analysis of anterior cruciate ligament deficient subjects. Gait Posture 4, 83–88.

Bennett, J.G., Stauber, W.T., 1986. Evaluation and treatment of anterior knee pain using eccentric exercise. Med. Sci. Sports Exerc. 18 (5), 526–530.

Berberich, P., Hoheisel, U., Mense, S., 1988. Effects of a carrageenan-induced myositis on the discharge properties of group III and IV muscle receptors in the cat. J. Neurophysiol. 59 (5), 1395–1409.

Berchuck, M., Andriacchi, T.P., Bach, B.R., et al., 1990. Gait adaptations by patients who have a deficient anterior cruciate ligament. J. Bone Joint Surg. 72A (6), 871–877.

Berg, H.E., Larsson, L., Tesch, P.A., 1997. Lower limb skeletal muscle function after 6 wk of bed rest. J. Appl. Physiol. 82, 182–188.

Bergmark, A., 1989. Stability of the lumbar spine. A study of mechanical engineering. Acta Orthop. Scand. 60 (Suppl. 230), 3–54.

Bodine, S.C., Roy, R.R., Meadows, D.A., et al., 1982. Architectural, histochemical, and contractile characteristics of a unique biarticular muscle: the cat semitendinosus. J. Neurophysiol. 48 (1), 192–201.

Bogduk, N., 1997. Clinical anatomy of the lumbar spine and sacrum, third ed. Churchill Livingstone, New York.

Bogduk, N., MacIntosh, J.E., 1984. The applied anatomy of the thoracolumbar fascia. Spine 9 (2), 164–170.

Borg, G.A.V., 1982. Psychophysical bases of perceived exertion. Med. Sci. Sports Exerc. 14 (5), 377–381.

Bors, E., 1926. Uber das Zahlenverhaltnis zwischen Nerven und Muskelfasern. Anat. Anz. 60, 415–420.

Bouisset, S., Zattara, M., 1981. A sequence of postural movements precedes voluntary movement. Neurosci. Lett. 22, 263–270.

Boyd, I.A., 1976. The mechanical properties of dynamic nuclear bag fibres, static nuclear bag fibres and nuclear chain fibres in isolated cat muscle spindles. Prog. Brain Res. 44, 33–50.

Branch, T.P., Hunter, R., Donath, M., 1989. Dynamic EMG analysis of anterior cruciate deficient legs with and without bracing during cutting. Am. J. Sports Med. 17 (1), 35–41.

Bredella, M.A., Tirman, P.F.J., Fritz, R.C., et al., 1999. MR imaging findings of lateral ulnar collateral ligament abnormalities in patients with lateral epicondylitis. Am. J. Roentgenol. 173, 1379–1382.

Brooke, M.H., Engel, W.K., 1969. The histographic analysis of human muscle biopsies with regard to fibre types. 1. Adult male and female. Neurology 19, 221–233.

Brooks, G.A., Fahey, T.D., 1987. Fundamentals of human performance. Macmillan, New York.

Brown, M.C., Hardman, V.J., 1987. Plasticity of vertebrate motoneurones. In: Winlow, W., McCrohan, C.R. (Eds.), Growth and plasticity of neural connections. Manchester University Press, Manchester, pp. 36–51.

Buller, A.J., Eccles, J.C., Eccles, R.M., 1960. Interactions between motoneurones and muscles in respect of the characteristic speeds of their responses. J. Physiol. 150, 417–439.

Burkholder, T.J., Fingado, B., Baron, S., et al., 1994. Relationship between muscle fiber types and sizes and muscle architectural properties in the mouse hindlimb. J. Morphol. 221, 177–190.

Butler, D.S., 2000. The sensitive nervous system. Noigroup, Adelaide.

Carr, A.J., Norris, S.H., 1989. The blood supply of the calcaneal tendon. J. Bone Joint Surg. 71B (1), 100–101.

Chansky, H.A., Iannottti, J.P., 1991. The vascularity of the rotator cuff. Clin. Sports Med. 10 (4), 807–822.

Ciccotti, M.G., Kerlan, R.K., Perry, J., et al., 1994. An electromyographic analysis of the knee during functional activities. II. The anterior cruciate ligament-deficient and -reconstructed profiles. Am. J. Sports Med. 22 (5), 651–658.

Clark, F.J., Horch, K.W., Bach, S.M., et al., 1979. Contributions of cutaneous and joint receptors to static knee-position sense in man. J. Neurophysiol. 42 (3), 877–888.

Clement, D.B., Taunton, J.E., Smart, G.W., 1984. Achilles tendonitis and peritendinitis: etiology and treatment. Am. J. Sports Med. 12 (3), 179–184.

Comerford, M.J., Mottram, S.L., 2001a. Functional stability re-training: principles and strategies for managing mechanical dysfunction. Man. Ther. 6 (1), 3–14.

Comerford, M.J., Mottram, S.L., 2001b. Movement and stability dysfunction – contemporary developments. Man. Ther. 6 (1), 15–26.

Coombs, R.R.H., Klenerman, L., Narcisi, P., et al., 1980. Collagen typing in Achilles tendon rupture. J. Bone Joint Surg. 62B (2), 258.

Cooper, S., Daniel, P.M., 1963. Muscles spindles in man; their morphology in the lumbricals and the deep muscles of the neck. Brain 86, 563–592.

Cooper, R.R., Misol, S., 1970. Tendon and ligament insertion: a light and electron microscopic study. J. Bone Joint Surg. 52A (1), 1–20.

Cordo, P.J., Nashner, L.M., 1982. Properties of postural adjustments associated with rapid arm movements. J. Neurophysiol. 47 (2), 287–302.

Corser, T., 1974. Temporal discrepancies in the electromyographic study of rapid movement. Ergonomics 17 (3), 389–400.

Cowan, S.M., Bennell, K.L., Crossley, K.M., et al., 2002. Physical therapy alters recruitment of the vasti in patellofemoral pain syndrome. Med. Sci. Sports Exerc. 34 (12), 1879–1885.

Cresswell, A.G., 1993. Responses of intra-abdominal pressure and abdominal muscle activity during dynamic trunk loading in man. Eur. J. Appl. Physiol. Occup. Physiol. 66, 315–320.

Cresswell, A.G., Thorstensson, A., 1994. Changes in intra-abdominal pressure, trunk muscle activation and force during isokinetic lifting and lowering. Eur. J. Appl. Physiol. Occup. Physiol. 68, 315–321.

Cresswell, A.G., Grundstrom, H., Thorstensson, A., 1992. Observations on intra-abdominal pressure and patterns of abdominal intra-muscular activity in man. Acta Physiol. Scand. 144, 409–418.

Crow, J.L., Haas, B.M., 2001. The neural control of human movement. In: Trew, M., Everett, T. (Eds.), Human movement, an introductory text, fourth ed. Churchill Livingstone, Edinburgh, p. 69.

David, G., Magarey, M.E., Jones, M.A., et al., 2000. EMG and strength correlates of selected shoulder muscles during rotations of the glenohumeral joint. Clin. Biomech. 15, 95–102.

deAndrade, J.R., Grant, C., Dixon St., A.J., 1965. Joint distension and reflex muscle inhibition in the knee. J. Bone Joint Surg. 47A (2), 313–322.

Descartes, R., 1985. Discourse on method and the meditations. Penguin, Middlesex, pp. 150–169, 6th meditation.

DeVita, P., Hortobagyi, T., Barrier, J., et al., 1997. Gait adaptations before and after anterior cruciate ligament reconstruction surgery. Med. Sci. Sports Exerc. 29 (7), 853–859.

De Vries, H.A., Housh, T.J., 1994. Physiology of exercise for physical education, athletics and sports science, fifth ed. Brown & Benchmark, Madison, Wisconsin.

Diehl, B., Hoheisel, U., Mense, S., 1988. Histological and neurophysiological changes induced by carrageenan in skeletal muscle of cat and rat. Agents Actions 25 (3/4), 210–213.

Edgerton, V.R., Zhou, M.-Y., Ohira, Y., et al., 1995. Human fiber size and enzymatic properties after 5 and 11 days of spaceflight. J. Appl. Physiol. 78, 1733–1739.

Eisenberg, B.R., Milton, R.L., 1984. Muscle fiber termination at the tendon in the frog's sartorius: a stereological study. Am. J. Anat. 171, 273–284.

Elftman, H., 1966. Biomechanics of muscle. J. Bone Joint Surg. 48A (2), 363–377.

Elliott, D.H., 1965. Structure and function of mammalian tendon. Biol. Rev. 40, 392–421.

Fahrer, H., Rentsch, H.U., Gerber, N.J., et al., 1988. Knee effusion and reflex inhibition of the quadriceps – a bar to effective retraining. J. Bone Joint Surg. 70B (4), 635–638.

Feinstein, B., Langton, J.N.K., Jameson, R.M., et al., 1954. Experiments on pain referred from deep somatic tissues. J. Bone Joint Surg. 36A (5), 981–997.

Ferrell, W.R., 1985. The response of slowly adapting mechanoreceptors in the cat knee joint to tetanic contraction of hind limb muscles. Q. J. Exp. Physiol. 70, 337–345.

Fitts, R.H., Riley, D.R., Widrick, J.J., 2000. Microgravity and skeletal muscle. J. Appl. Physiol. 89, 823–839.

Fitts, R.H., Riley, D.R., Widrick, J.J., 2001. Functional and structural adaptations of skeletal muscle to microgravity. J. Exp. Biol. 204, 3201–3208.

Foreman, R.D., Schmidt, R.F., Willis, W.D., 1979. Effects of mechanical and chemical stimulation of fine muscle afferents upon primate spinothalamic tract cells. J. Physiol. (Lond.) 286, 215–231.

Frank, C.B., Loitz, B., Bray, R., et al., 1994. Abnormality of the contralateral ligament after injuries of the medial collateral ligament – an experimental study in rabbits. J. Bone Joint Surg. 76A (3), 403–412.

Franz, M., Mense, S., 1975. Muscle receptors with group IV afferent fibres responding to application of bradykinin. Brain Res. 92, 369–383.

Freeman, M.A.R., Wyke, B., 1967. Articular reflexes at the ankle joint: an electromyographic study of normal and abnormal influences of ankle joint mechanoreceptors upon reflex activity in the leg muscles. Br. J. Surg. 54 (12), 990–1001.

Frey, C., Shereff, M., Greenidge, N., 1990. Vascularity of the posterior tibial tendon. J. Bone Joint Surg. 72A (6), 884–888.

Friden, J., Sjostrom, M., Ekblom, B., 1983. Myofibrillar damage following intense eccentric exercise in man. Int. J. Sports Med. 4, 170–176.

Friedli, W.G., Hallett, M., Simon, S.R., 1984. Postural adjustments associated with rapid voluntary arm movements. 1. Electromyographic data. J. Neurol. Neurosurg. Psychiatry 47, 611–622.

Fukunaga, T., Ichinose, Y., Ito, M., et al., 1997. Determination of fascicle length and pennation in a contracting human muscle in vivo. J. Appl. Physiol. 82 (1), 354–358.

Fung, Y.C., 1993. Biomechanics, biomechanical properties of living tissues, second ed. Springer-Verlag, New York.

Gajdosik, R.L., Linden, D.W.V., Williams, A.K., 1996. Influence of age on concentric isokinetic torque and passive extensibility variables of the calf muscles of women. Eur. J. Appl. Physiol. 74, 279–286.

Gandevia, S.C., McClosky, D.I., 1976. Joint sense, muscle sense, and their combination as position sense, measured at the distal interphalangeal joint of the middle finger. J. Physiol. (Lond.) 260, 387–407.

Gandevia, S.C., Hall, L.A., McCloskey, D.I., et al., 1983. Proprioceptive sensation at the terminal joint of the middle finger. J. Physiol. (Lond.) 335, 507–517.

Gandevia, S.C., Herbert, R.D., Leeper, J.B., 1998. Voluntary activation of human elbow flexor muscles during maximal concentric contractions. J. Physiol. 512 (2), 595–602.

Garell, P.C., McGillis, S.L.B., Greenspan, J.D., 1996. Mechanical response properties of nociceptors innervating feline hairy skin. J. Neurophysiol. 75 (3), 1177–1189.

Garfin, S.R., Tipton, C.M., Mubarak, S.J., et al., 1981. Role of fascia in maintenance of muscle tension and pressure. J. Appl. Physiol. 51 (2), 317–320.

Garrett, W.E., 1990. Muscle strain injuries: clinical and basic aspects. Med. Sci. Sports Exerc. 22 (4), 436–443.

Garrett, W.E., Rich, F.R., Nikolaou, P.K., et al., 1989. Computed tomography of hamstring muscle strains. Med. Sci. Sports Exerc. 21 (5), 506–514.

Ghez, C., 1991. Muscles: effectors of the motor systems. In: Kandel, E.R., Schwartz, J.H., Jessell, T.M. (Eds.), Principles of neural science. third ed. Elsevier, New York, pp. 548–563.

Gifford, L., 1998. Pain. In: Pitt-Brooke, J., Reid, H., Lockwood, J., Kerr, K. (Eds.), Rehabilitation of movement, theoretical basis of clinical practice. W B Saunders, London, pp. 196–232.

Glousman, R., Jobe, F., Tibone, J., et al., 1988. Dynamic electromyographic analysis of the throwing shoulder with glenohumeral instability. J. Bone Joint Surg. 70A (2), 220–226.

Glousman, R.E., Barron, J., Jobe, F.W., et al., 1992. An electromyographic analysis of the elbow in normal and injured pitchers with medial collateral ligament insufficiency. Am. J. Sports Med. 20 (3), 311–317.

Goldspink, G., 1976. The adaptation of muscle to a new functional length. In: Anderson, D.J., Matthews, B. (Eds.), Mastication. Wright, Bristol, pp. 90–99.

Goldspink, G., Williams, P.E., 1979. The nature of the increased passive resistance in muscle following immobilization of the mouse soleus muscle. J. Physiol. 289, 55P (Proceedings of the Physiological Society December 15/16th 1978).

Gombrich, E., Biancheri, B., Thomas, D., et al., 1989. Leonardo da Vinci. South Bank Centre, London.

Goodwin, G.M., McCloskey, D.I., Matthews, P.B.C., 1972. The contribution of muscle afferents to kinaesthesia shown by vibration induced illusions of movement and by

the effects of paralysing joint afferents. Brain 95, 705–748.

Granata, K.P., Marras, W.S., 1995. The influence of trunk muscle coactivity on dynamic spinal loads. Spine 20 (8), 913–919.

Granit, R., Phillips, C.G., Skoglund, S., et al., 1957. Differentiation of tonic from phasic alpha ventral horn cells by stretch, pinna and crossed extensor reflexes. J. Neurophysiol. 20 (5), 470–481.

Greenleaf, J.E., Bulbulian, R., Bernauer, E.M., et al., 1989. Exercise-training protocols for astronauts in microgravity. J. Appl. Physiol. 67, 2191–2204.

Grigg, P., 1994. Peripheral neural mechanisms in proprioception. J. Sport Rehabil. 3, 2–17.

Grimby, G., 1995. Muscle performance and structure in the elderly as studied cross-sectionally and longitudinally. J. Gerontol. 50A, 17–22 (special issue).

Gydikov, A.A., 1976. Pattern of discharge of different types of alpha motoneurones and motor units during voluntary and reflex activities under normal physiological conditions. In: Komi, P.V. (Ed.), Biomechanics V-A. University Park, Baltimore, p. 45–57.

Haggmark, T., Jansson, E., Eriksson, E., 1981. Fibre type area and metabolic potential of the thigh muscle in man after knee surgery and immobilization. Int. J. Sports Med. 2, 12–17.

Hales, J.P., Gandevia, S.C., 1988. Assessment of maximal voluntary contraction with twitch interpolation: an instrument to measure twitch responses. J. Neurosci. Methods 25, 97–102.

Harpuder, K., Stein, I.D., 1943. Studies on the nature of pain arising from an ischaemic limb. II. Biochemical studies. Am. Heart J. 25 (4), 438–448.

Hasan, Z., Houk, J.C., 1975. Transition in sensitivity of spindle receptors that occurs when muscle is stretched more than a fraction of a millimeter. J. Neurophysiol. 38, 673–689.

Henneman, E., Olson, C.B., 1965. Relations between structure and function in the design of skeletal muscles. J. Neurophysiol. 28, 581–598.

Henneman, E., Somjen, G., Carpenter, D.O., 1965. Functional significance of cell size in spinal motoneurons. J. Neurophysiol. 28, 560–580.

Herzog, W., 1999. Muscle. In: Nigg, B.M., Herzog, W. (Eds.), Biomechanics of the musculo-skeletal system. second ed. John Wiley, Chichester, pp. 148–188.

Herzog, W., Gal, J., 1999. Tendon. In: Nigg, B.M., Herzog, W. (Eds.), Biomechanics of the musculo-skeletal system. second ed. John Wiley, Chichester, pp. 127–147.

Hess, G.P., Cappiello, W.L., Poole, R.M., et al., 1989. Prevention and treatment of overuse tendon injuries. Sports Med. 8 (6), 371–384.

Heyley, M.V., Rees, J., Newham, D.J., 1998. Quadriceps function, proprioceptive acuity and functional performance in healthy young, middle-aged and elderly subjects. Age Ageing 27 (1), 55–62.

Hides, J., Richardson, C., Jull, G., et al., 1995. Ultrasound imaging in rehabilitation. Aust. J. Physiother. 41 (3), 187–193.

Hill, A.V., 1938. The heat of shortening and the dynamic constants of muscle. Proc. R. Soc. Lond. (Biol.) 126, 136–195.

Hirsch, C., 1974. Tensile properties during tendon healing. A comparative study of intact and sutured rabbit peroneus brevis tendons. Acta Orthop. Scand. 153 (Suppl.), 11.

Hodges, P.W., Richardson, C.A., 1996. Inefficient muscular stabilization of the lumbar spine associated with low back pain. A motor control evaluation of transversus abdominis. Spine 21 (22), 2640–2650.

Hodges, P.W., Richardson, C.A., 1997a. Contraction of the abdominal muscles associated with movements of the lower limb. Phys. Ther. 77 (2), 132–144.

Hodges, P.W., Richardson, C.A., 1997b. Feedforward contraction of transversus abdominis is not influenced by the direction of arm movement. Exp. Brain Res. 114, 362–370.

Hodges, P.W., Richardson, C.A., 1997c. Relationship between limb movement speed and associated contraction of the trunk muscles. Ergonomics 40 (11), 1220–1230.

Horak, F.B., Esselman, P., Anderson, M.E., et al., 1984. The effects of movement velocity, mass displaced, and task certainty on associated postural adjustments made by normal and hemiplegic individuals. J. Neurol. Neurosurg. Psychiatry 47, 1020–1028.

Horowits, R., Maruyama, K., Podolsky, R.J., 1989. Elastic behavior of connectin filaments during thick filament movement in activated skeletal muscle. J. Cell Biol. 109, 2169–2176.

Hortobagyi, T., DeVita, P., 2000. Muscle pre- and coactivity during downward stepping are associated with leg stiffness in aging. J. Electromyogr. Kinesiol. 10, 117–126.

Hortobagyi, T., Zheng, D., Weidner, M., et al., 1995. The influence of aging on muscle strength and muscle fiber characteristics with special reference to eccentric strength. J. Gerontol. 50A (6), B399–B406.

Hortobagyi, T., Dempsey, L., Fraser, D., et al., 2000. Changes in muscle strength, muscle fibre size and myofibrillar gene expression after immobilization and retraining in humans. J. Physiol. 524 (1), 293–304.

Houk, J., Henneman, E., 1967. Responses of Golgi tendon organs to active contractions of the soleus muscle of the cat. J. Neurophysiol. 30, 466–481.

Houk, J.C., Singer, J.J., Henneman, E., 1971. Adequate stimulus for tendon organs with observations on mechanics of ankle joint. J. Neurophysiol. 34, 1051–1065.

Hughes, V.A., Frontera, W.R., Wood, M., et al., 2001. Longitudinal muscle strength changes in older adults: influence of muscle mass, physical activity, and health. J. Gerontol. 56A (5), B209–B217.

Hughston, J.C., Walsh, W.M., Puddu, G., 1984. Patellar subluxation and dislocation, vol. 5. W B Saunders, Philadelphia.

Hukins, D.W.L., Aspden, R.M., Hickey, D.S., 1990. Thoracolumbar fascia can increase the efficiency of the erector spinae muscles. Clin. Biomech. 5, 30–34.

Hunt, C.C., 1990. Mammalian muscle spindle: peripheral mechanisms. Physiol. Rev. 70 (3), 643–663.

Hurley, M.V., Newham, D.J., 1993. The influence of arthrogenous muscle inhibition on quadriceps rehabilitation of patients with early, unilateral osteoarthritic knees. Br. J. Rheumatol. 32, 127–131.

Hurley, M.V., O'Flanagan, S.J., Newham, D.J., 1991. Isokinetic and isometric muscle strength and inhibition after elbow arthroplasty. J. Orthop. Rheumatol. 4, 83–95.

Hurley, M.V., Jones, D.W., Wilson, D., et al., 1992. Rehabilitation of quadriceps inhibited due to isolated rupture of the anterior cruciate ligament. J. Orthop. Rheumatol. 5, 145–154.

Hurley, M.V., Jones, D.W., Newham, D.J., 1994. Arthrogenic quadriceps inhibition and rehabilitation of patients with extensive traumatic knee injuries. Clin. Sci. 86, 305–310.

Huxley, A.F., 2000. Cross-bridge action: present views, prospects, and unknowns. In: Herzog, W. (Ed.), Skeletal muscle mechanics: from mechanisms to function. John Wiley, Chichester, pp. 7–31.

Iggo, A., 1961. Non-myelinated afferent fibres from mammalian skeletal muscle. J. Physiol. 155, 52P–53P.

Iles, J.F., Stokes, M., Young, A., 1990. Reflex actions of knee joint afferents during contraction of the human quadriceps. Clin. Physiol. 10, 489–500.

Indahl, A., Kaigle, A., Reikeras, O., et al., 1995. Electromyographic response of the porcine multifidus musculature after nerve stimulation. Spine 20 (24), 2652–2658.

Indahl, A., Kaigle, A., Reikeras, O., et al., 1997. Interaction between the porcine lumbar intervertebral disc, zygapophysial joints, and paraspinal muscles. Spine 22 (24), 2834–2840.

Ingelmark, B.O.E., 1948. The structure of tendons at various ages and under different functional conditions. II. An electron-microscopic investigation of Achilles tendons from white rats. Acta Anat. (Basel) 6 (3), 193–225.

Inman, V.T., Saunders DeC, J.B.M., 1944. Referred pain from skeletal structures. J. Nerv. Ment. Dis. 99, 660–667.

Jami, L., 1992. Golgi tendon organs in mammalian skeletal muscle: functional properties and central actions. Physiol. Rev. 72 (3), 623–666.

Janda, V., 1985. Pain in the locomotor system – a broad approach. In:

Glasgow, E.F., Twomey, L.T., Scull, E.R., et al. (Eds.), Aspects of manipulative therapy. Churchill Livingstone, Melbourne, pp. 148–151.

Johns, R.J., Wright, V., 1962. Relative importance of various tissues in joint stiffness. J. Appl. Physiol. 17 (5), 824–828.

Johnson, M.A., Polgar, J., Weightman, D., et al., 1973. Data on the distribution of fibre types in thirty-six human muscles: an autopsy study. J. Neurol. Sci. 18, 111–129.

Jones, D.A., Newham, D.J., Round, J.M., et al., 1986. Experimental human muscle damage: morphological changes in relation to other indices of damage. J. Physiol. 375, 435–448.

Jones, D.W., Jones, D.A., Newham, D.J., 1987. Chronic knee effusion and aspiration: the effect on quadriceps inhibition. Br. J. Rheumatol. 26, 370–374.

Jozsa, L., Kannus, P., 1997. Human tendons: anatomy, physiology and pathology. Human Kinetics, Champaign, Illinois.

Jozsa, L., Kvist, M., Kannus, P., et al., 1988. The effect of tenotomy and immobilization on muscle spindles and tendon organs of the rat calf muscles. Acta Neuropathol. (Berl.) 76, 465–470.

Jozsa, L., Lehto, M., Kvist, M., et al., 1989a. Alterations in dry mass content of collagen fibers in degenerative tendinopathy and tendon-rupture. Matrix 9, 140–146.

Jozsa, L., Kvist, M., Balint, B.J., et al., 1989b. The role of recreational sport activity in Achilles tendon rupture, a clinical, pathoanatomical, and sociological study of 292 cases. Am. J. Sports Med. 17 (3), 338–343.

Jozsa, L., Kannus, P., Balint, J.B., et al., 1991. Three-dimensional ultrastructure of human tendons. Acta Anat. (Basel) 142, 306–312.

Jozsa, K., Kannus, P., Jarvinen, M., et al., 1992. Denervation and immobilization induced changes in the myotendinous junction. Eur. J. Exp. Musculoskeletal Res. 1, 105–112.

Kalund, S., Sinkjaer, T., Arendt-Nielsen, L., et al., 1990. Altered timing of hamstring muscle action in anterior cruciate ligament deficient patients. Am. J. Sports Med. 18 (3), 245–248.

Kannus, P., Jozsa, L., 1991. Histopathological changes preceding spontaneous rupture of a tendon. J. Bone Joint Surg. 73A (10), 1507–1525.

Kannus, P., Jozsa, L., Kvist, M., et al., 1992. The effect of immobilization on myotendinous junction: an ultrastructural, histochemical and immunohistochemical study. Acta Physiol. Scand. 144, 387–394.

Kao, F.F., 1963. An experimental study of the pathways involved in exercise hyperpnoea employing cross-circulation techniques. In: Cunningham, D.J.C., Lloyd, B.B. (Eds.), The regulation of human respiration. Blackwell, Oxford, pp. 461–502.

Karpakka, J., Vaananen, K., Virtanen, P., et al., 1990. The effects of remobilization and exercise on collagen biosynthesis in rat tendon. Acta Physiol. Scand. 139, 139–145.

Katz, B., 1939. The relation between force and speed in muscular contraction. J. Physiol. 96, 45–64.

Kaufman, M.P., Iwamoto, G.A., Longhurst, J.C., et al., 1982. Effects of capsaicin and bradykinin on afferent fibers with endings in skeletal muscle. Circ. Res. 50, 133–139.

Kaufman, M.P., Longhurst, J.C., Rybicki, K.J., et al., 1983. Effects of static muscular contraction on impulse activity of groups III and IV afferents in cats. J. Appl. Physiol. 55, 105–112.

Kaufman, M.P., Waldrop, T.G., Rybicki, K.J., et al., 1984a. Effects of static and rhythmic twitch contractions on the discharge of group III and IV muscle afferents. Cardiovasc. Res. 18, 663–668.

Kaufman, M.P., Rybicki, K.J., Waldrop, T.G., et al., 1984b. Effect of ischaemia on responses of group III and IV afferents to contraction. J. Appl. Physiol. 57, 644–650.

Kawakami, Y., Ichinose, Y., Fukunaga, T., 1998. Architectural and functional features of human triceps surae muscles during contraction. J. Appl. Physiol. 85 (2), 398–404.

Keating, J.F., Crossan, J.F., 1992. Evaluation of rotator cuff function following anterior dislocation of the shoulder. J. Orthop. Rheumatol. 5, 135–140.

Kellgren, J.H., 1938. Observations on referred pain arising from muscle. Clin. Sci. 3, 175–190.

Kellgren, J.H., 1939. On the distribution of pain arising from deep somatic structures with charts of segmental pain areas. Clin. Sci. 4, 35–46.

Kennedy, J.C., Alexander, I.J., Hayes, K.C., 1982. Nerve supply of the human knee and its functional importance. Am. J. Sports Med. 10 (6), 329–335.

Kent-Braun, J.A., Le Blanc, R., 1996. Quantification of central activation failure during maximal voluntary contractions in humans. Muscle and Nerve 19, 861–869.

Kerr, K., 1998. Exercise in rehabilitation. In: Pitt-Brooke, J., Reid, H., Lockwood, J. et al., (Eds.), Rehabilitation of movement, theoretical basis of clinical practice. W B Saunders, London, pp. 423–457.

Kidd, G., Lawes, N., Musa, I., 1992. Understanding neuromuscular plasticity a basis for clinical rehabilitation. Edward Arnold, London.

Kieschke, J., Mense, S., Prabhakar, N.R., 1988. Influence of adrenaline and hypoxia on rat muscle receptors in vitro. In: Hamann, W., Iggo, A. (Eds.), Progress in brain research, vol. 74. Elsevier, Amsterdam, pp. 91–97.

Knatt, T., Guanche, C., Solomonow, M., et al., 1995. The glenohumeral-biceps reflex in the feline. Clin. Orthop. Relat. Res. 314, 247–252.

Kniffki, K.-D., Mense, S., Schmidt, R.F., 1978. Responses of group IV afferent units from skeletal muscle to stretch, contraction and chemical stimulation. Exp. Brain Res. 31, 511–522.

Kojima, T., 1991. Force–velocity relationship of human elbow flexors in voluntary isotonic contraction under heavy loads. Int. J. Sports Med. 12, 208–213.

Krebs, D.E., Staples, W.H., Cuttita, D., et al., 1983. Knee joint angle: its relationship to quadriceps femoris activity in normal and postarthrotomy limbs. Arch. Phys. Med. Rehabil. 64, 441–447.

Kumazawa, T., Mizumura, K., 1977. Thin-fibre receptors responding to mechanical, chemical, and thermal stimulation in the skeletal muscle of the dog. J. Physiol. 273, 179–194.

Kvist, H., Kvist, M., 1980. The operative treatment of chronic calcaneal paratenonitis. J. Bone Joint Surg. 62B (3), 353–357.

Kvist, M., Jozsa, L., Kannus, P., et al., 1991. Morphology and histochemistry of the myotendineal junction of the rat calf muscles. Histochemical, immunohistochemical and electron-microscopic study. Acta Anat. (Basel) 141, 199–205.

Kvist, M., Hurme, T., Kannus, P., et al., 1995. Vascular density at the myotendinous junction of the rat gastrocnemius muscle after immobilization and remobilization. Am. J. Sports Med. 23 (3), 359–364.

Labarque, V.L., Eijnde Op't, B., Van Leemputte, M., 2002. Effect of immobilization and retraining on torque–velocity relationship of human knee flexor and extensor muscles. Eur. J. Appl. Physiol. 86, 251–257.

Larsson, L., Grimby, G., Karlsson, J., 1979. Muscle strength and speed of movement in relation to age and muscle morphology. J. Appl. Physiol. 46 (3), 451–456.

Laughlin, M.H., Korthuis, R.J., 1987. Control of muscle blood flow during sustained physiological exercise. Can. J. Sport Sci. 12 (Suppl.), 77S–83S.

Levick, J.R., 1983. Joint pressure–volume studies: their importance, design and interpretation. J. Rheumatol. 10, 353–357.

Levine, J.D., Dardick, S.J., Basbaum, A.I., et al., 1985a. Reflex neurogenic inflammation. 1. Contribution of the peripheral nervous system to spatially remote inflammatory responses following injury. J. Neurosci. 5 (5), 1380–1386.

Levine, J.D., Moskowitz, M.A., Basbaum, A.I., 1985b. The contribution of neurogenic inflammation in experimental arthritis. J. Immunol. 135 (2), 843s–847s.

Lieb, F.J., Perry, J., 1968. Quadriceps function. An anatomical and mechanical study using amputated limbs. J. Bone Joint Surg. 50A (8), 1535–1548.

Lockwood, J., 1998. Musculoskeletal requirements for normal movement. In: Pitt-Brooke, J., Reid, H., Lockwood, J. et al., (Eds.), Rehabilitation of movement, theoretical basis of clinical practice. W B Saunders, London, p. 107.

Lohr, J.F., Uhthoff, H.K., 1990. The microvascular pattern of the supraspinatus tendon. Clin. Orthop. Relat. Res. 254, 35–38.

Lomo, T., Westgaard, R.H., Engebretsen, L., 1980. Different stimulation patterns affect contractile properties of denervated rat soleus muscles. In: Pette, D. (Ed.), Plasticity of muscle. Walter de Gruyter, Berlin.

Louie, J.K., Mote, C.D., 1987. Contribution of the musculature to rotatory laxity and torsional stiffness at the knee. J. Biomech. 20 (3), 281–300.

Louie, J.K., Kuo, C.Y., Gutierrez, M.D., et al., 1984. Surface EMG and torsion measurements during snow skiing: laboratory and field tests. J. Biomech. 17 (10), 713–724.

Lundborg, G., 1976. Experimental flexor tendon healing without adhesion formation – a new concept of tendon nutrition and intrinsic healing mechanisms. Hand 8 (3), 235–238.

MacDougall, J.D., 1986. Morphological changes in human skeletal muscle following strength training and immobilization. In: Jones, N.L., McCartney, N., McComas, A.J. (Eds.), Human muscle power. Human Kinetics, Champaign, Illinois, pp. 269–288.

MacDougall, J.D., Elder, G.C.B., Sale, D.G., et al., 1980. Effects of strength training and immobilisation on human muscle fibres. Eur. J. Appl. Physiol. Occup. Physiol. 43, 25–34.

Macefield, G., Gandevia, S.C., Burke, D., 1990. Perceptual responses to microstimulation of single afferents innervating joints, muscles and skin of the human hand. J. Physiol. (Lond.) 429, 113–129.

Maganaris, C.N., Baltzopoulos, V., Sargeant, A.J., 1998. In vivo measurements of the triceps surae complex architecture in man: implications for muscle function. J. Physiol. 512 (2), 603–614.

Maier, A., Crockett, J.L., Simpson, D.R., et al., 1976. Properties of immobilized guinea pig hindlimb muscles. Am. J. Physiol. 231 (5), 1520–1526.

Matthews, P., 1976. The fate of isolated segments of flexor tendons within the digital sheath – a study in synovial nutrition. Br. J. Plast. Surg. 29, 216–224.

Matthews, P.B.C., Simmonds, A., 1974. Sensations of finger movement elicited by pulling upon flexor tendons in man. J. Physiol. (Lond.) 239, 27P–28P.

Matre, D.A., Sinkjaer, T., Svensson, P., et al., 1998. Experimental muscle pain increases the human stretch reflex. Pain 75, 331–339.

Matre, D.A., Sinkjaer, T., Knardahl, S., et al., 1999. The influence of experimental muscle pain on the human soleus stretch reflex during sitting and walking. Clin. Neurophysiol. 110, 2033–2043.

McArdle, W.D., Katch, F.I., Katch, V.L., 2000. Essentials of exercise physiology, second ed. Lippincott Williams & Wilkins, Philadelphia.

McBryde, A.M., Anderson, R.B., 1988. Sesamoid foot problems in the athlete. Clin. Sports Med. 7 (1), 51–60.

McCloskey, D.I., Mitchell, J.H., 1972. Reflex cardiovascular and respiratory responses originating in exercising muscle. J. Physiol. 224, 173–186.

McCloskey, D.I., Macefield, G., Gandevia, S.C., et al., 1987. Sensing position and movements of the fingers. News Physiol. Sci. 2, 226–230.

McComas, A.J., 1996. Skeletal muscle: form and function. Human Kinetics, Champaign, Illinois.

McGill, S.M., Norman, R.W., 1986. Partitioning of the L4–L5 dynamic moment into disc, ligamentous, and muscular components during lifting. Spine 11 (7), 666–678.

McGuire, D.B., 1995. The multiple dimensions of cancer pain: a framework for assessment and management. In: McGuire, D.B., Yarbro, C.H., Ferrell, B.R. (Eds.), Cancer pain management. second ed. Jones and Bartlett, Boston, pp. 1–17.

McNair, P.J., Marshall, R.N., Maguire, K., 1994. Knee effusion and quadriceps muscle strength. Clin. Biomech. 9 (6), 331–334.

Mense, S., 1981. Sensitization of group IV muscle receptors to bradykinin by 5-hyroxytryptamine and prostaglandin E$_2$. Brain Res. 225, 95–105.

Mense, S., 1996. Group III and IV receptors in skeletal muscle: are they specific or polymodal? In: Kumazawa, T., Kruger, L., Mizumura, K. (Eds.), Progress in brain research Elsevier Science Amsterdam 113, pp. 83–100.

Mense, S., Meyer, H., 1985. Different types of slowly conducting afferent

units in cat skeletal muscle and tendon. J. Physiol. 363, 403–417.

Mense, S., Stahnke, M., 1983. Responses in muscle afferent fibres of slow conduction velocity to contractions and ischaemia in the cat. J. Physiol. 342, 383–397.

Milner-Brown, H.S., Stein, R.B., Yemm, R., 1973. The orderly recruitment of human motor units during voluntary isometric contractions. J. Physiol. (Lond.) 230, 359–370.

Mitchell, F.L., 1993. Elements of muscle energy technique. In: Basmajian, J.V., Nyberg, R. (Eds.), Rational manual therapies. Williams & Wilkins, Baltimore, p. 297.

Moberg, E., 1983. The role of cutaneous afferents in position sense, kinaesthesia, and motor function of the hand. Brain 106, 1–19.

Mooney, V., Robertson, J., 1976. The facet syndrome. Clin. Orthop. Relat. Res. 115, 149–156.

Moore, R.M., Moore, R.E., Singleton, A.O., 1934. Experiments on the chemical stimulation of pain-endings associated with small blood-vessels. Am. J. Physiol. 107, 594–602.

Muller, E.A., 1970. Influence of training and of inactivity on muscle strength. Arch. Phys. Med. Rehabil. 51, 449–462.

Myers, T.W., 2001. Anatomy trains: myofascial meridians for manual and movement therapists. Churchill Livingstone, Edinburgh.

Nakagawa, Y., Totsuka, M., Sato, T., et al., 1989. Effect of disuse on the ultrastructure of the achilles tendon in rats. Eur. J. Appl. Physiol. 59, 239–242.

Nakahara, M., 1971. The effect of a tourniquet on the kinin–kininogen system in blood and muscle. Thromb. Diath. Haemorrh. 26, 264–274.

Newham, D.J., 1993. Eccentric muscle activity in theory and practice. In: Harms-Ringdahl, K. (Ed.), Muscle strength. Churchill Livingstone, Edinburgh, p. 63.

Newham, D.J., 2001. Strength, power and endurance. In: Trew, M., Everett, T. (Eds.), Human movement, fourth ed. Churchill Livingstone, Edinburgh, pp. 105–128.

Newham, D.J., Ainscough-Potts, A.-M., 2001. Musculoskeletal basis for movement. In: Trew, M., Everett, T.

(Eds.), Human movement, fourth ed. Churchill Livingstone, Edinburgh, pp. 105–128.

Newham, D.J., Hurley, M.V., Jones, D.W., 1989. Ligamentous knee injuries and muscle inhibition. J. Orthop. Rheumatol. 2, 163–173.

Newman, P.H., 1968. The spine, the wood and the trees. Proc. R. Soc. Med. 61, 35–41.

Nicholls, S.P., Gathercole, L.J., Keller, A., et al., 1983. Crimping in rat tail tendon collagen: morphology and transverse mechanical anisotrophy. Int. J. Biol. Macromol. 5, 283–288.

Nikolaou, P.K., MacDonald, B.L., Glisson, R.R., et al., 1987. Biomechanical and histological evaluation of muscle after controlled strain injury. Am. J. Sports Med. 15 (1), 9–14.

Nordin, M., Frankel, V.H., 1989. Basic biomechanics of the musculoskeletal system, second ed. Lea & Febiger, Philadelphia.

Norkin, C.C., Levangie, P.K., 1992. Joint structure and function, a comprehensive analysis, second ed. F A Davis, Philadelphia, pp. 101, 115.

Norman, R.W., Komi, P.V., 1979. Electromechanical delay in skeletal muscle under normal movement conditions. Acta Physiol. Scand. 106, 241–248.

Osu, R., Franklin, D.W., Kato, H., et al., 2002. Short- and long-term changes in joint co-contraction associated with motor learning as revealed from surface EMG. J. Neurophysiol. 88 (8), 991–1004.

Paintal, A.S., 1960. Functional analysis of group III afferent fibres of mammalian muscles. J. Physiol. 152, 250–270.

Palastanga, N., Field, D., Soames, R., 2002. Anatomy and human movement – structure and function, fourth ed. Butterworth-Heinemann, Oxford.

Panjabi, M.M., 1992. The stabilizing system of the spine. Part 1. Function, dysfunction, adaptation, and enhancement. J. Spinal Disord. 5 (4), 383–389.

Panjabi, M.M., White, A.A., 2001. Biomechanics in the musculoskeletal system. Churchill Livingstone, New York.

Panjabi, M., Abumi, K., Duranceau, J., et al., 1989. Spinal stability and intersegmental muscle forces: a biomechanical model. Spine 14 (2), 194–200.

Passatore, M., Grassi, C., Filippi, G.M., 1985. Sympathetically-induced development of tension in jaw muscles: the possible contraction of intrafusal muscle fibres. Pflügers Arch. 405, 297–304.

Peacock, E.E., 1959. A study of the circulation in normal tendons and healing grafts. Ann. Surg. 149 (3), 415–428.

Peck, D., Buxton, D.F., Nitz, A., 1984. A comparison of spindle concentrations in large and small muscles acting in parallel combinations. J. Morphol. 180, 243–252.

Perry, J., Antonelli, D., Ford, W., 1975. Analysis of knee-joint forces during flexed-knee stance. J. Bone Joint Surg. 57A (7), 961–967.

Pette, D., Staron, R.S., 1990. Cellular and molecular diversities of mammalian skeletal muscle fibres. Rev. Physiol. Biochem. Pharmacol. 116, 1–76.

Pette, D., Peuker, H., Staron, R.S., 1999. The impact of biochemical methods for single muscle fibre analysis. Acta Physiol. Scand. 166, 261–277.

Petty, R., 2003. Evaluating muscle symptoms. J. Neurol. Neurosurg. Psychiatry 74 (Suppl. 11), ii38–ii42.

Petty, N.J., 2011. Neuromusculoskeletal examination and assessment, a handbook for therapists, fourth ed. Churchill Livingstone, Edinburgh.

Phillips, D., Petrie, S., Solomonow, M., et al., 1997. Ligamentomuscular protective reflex in the elbow. J. Hand Surg. 22A (3), 473–478.

Pickering, G.W., Wayne, E.J., 1933–1934. Observations on angina pectoris and intermittent claudication in anaemia. Clin. Sci. 1, 305–325.

Pope, M.H., Johnson, R.J., Brown, D.W., et al., 1979. The role of musculature in injuries to the medial collateral ligament. J. Bone Joint Surg. 61A (3), 398–402.

Powers, S.K., Howley, E.T., 1997. Exercise physiology: theory and application to fitness and performance, third ed. McGraw-Hill, Boston.

Raja, S.N., Meyer, R.A., Ringkamp, M., et al., 1999. Peripheral neural mechanisms of nociception. In: Wall, P.D., Melzack, R. (Eds.), Textbook of pain, fourth ed. Churchill Livingstone, Edinburgh.

Rantanen, J., Rissanen, A., Kalimo, H., 1994. Lumbar muscle fiber size and type distribution in normal subjects. Eur. Spine J. 3, 331–335.

Rees, J.D., Wilson, A.M., Wolman, R.L., 2006. Current concepts in the management of tendon disorders. Rheumatology 45, 508–521.

Reinert, A., Mense, S., 1992. Free nerve endings in the skeletal muscle of the rat exhibiting immunoreactivity to substance P and calcitonin gene-related peptide. Pflügers Arch. 420 (Suppl. 1), R54.

Reinert, A., Vitek, M., Mense, S., 1992. Effects of substance P on the activity of high- and low-threshold mechanosensitive receptors of the rat diaphragm in-vitro. Pflügers Arch. 420, R47.

Renstrom, P., Arms, S.W., Stanwyck, T.S., 1986. Strain within the anterior cruciate ligament during hamstring and quadriceps activity. Am. J. Sports Med. 14 (1), 83–87.

Reynolds, N.L., Worrell, T.W., 1991. Chronic achilles peritendinitis: etiology, pathophysiology, and treatment. J. Orthop. Sports Phys. Ther. 13 (4), 171–176.

Richardson, C., Bullock, M.I., 1986. Changes in muscle activity during fast, alternating flexion–extension movements of the knee. Scand. J. Rehabil. Med. 18, 51–58.

Richardson, C., Jull, G., Hodges, P., et al., 1999. Therapeutic exercise for spinal segmental stabilization in low back pain, scientific basis and clinical approach. Churchill Livingstone, Edinburgh.

Rigby, B.J., Hirai, N., Spikes, J.D., et al., 1959. The mechanical properties of rat tail tendon. J. Gen. Physiol. 43, 265–283.

Rowe, R.W.D., 1985. The structure of rat tail tendon fascicles. Connect. Tissue Res. 14, 21–30.

Royce, J., 1958. Isometric fatigue curves in human muscle with normal and occluded circulation. Res. Q. 29 (2), 204–212.

Rutherford, O.M., Jones, D.A., Newham, D.J., 1986. Clinical and experimental application of the percutaneous twitch superimposition technique for the study of human muscle activation. J. Neurol.

Neurosurg. Psychiatry 49, 1288–1291.

Sacks, R.D., Roy, R.R., 1982. Architecture of the hind limb muscles of cats: functional significance. J. Morphol. 173, 185–195.

Saltin, B., Henriksson, J., Nygaard, E., et al., 1977. Fiber types and metabolic potentials of skeletal muscles in sedentary man and endurance runners. Ann. N. Y. Acad. Sci. 301, 3–29.

Sargeant, A.J., Davies, C.T.M., Edwards, R.H.T., et al., 1977. Functional and structural changes after disuse of human muscle. Clin. Sci. Mol. Med. 52, 337–342.

Schmid, H., Spring, H., 1985. Muscular imbalance in skiers. Man. Med. 2, 23–26.

Scott, W., Stevens, J., Binder-Macleod, S.A., 2001. Human skeletal muscle fiber type classifications. Phys. Ther. 81 (11), 1810–1816.

Seki, K., Taniguchi, Y., Narusawa, M., 2001. Effects of joint immobilization on firing rate modulation of human motor units. J. Physiol. 530 (3), 507–519.

Shakespeare, D., Stokes, M., Sherman, K.P., et al., 1983. The effect of knee flexion on quadriceps inhibition after meniscectomy. Clin. Sci. 65, 64P.

Shakespeare, D.T., Stokes, M., Sherman, K.P., et al., 1985. Reflex inhibition of the quadriceps after meniscectomy: lack of association with pain. Clin. Physiol. 5, 137–144.

Shoemaker, S.C., Markolf, K.L., 1982. In vivo rotary knee stability: ligamentous and muscular contributions. J. Bone Joint Surg. 64A (2), 208–216.

Shumway-Cook, A., Woollacott, M.H., 1995. Motor control, theory and practical applications. Williams & Wilkins, Baltimore.

Simone, D.A., Marchettini, P., Caputi, G., et al., 1994. Identification of muscle afferents subserving sensation of deep pain in humans. J. Neurophysiol. 72 (2), 883–889.

Simoneau, J.A., Lortie, G., Boulay, M.R., et al., 1986. Inheritance of human skeletal muscle and anaerobic capacity adaptation to high-intensity intermittent training. Int. J. Sports Med. 7, 167–171.

Sirca, A., Kostevc, V., 1985. The fibre type composition of thoracic and lumbar paravertebral muscles in man. J. Anat. 141, 131–137.

Skinner, H.B., Barrack, R.L., Cook, S.D., 1984. Age-related decline in proprioception. Clin. Orthop. Relat. Res. 184, 208–211.

Snyder-Mackler, L., De Luca, P.F., Williams, P.R., et al., 1994. Reflex inhibition of the quadriceps femoris muscle after injury or reconstruction of the anterior cruciate ligament. J. Bone Joint Surg. 76-A (4), 555–560.

Solomonow, M., Guzzi, A., Baratta, R., et al., 1986. EMG-force model of the elbows antagonistic muscle pair: the effect of joint position, gravity and recruitment. Am. J. Phys. Med. 65 (5), 223–244.

Solomonow, M., Baratta, R., Zhou, B.-H., et al., 1987. The synergistic action of the anterior cruciate ligament and thigh muscles in maintaining joint stability. Am. J. Sports Med. 15 (3), 207–213.

Solomonow, M., Zhou, B.-H., Harris, M., et al., 1998. The ligamento-muscular stabilizing system of the spine. Spine 23 (23), 2552–2562.

Speers, R.A., Kuo, A.D., Horak, F.B., 2002. Contributions of altered sensation and feedback responses to changes in coordination of postural control due to aging. Gait Posture 16, 20–30.

Spencer, J.D., Hayes, K.C., Alexander, I.J., 1984. Knee joint effusion and quadriceps reflex inhibition in man. Arch. Phys. Med. Rehabil. 65, 171–177.

Stacey, M.J., 1969. Free nerve endings in skeletal muscle of the cat. J. Anat. 105 (2), 231–254.

Staron, R.S., 1997. Human skeletal muscle fiber types: delineation, development, and distribution. Can. J. Appl. Physiol. 22 (4), 307–327.

Stauber, W.T., 1989. Eccentric action of muscles: physiology, injury, and adaptation. Exerc. Sport Sci. Rev. 17, 157–185.

Stener, B., 1969. Reflex inhibition of the quadriceps elicited from a subperiosteal tumour of the femur. Acta Orthop. Scand. 40, 86–91.

Stener, B., Petersen, I., 1963. Excitatory and inhibitory reflex motor effects from the partially ruptured medial collateral ligament of the knee joint. Acta Orthop. Scand. 33, 359.

Stokes, M., Young, A., 1984. The contribution of reflex inhibition to arthrogenous muscle weakness. Clin. Sci. 67, 7–14.

Strasmann, T., van der Wal, J.C., Halata, Z., et al., 1990. Functional topography and ultrastructure of periarticular mechanoreceptors in the lateral elbow region of the rat. Acta Anat. (Basel) 138, 1–14.

Stratford, P., 1981. Electromyography of the quadriceps femoris muscles in subjects with normal knees and acutely effused knees. Phys. Ther. 62 (3), 279–283.

Stuart, A., McComas, A.J., Goldspink, G., et al., 1981. Electrophysiologic features of muscle regeneration. Exp. Neurol. 74, 148–159.

Suter, E., Herzog, W., 1997. Extent of muscle inhibition as a function of knee angle. J. Electromyogr. Kinesiol. 7 (2), 123–130.

Suter, E., Herzog, W., 2000. Muscle inhibition and functional deficiencies associated with knee pathologies. In: Herzog, W. (Ed.), Skeletal muscle mechanics, from mechanisms to function. Wiley, Chichester, p. 365.

Suter, E., Herzog, W., Huber, A., 1996. Extent of motor unit activation in the quadriceps muscles of healthy subjects. Muscle Nerve 19, 1046–1048.

Suter, E., Herzog, W., Bray, R.C., 1998a. Quadriceps inhibition following arthroscopy in patients with anterior knee pain. Clin. Biomech. 13, 314–319.

Suter, E., Herzog, W., De Souza, K.D., et al., 1998b. Inhibition of the quadriceps muscles in patients with anterior knee pain. J. Appl. Biomech. 14, 360–373.

Tabary, J.C., Tabary, C., Tardieu, C., et al., 1972. Physiological and structural changes in the cat's soleus muscle due to immobilization at different lengths by plaster casts. J. Physiol. 224 (1), 231–244.

Talishev, F.M., Fedina, T.I., 1976. Influence of muscle viscoelastic characteristics on the accuracy of movement control. In: Komi, P.V. (Ed.), Biomechanics V-A. University Park, Baltimore, pp. 124–128.

Taylor, D.C., Dalton, J.D., Seaber, A.V., et al., 1990. Viscoelastic properties of muscle–tendon units, the biomechanical effects of stretching. Am. J. Sports Med. 18 (3), 300–309.

Thelen, D.G., Shultz, A.B., Alexander, N.B., et al., 1996. Effects of age on rapid ankle torque development. J. Gerontol. 51A (5), M226–M232.

Thelen, D.G., Muriuki, M., James, J., et al., 2000. Muscle activities used by young and old adults when stepping to regain balance during a forward fall. J. Electromyogr. Kinesiol. 10, 93–101.

Threlkeld, A.J., 1992. The effects of manual therapy on connective tissue. Phys. Ther. 72 (12), 893–902.

Tidball, J.G., 1991. Myotendinous junction injury in relation to junction structure and molecular composition. Exerc. Sport Sci. Rev. 19, 419–445.

Torebjork, H.E., Ochoa, J.L., Schady, W., 1984. Referred pain from intraneural stimulation of muscle fascicles in the median nerve. Pain 18, 145–156.

Torry, M.R., Decker, M.J., Viola, R.W., et al., 2000. Intra-articular knee joint effusion induces quadriceps avoidance gait patterns. Clin. Biomech. 15, 147–159.

Tracy, B.L., Enoka, R.M., 2002. Older adults are less steady during submaximal isometric contractions with the knee extensor muscles. J. Appl. Physiol. 92, 1004–1012.

Trappe, T.A., Lindquist, D.M., Carrithers, J.A., 2001. Muscle-specific atrophy of the quadriceps femoris with aging. J. Appl. Physiol. 90, 2070–2074.

Urbach, D., Awiszus, F., 2002. Impaired ability of voluntary quadriceps activation bilaterally interferes with function testing after knee injuries. A twitch interpolation study. Int. J. Sports Med. 23 (4), 231–236.

van der Heide, B., Allison, G.T., Zusman, M., 2001. Pain and muscular responses to a neural tissue provocation test in the upper limb. Man. Ther. 6 (3), 154–162.

Van Vlieta, P., Heneghan, N.R., 2006. Motor control and the management of musculoskeletal dysfunction. Man. Ther. 11, 208–213.

Vaughan, V.G., 1989. Effects of upper limb immobilization on isometric muscle strength, movement time, and triphasic electromyographic characteristics. Phys. Ther. 69 (2), 36–46.

Vleeming, A., Mooney, V., Snijders, C.J., et al., 1997. Movement, stability and low back pain, the essential role of the pelvis. Churchill Livingstone, New York.

Voight, M.L., Wieder, D.L., 1991. Comparative reflex response times of vastus medialis obliquus and vastus lateralis in normal subjects and subjects with extensor mechanism dysfunction, an electromyographic study. Am. J. Sports Med. 19 (2), 131–137.

Wainwright, S.A., Biggs, W.D., Currey, J. D., et al., 1982. Mechanical design in organisms. Princeton University Press, Princeton, New Jersey.

Walla, D.J., Albright, J.P., McAuley, E., et al., 1985. Hamstring control and the unstable anterior cruciate ligament-deficient knee. Am. J. Sports Med. 13 (1), 34–39.

Watkins, M.P., Harris, B.A., Kozlowski, B.A., 1984. Isokinetic testing in patients with hemiparesis. A pilot study. Phys. Ther. 64, 184–189.

Watson, D.H., 1994. Cervical headache: an investigation of natural head posture and upper cervical flexor muscle performance. In: Boyling, J.D., Palastanga, N. (Eds.), Grieve's modern manual therapy, the vertebral column, second ed. Churchill Livingstone, Edinburgh, pp. 349–360.

Wells, P.E., Frampton, V., Bowsher, D., 1994. Pain management by physiotherapy, second ed. Butterworth-Heinemann, Oxford.

Widrick, J.J., Romatowski, J.G., Norenberg, K.M., et al., 2001. Functional properties of slow and fast gastrocnemius muscle fibers after a 17-day spaceflight. J. Appl. Physiol. 90, 2203–2211.

Wilke, H.-J., Wolf, S., Claes, L.E., et al., 1995. Stability increase of the lumbar spine with different muscle groups: a biomechanical in vitro study. Spine 20 (2), 192–198.

Wilkie, D.R., 1950. The relation between force and velocity in human muscle. J. Physiol. 110, 249–280.

Williams, P.E., 1988. Effect of intermittent stretch on immobilised muscle. Ann. Rheum. Dis. 47 (12), 1014–1016.

Williams, P.E., Goldspink, G., 1973. The effect of immobilization on the longitudinal growth of striated muscle fibres. J. Anat. 116 (1), 45–55.

Williams, P.E., Goldspink, G., 1976. The effect of denervation and dystrophy on the adaptation of sarcomere number to the functional length of the muscle in young and adult mice. J. Anat. 122 (2), 455–465.

Williams, P.E., Goldspink, G., 1978. Changes in sarcomere length and physiological properties in immobilized muscle. J. Anat. 127 (3), 459–468.

Williams, P.E., Goldspink, G., 1984. Connective tissue changes in immobilized muscle. J. Anat. 138 (2), 343–350.

Williams, P.L., Bannister, L.H., Berry, M.M., et al., 1995. Gray's anatomy, thirty-eighth ed. Churchill Livingstone, New York.

Witvrouw, E., Sneyers, C., Lysens, R., et al., 1996. Reflex response times of vastus medialis oblique and vastus lateralis in normal subjects and in subjects with patellofemoral pain syndrome. J. Orthop. Sports Phys. Ther. 24 (3), 160–165.

Witzmann, F.A., 1988. Soleus muscle atrophy in rats induced by cast immobilization: lack of effect by anabolic steroids. Arch. Phys. Med. Rehabil. 69 (2), 81–85.

Woo, S., Maynard, J., Butler, D., et al., 1988. Ligament, tendon, and joint capsule insertions to bone. In: Woo, S. L.-Y., Buckwalter, J. (Eds.), Injury and repair of the musculoskeletal soft tissues. American Academy of Orthopaedic Surgeons, Park Ridge, Illinois, pp. 133–166.

Wood, L., Ferrell, W.R., Baxendale, R.H., 1988. Pressures in normal and acutely distended human knee joints and effects on quadriceps maximal voluntary contractions. Q. J. Exp. Physiol. 73, 305–314.

Wood, T.O., Cooke, P.H., Goodship, A.E., 1988. The effect of exercise and anabolic steroids on the mechanical properties and crimp morphology of the rat tendon. Am. J. Sports Med. 16 (2), 153–158.

Woodley, B.L., Newsham-West, R.J., Baxter, D., et al., 2007. Chronic tendinopathy: effectiveness of eccentric exercise. Br. J. Sports Med. 41, 188–198.

Wuerker, R.B., McPhedran, A.M., Henneman, E., 1965. Properties of motor units in a heterogeneous pale muscle (m. gastrocnemius) of the cat. J. Neurophysiol. 28, 85–99.

Wyke, B.D., Polacek, P., 1975. Articular neurology: the present position. J. Bone Joint Surg. 57B (3), 401.

Yamashita, T., Minaki, Y., Ozaktay, A.C., et al., 1996. A morphological study of the fibrous capsule of the human lumbar facet joint. Spine 21 (5), 538–543.

Yoshihara, K., Shirai, Y., Nakayama, Y., et al., 2001. Histochemical changes in the multifidus muscle in patients with lumbar intervertebral disc herniation. Spine 26 (6), 622–626.

Young, A., Hughes, I., Russell, P., et al., 1980. Measurement of quadriceps muscle wasting by ultrasonography. Rheumatol. Rehabil. 19 (3), 141–148.

Young, A., Stokes, M., Crowe, M., 1982a. The relationship between quadriceps size and strength in elderly women. Clin. Sci. 63 (3), 35P–36P.

Young, A., Hughes, I., Round, J.M., et al., 1982b. The effect of knee injury on the number of muscle fibres in the human quadriceps femoris. Clin. Sci. 62, 227–234.

Young, A., Stokes, M., Round, J.M., et al., 1983. The effect of high-resistance training on the strength and cross-sectional area of the human quadriceps. Eur. J. Clin. Invest. 13, 411–417.

Young, A., Stokes, M., Iles, J.F., 1987. Effects of joint pathology on muscle. Clin. Orthop. Relat. Res. 219, 21–27.

Zattara, M., Bouisset, S., 1988. Posturo-kinetic organisation during the early phase of voluntary upper limb movement. 1. Normal subjects. J. Neurol. Neurosurg. Psychiatry 51, 956–965.

Zhang, L.-Q., Nuber, G., Butler, J., et al., 1998. In vivo human knee joint dynamic properties as functions of muscle contraction and joint position. J. Biomech. 31, 71–76.

Zhao, W.-P., Kawaguchi, Y., Matsui, H., et al., 2000. Histochemistry and morphology of the multifidus muscle in lumbar disc herniation comparative study between diseased and normal sides. Spine 25 (17), 2191–2199.

Principles of muscle treatment

5

Laura Finucane

CHAPTER CONTENTS

There is no pure treatment for muscle, that is, treatment cannot be isolated to muscle alone; it will always to a greater or lesser extent affect joint and/or nerve tissue. Some sort of classification system for treatment is needed in order to have meaningful communication between clinicians, and this text follows the traditional classification of muscle, joint and nerve treatment. In this text a 'muscle treatment' is defined as a 'treatment to effect a change in muscle'; that is, the intention of the clinician is to produce a change in muscle and therefore it is described as a muscle treatment. Similarly, where a technique is used to effect a change in a joint, it will be referred to as a 'joint treatment', and where a technique is used to effect a change in nerve, it will be referred to as a 'nerve treatment'. Thus, treatments are classified according to which tissue the clinician is predominantly attempting to affect. This relationship of treatment of muscle, joint and nerve is depicted in Figure 5.1.

An example may help to illustrate the impurity of a muscle treatment technique. With the patient sitting over the edge of the couch, the patient is asked to contract the knee extensors against the manual resistance of the clinician. After maximal contraction there is relaxation of the muscle and the clinician is able to move the knee into more flexion. This is a hold–relax technique for the knee extensors. Further analysis reveals that this technique is not purely a muscle treatment: it also involves joints and nerves. The quadriceps muscle contains the patella and so

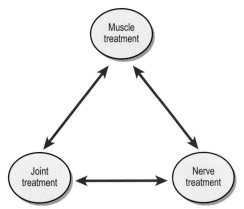

Figure 5.1 • Relationship of treatment techniques of muscle, joint and nerve. Treatment of muscle will also affect joint and nerve.

muscle contraction will cause movement of the patellofemoral joint and may cause some change to the tibiofemoral joint. Following muscle relaxation, the clinician moves the knee joint further into flexion, which will affect the tibiofemoral joint and patellofemoral joint. Throughout this technique there will

be neural activity in the form of afferent information from skin, joint and muscle, and efferent activity to muscle. In addition, the movement of the knee into further flexion will lengthen the femoral nerve. It can be readily seen that a simple hold–relax technique, which might be described as a muscle treatment, also affects joint and nerve. For this reason the hold–relax technique could be used to effect a change in muscle, joint and/or nerve tissue. The therapeutic effect of the hold–relax technique is likely to be a combined effect on muscle, joint and nerve.

There are a variety of muscle treatments. Treatments are categorised in this text from the dysfunctions identified in the previous chapter, namely, reduced strength, power and endurance, altered motor control (muscle inhibition, increased muscle activation, delayed timing of onset, altered activation of agonist and antagonist), reduced length and production of symptoms (Table 5.1). From this, a classification of muscle treatment can be identified: to increase muscle strength, power and endurance, alter motor control (increase muscle activation, reduce muscle activation, increase timing of onset, alter activation of agonist and antagonist), increase muscle

Table 5.1 Muscle dysfunction, aims of muscle treatment and treatment techniques

Muscle dysfunction	Aims of muscle treatment	Treatment techniques
Reduced strength, power and endurance	Increase strength, power and endurance	Training regimes using free weights, springs, pulleys, theraband, dynamometers, PNF
Altered motor control:	Increase muscle activation	Active assisted movements, rapid stretch mechanical vibration, PNF, touch, use of overflow, ice and taping
muscle inhibition delayed timing of onset	Increase time of onset	Challenge posture and balance using, for example, sit fit, gym ball
increased muscle activation	Reduce muscle activation	Made aware of the unwanted muscle activity using a mirror, verbal feedback, touch, electromyogram feedback. Positioning, PNF, trigger points, deep inhibitory massage and taping
Reduced length	Increase length	Stretching: ballistic or static, passively by clinician or actively by patient PNF
Symptom production	Reduce symptoms	Soft-tissue mobilisation: massage, connective tissue massage, specific soft-tissue mobilisations, trigger points, frictions Joint mobilisations Taping Electrotherapy

PNF, proprioceptive neuromuscular facilitation.

length and reduce muscle-related symptoms. A variety of techniques to address each of these treatments is also given in Table 5.1.

Principles of increasing muscle strength, power and endurance

There are a variety of exercise regimes used to increase muscle strength, power and endurance and the reader is referred to the numerous exercise physiology textbooks for further details on these.

This text reviews the principles involved in increasing muscle strength, power and endurance. The principles are overload, specificity, individuality, motivation, learning, reversibility and diminishing returns (Newham 2001); these principles are summarised in Box 5.1.

Overload

To improve the strength or endurance of a muscle it must be progressively overloaded (Bruton 2002). When strengthening a muscle, the resistance must be greater than that during everyday activities, and as the muscle gains strength the resistance must be progressively increased. When increasing muscle endurance, there must be a progressive increase in duration and frequency.

Specificity

This relates to the specific adaptation of muscle to the imposed demands (DiNubile 1991). The effect on muscle is specific to the nature of the exercise:

1. High resistance and low repetition will result in an increase in muscle strength (Staron et al. 1994; Hakkinen et al. 1998); there will be little to no improvement in endurance (Newham 2001).
2. Low resistance and high repetition will result in an increase in muscle endurance; there will be little to no improvement in strength (Newham 2001).
3. Low resistance at high speed will increase muscle power, that is, an increase in the speed of contraction.
4. High resistance at slow speed will result in an increase in muscle strength (and will not improve the speed of contraction).

The implication of specificity is that the prescribed exercise needs to mirror the functional activity it aims to improve.

Individuality

Individuals will respond differently to the same exercise; this response is determined by genetics, cellular growth rates, metabolism and neural and endocrine regulation (Wilmore & Costill 1999). For example, over the age of 60 years the number of fast-twitch fibres diminishes; therefore, an exercise given to an 80-year-old and a 26-year-old will have different effects. The training response may also be limited because of acquired damage to the neuromusculo-skeletal system.

Motivation

Only those motivated enough will make the physical and mental effort of following a training programme. The clinician can help to motivate the patient by the use of voice, explanation and enthusiasm.

Learning

The clinician educates the patient about the required exercise so that it is carried out effectively. Where the movement is unfamiliar, motor learning may need to occur.

Diminishing returns

An exercise regime will produce a greater improvement in people in poor physical condition than in those already in a good physical condition (Newham 2001).

Box 5.1

Principles of increasing muscle strength, power and endurance (Newham 2001)

- Overload
- Specificity
- Individuality
- Motivation
- Learning
- Reversibility
- Diminishing returns

Endurance training gains take longer to have an effect but are longer-lasting, whereas power can be achieved more quickly but tends to diminish faster.

Reversibility

This rather disappointing principle states that, when training stops, any strength or endurance gains will be lost (Bruton 2002).

Increasing muscle strength

The above principles need to be applied when attempting to increase muscle strength. The resistance to a muscle contraction needed to strengthen a muscle can be provided by: gravity, the clinician, the patient, a wall or piece of furniture, free weights, pulleys, springs, theraband and dynamometers such as the Cybex machine (Cybex, Bay Shore, NY). Interestingly, an isotonic exercise programme using free weights has been found to be as effective in strengthening the quadricep femoris muscle as the more expensive Cybex machine (DeLateur et al. 1972a).

Recommended strengthening regimes for healthy sedentary adults have been advocated by the American College of Sports Medicine (ACSM). This programme involves a minimum of 8–10 repetition maximum (RM) at least twice a week using the major muscle groups. An 8 RM would be the maximum amount of weight that could be lifted eight times before fatigue or loss of technique occurs. More importantly, recommendations are described for the older adult (over the age of 65 years) and for those adults aged 50–64 years with clinically significant chronic conditions and/or functional limitations, such as osteoarthritis (Nelson et al. 2007). These recommendations suggest a 10–15 RM where the level of effort for muscle-strengthening activity should be moderate to high. The Borg scale is used as a guide: this is a 10-point scale where 10 is maximum effort. Five to six on the scale would constitute moderate intensity and 7–8 high intensity. These recommendations are supported by research findings. The majority of studies have found that one set is as effective as two or three sets of resisted exercises (Westcott 1986; Westcott et al. 1989; Graves et al. 1990; Pollock et al. 1993; Starkey et al. 1996). In one study, the optimum number for strengthening muscle was found to be three sets (Berger 1962).

The optimum frequency of exercise has also been investigated by a number of studies with varying results. An optimum frequency for strengthening the muscles around the chest, arms and legs has been found to be three or more times a week (Gillam 1981; Braith et al. 1989), one, two or three times a week for spinal muscles (Graves et al. 1990; Leggett et al. 1991; Pollock et al. 1993; DeMichele et al. 1997) and trunk flexion and extension muscle strength has been found to increase following two or three sessions a week (Parkkola et al. 1992). A reasonable guideline for frequency would be a minimum of twice a week (Feigenbaum & Pollock 1999).

A strengthening regime would normally start slowly with a low intensity of exercise (American College of Sports Medicine 1998; Feigenbaum & Pollock 1999). Following assessment of 1 RM, the upper body should train at 30–40% of 1 RM and the lower body at 50–60%. Once the weight can be lifted well 12 times with a rating of perceived exertion (RPE) of 12–14 RPE (Borg 1982), 5% can be added to the next training session (Figure 5.2). Exercising to maximal effort, that is, to 19–20 RPE, will produce the greatest gains in strength (American College of Sports Medicine 1998), with progression of weight every 1–2 weeks.

It is recommended that, for the elderly and those with clinically significant chronic conditions, the intensity be reduced to one set of 10–15 RM, increasing the weight every 2–4 weeks (Feigenbaum & Pollock 1999; Nelson et al. 2007). Using 1 RM to

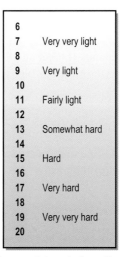

Figure 5.2 • Fifteen-point scale for ratings of perceived exertion, the RPE scale (reproduced from Borg 1982, with permission).

assess strength in those with musculoskeletal injuries and chronic diseases can risk injury, so 10 RM is an appropriate calculation. While muscle strength is less in the older person, the potential to strengthen muscle with a training programme is much the same as with a young person (Grimby 1995).

In conformity with the principle of specificity, the type of muscle contraction used in an exercise regime affects the change in muscle strength.

Eccentric muscle contraction appears to be more effective and efficient in increasing muscle strength as this type of exercise is more functional. Eccentric exercises have been found to cause a greater increase in eccentric, isometric and concentric muscle strength than either concentric exercises or a mixed exercise regime (Hortobagyi et al. 2000). Eccentric exercises three times a week for 12 weeks have been found to increase eccentric strength three and a half times more than concentric exercises increase concentric strength (Hortobagyi et al. 1996).

Isotonic exercise with free weights increases isotonic strength of quadriceps but not isometric strength, even after a few days of isometric exercises (DeLateur et al. 1972b). Isometric exercises, on the other hand, increase isometric strength and after 4 days of isotonic exercises produce a rapid increase in isotonic strength (DeLateur et al. 1972b). The clinical implication of this is that if movement is not possible due to some pathological process or injury, isometric exercises will improve isometric strength and enhance isotonic strength gains when movement is allowed (DeLateur et al. 1972b). However, research suggests that to have an effect the individual must perform multiples of 50–100 isometric contractions per day for 5–10 seconds each and as hard as pain allows (Morrissey et al. 1995).

The value of isometric exercises is further highlighted in another study, exploring the optimal exercise regime to produce hypertrophy of multifidus in patients with chronic low-back pain (Danneels et al. 2001). General stabilisation exercises, isometric contractions and concentric and eccentric muscle contractions at 70% of 1 RM (15–18 repetitions) three times a week for 10 weeks resulted in hypertrophy of multifidus. However, the group of patients who carried out only general stabilisation exercises, and the group of patients who carried out only general stabilisation exercises and the concentric and eccentric exercises, failed to produce a significant hypertrophy of multifidus. It was therefore concluded that the isometric exercises were critical in producing hypertrophy of multifidus in patients with chronic low-back pain. However, it is worth mentioning that isometric exercises produce strength gains only in the range within which the exercise is carried out.

The speed of isotonic muscle contractions can affect the strength changes in muscle. A high speed of contraction has been found to eliminate muscle inhibition, so fast dynamic work may be the best form of strength training (Newham et al. 1989).

The clinician can provide manual resistance to a concentric or isometric muscle contraction and this has been most fully explored with proprioceptive neuromuscular facilitation (PNF). PNF is thought to be useful when a muscle is very weak; once active contraction is possible equipment to provide resistance is more effective (Newham 2001). The advantages of PNF include a reduced need for equipment; PNF also allows tactile encouragement by the clinician and versatile movement patterns can be incorporated. The disadvantages of PNF are the time and effort required by the clinician and the imprecise measurement of the resistance applied and the muscle torque produced. Further information about PNF can be found elsewhere (Knott & Voss 1968; Waddington 1999).

Underlying effect of strengthening a muscle

A small number of repetitions against a high resistance will strengthen muscle (Staron et al. 1994; Hakkinen et al. 1998); the underlying effects are, first, a change in neural tissue, so that motor learning occurs, and, second, a change in muscle tissue, so that there is muscle hypertrophy (Figure 5.3). The stimulus for a strength change is the force of contraction, and this is reflected in the nature of the changes.

Motor learning

The first stage, which lasts for 6–8 weeks, is where motor learning occurs; performance improves but strength remains the same.

The changes include:

- Increased neural activation to the muscle (Moritani & DeVries 1979; Sale et al. 1983; Komi 1986). The amount of increase parallels the amount of increase in muscle strength
- Increased activation of prime movers (Sale 1988)
- Improved coordination (Sale 1988).

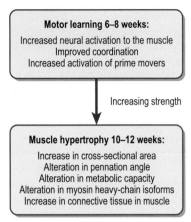

Figure 5.3 • The underlying effects of strengthening muscle (Newham 2001).

It has been proposed that neural changes alone can produce an increase in muscle strength (Enoka 1988). During an 8-week training programme neural changes were responsible for almost all the strength gains in subjects with a mean age of 70 years. In subjects with a mean age of 22 years, neural changes were responsible for most of the strength changes in the first 4 weeks, with muscle hypertrophy after 4–6 weeks (Moritani & DeVries 1979). It appears from this study that the timing of the changes in nerve and muscle varies with age.

Neural activation may be responsible for improved muscle activation, strength and endurance beyond the suggested 6–8 weeks (Kaser et al. 2001; Mannion et al. 2001). Patients with chronic low-back pain followed a 3-month back exercise programme (Mannion et al. 2001), and, although activation, strength and endurance improved, this was not accompanied by any change in the size of the muscle fibres or proportion of muscle fibre type (Kaser et al. 2001).

Muscle hypertrophy

The final stage after about 10–12 weeks is muscle hypertrophy, where muscle increases in size and strength (Newham 2001). The changes are:

1. An increase in the cross-sectional area of the muscle, mainly at the proximal and distal parts of the muscle belly; this is visible after a few weeks of training (Housh et al. 1992; Narici et al. 1996). The increase in cross-sectional area of the muscle is due to hypertrophy of muscle fibres (see below) and an increase in the connective tissue in muscle (MacDougall 1986). In addition, where the strength training involves a group of muscles, the increase in cross-sectional area is not equal in each muscle (Housh et al. 1992; Narici et al. 1996). For example, with quadriceps strength training, greatest hypertrophy was seen in rectus femoris and least hypertrophy in vastus intermedius (Narici et al. 1996).

2. An increase in the cross-sectional area of the muscle fibres (MacDougall et al. 1980; Hortobagyi et al. 1996; Melissa et al. 1997; Andersen & Aagaard 2000). It is unclear whether fibre types respond differently to strength training; two studies found an increase in cross-sectional area in type II fibres (Melissa et al. 1997; Andersen & Aagaard 2000), and two studies found type II fibres increased in cross-sectional area at a faster rate than type I fibres (MacDougall et al. 1980; Hortobagyi et al. 1996). Yet another study found equal increases between type I and II fibres (Young et al. 1983). Differences in methodology such as upper- or lower-limb muscle, exercise regime and type of muscle contraction may, in part, be responsible for the conflicting results. The most distinctive difference was found within one study which found that eccentric exercises produced a 10-fold greater increase in type II cross-sectional area than concentric exercises (Hortobagyi et al. 1996).

3. Alteration in muscle fibre types. Some studies have found no change in proportion of type I or type II fibres (Terrados et al. 1990; Labarque et al. 2002), whereas other studies have found an increase in the proportion of type IIa fibres and a decrease in type IIb fibres following strength training (Hortobagyi et al. 1996; Andersen & Aagaard 2000).

4. An alteration in pennation angles has been demonstrated in hypertrophied muscle (Kawakami et al. 1993, 1995).

5. An alteration in metabolic capacity of muscle has been demonstrated; this effect appears to be genetically determined (Simoneau et al. 1986).

6. An alteration in myosin heavy-chain (MHC) isoforms (Gea 1997; Andersen & Aagaard 2000). The myosin head, which binds with actin during a muscle contraction, contains the MHC isoforms (Scott et al. 2001).

7. There is an increase in the amount of connective tissue found in muscle structures proportional to muscle hypertrophy (MacDougall 1986).

Increasing muscle power

The principles of overload, specificity, individuality, motivation, learning, reversibility and diminishing returns (Newham 2001) need to be considered when attempting to increase muscle power. Because muscle power is a function of muscle force and velocity of contraction, improvement in either or both of these aspects will result in an increase in muscle power. Increasing muscle strength has been discussed in the previous section; increasing speed of contraction involves active contraction at speed. Repeated practice of the movement, or a component of the movement, at speed, is thought to produce an improvement in muscle power (deVries & Housh 1994). It is suggested that the whole movement, or a component of the movement, should be carried out as fast as possible against a resistance of 30% maximal isometric strength (Kerr 1998), although one study has found that exercises carried out at high speed caused improvement in power at only high speed, whereas exercises at slow or intermediate speed increased power at slow, intermediate and high speed (Kanehisa & Miyashita 1983). In line with the principle of specificity, the speed at which the muscle needs to contract for a specific functional task is the ideal speed at which the exercises should be carried out. Many functional activities are carried out at speed and require power training, for example stairs, sit to stand, and running.

Increasing muscle endurance

Muscle endurance can refer to the ability of a muscle to contract repetitively or to sustain a contraction for a period of time (Bruton 2002). The principles of overload, specificity, individuality, motivation, learning, reversibility and diminishing returns (Newham 2001) also need to be applied when attempting to increase muscle endurance.

The differing effect of exercise, between individuals, to improve endurance is beginning to emerge. The effect of exercises on muscle endurance training has been found to be related to an 'insertion' gene encoding angiotensin-converting enzyme which has been found in significantly ($P < 0.05$) greater frequency in elite high-altitude mountaineers than in control subjects (Montgomery et al. 1998). In addition, the same researchers found that subjects with the 'insertion' allele had an 11-fold greater improvement than those with the 'deletion' allele following a 10-week endurance training programme. The underlying mechanism is unclear but may affect the circulation system, hormone concentration and/or metabolism (Montgomery et al. 1998).

To increase muscle endurance a muscle must contract at 30–50% of its maximum contraction, for 20–30 minutes three times a week (McArdle et al. 1996) and 25–35 repetitions need to occur at each session (Berger 1982; Kerr 1998). Where endurance training incorporates general cardiorespiratory exercises, such as walking, running, swimming and cycling, the ACSM provides guidance for healthy adults recommending moderate exercise intensity sufficient to raise the heart rate to 60–90% of maximal, and it should be carried out for 30 minutes five times a week, or 20 minutes of vigorous intensity three times per week (Haskell et al. 2007). For the older adult and those with clinically significant chronic conditions the recommendations are similar except the heart rate should be raised to 50–85%, where 5–6 is moderate (50%) and 7–8 (80%) is vigorous intensity on a 10-point scale. Recommended maximal heart rates during training for different age groups are shown in Table 5.2 (Newham 2001).

Underlying effects of increasing muscle endurance

A high number of repetitions of muscle contractions against a low resistance will increase muscle endurance (Newham 2001) by effecting a change in muscle. The stimulus is the metabolic demand of the muscle and this is reflected in the nature of the changes (Box 5.2) and includes:

- an increase in the number of type I and IIa fibres and a decrease in type IIb fibres (Ingjer 1979; Demirel et al. 1999)

Table 5.2 The maximal heart rate recommended during training at different ages (Newham 2001)

Age (years)	Upper limit (beats per minute)
20–29	170
30–39	160
40–49	150
50–59	140
60 and over	130

Box 5.2

Underlying effect of increasing muscle endurance

- Increase in number of I and IIa fibres, and a decrease in type IIb fibres
- Increase in cross-sectional area of type I fibres
- Increase in number of capillaries
- Increase in myoglobin content
- Increase in oxidative power and enzyme activity of mitochondria
- Increase in oxidative enzymes
- Increased store of muscle glycogen and fat
- Increased activity of enzymes
- Higher threshold level of lactate
- Altered myosin heavy-chain isoforms

- an increase in the cross-sectional area of type I fibres (Ingjer 1979)
- an increase in number of capillaries surrounding each muscle fibre (Hermansen & Wachtlova 1971; Ingjer 1979)
- an increase in blood flow in muscle (Vanderhoof et al. 1961; Rohter et al. 1963)
- an increase in myoglobin content, which increases oxidative power of muscle (Holloszy 1976)
- an increase in oxidative power and enzyme activity of mitochondria. An endurance training programme resulted in a 40% increase in the mitochondrial oxidative power (Tonkonogi et al. 2000)
- an increase in oxidative enzymes (Holloszy 1976; Fitts & Widrick 1996)
- an increase in glycogen and fat storage in muscle (Holloszy 1976)
- an increase in activity of enzymes involved in beta-oxidation of fat (Holloszy 1976)
- a higher threshold level of lactate (Holloszy 1976)
- an alteration in MHC isoforms (Demirel et al. 1999; O'Neill et al. 1999).

Clinical implications of strength power and endurance training

Exercise prescription is a core skill of therapists that combines management of disorders of movement, knowledge of exercise regimens and clinical reasoning skills to ensure that the exercises prescribed are optimal for the individual (Taylor et al. 2007). For example, there is strong evidence that strengthening and aerobic exercises reduce pain and improve activity level in people with osteoarthritis of the knee (Brosseau et al. 2004; Hurley et al. 2007). A patient with osteoarthritis of the knee is likely to have weak quadriceps and pain, and may be unable to achieve a functional activity such as sit to stand, stair-climbing and walking for more than 10 minutes. Therefore a training programme needs to reflect each of these elements. It requires power training to enable the patient to carry out sit to stand, endurance strengthening to carry out stairs and cardiovascular endurance to enable the patient to walk. Consideration needs to be taken for the load, repetition, rest period and order of exercise.

Altering motor control

Signs of altered motor control have been considered in the previous chapter as muscle inhibition, delayed timing of onset, increased muscle activation and altered relative activation of agonist and antagonist. The aim of treatment, in this case, would therefore be to increase muscle activation, increase the speed of onset of muscle contraction, reduce muscle activation or alter relative activation of agonist and antagonist. The common theme for each of these aims is to alter the pattern of muscle activation, which is to alter motor control. The principles of altering motor control are largely provided by the theory of motor learning and have been applied in patients with neurological problems and neuromusculoskeletal dysfunction; the underlying processes involved are thought to be similar (Carr & Shepherd 1998).

As in any learning environment, the learner – in this case the patient – is the key player. Patients come with a unique set of abilities and past experience which can influence their ability to learn new motor patterns; these factors include attitude to new experiences, body type, cultural background, emotional make-up, fitness level, dexterity, stamina, strength, learning style (visual, verbal or kinaesthetic), maturity, motivation, previous social and therapeutic experiences, prior movement experiences and stage of learning (Schmidt & Wrisberg 2000). These are summarised in Box 5.3. Patient motivation is critical and can be enhanced by fully involving the patient with the treatment, allowing them to set and evaluate their own goals of treatment. The patient needs to be motivated to practise because the improvement of performance is directly related to the amount of practice (Carr & Shepherd 1998).

Box 5.3

Factors affecting the ability of a person to learn a new movement pattern (Schmidt & Wrisberg 2000)

- Attitude to new experiences
- Body type
- Cultural background
- Emotional make-up
- Fitness level
- Dexterity
- Stamina
- Strength
- Learning style (visual, verbal or kinaesthetic)
- Maturity
- Motivation
- Previous social and therapeutic experiences
- Prior movement experiences
- Stage of learning

Motor learning can be divided into three stages: verbal–cognitive, motor and autonomous (Schmidt & Wrisberg 2000); these stages are summarised in Figure 5.4. The verbal–cognitive stage is where patients are being asked to do a new unfamiliar movement and is characterised by patients thinking and perhaps talking about the movement they want to achieve. Any past experience of something similar will help patients in this stage. Their ability to achieve the movement is likely to be jerky and uncertain.

The effects of mental practice compared with physical practice have been investigated in an interesting study on piano-playing (Pascual-Leone et al. 1995). One subject group undertook mental practice, and another group physical practice, for 2 hours a day over a 5-day period. Both groups demonstrated

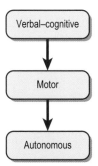

Figure 5.4 • Stages in motor learning (Schmidt & Wrisberg 2000).

similar cortical changes in the motor system. The mental practice group were not as good as the physical practice group in performing the actual physical task; however, they did become equivalent in their ability after just one 2-hour physical practice session. This suggests that mental practice can be used to minimise the time needed for physical practice and is of equal value to physical practice (Pascual-Leone et al. 1995). The clinician can enhance learning by being aware of patients' learning style (Honey & Mumford 1986) and emphasising their preferred cue, whether that be a visual, verbal or kinaesthetic cue. Thus, the clinician will explain, demonstrate and use touch to help teach the patient a new movement strategy.

The motor stage is where the learner refines the movement pattern so that it is smoother and more certain. If the required movement or muscular control is slow, for example, challenging balance and posture, then the patient will focus on any internal or external feedback to improve motor control. If, on the other hand, the required movement is fast, the patient will focus on the movement itself. Whichever feedback is used, patients can be encouraged to reflect on their performance, and any errors they may have made, as this has been found to promote development of skill (Liu & Wrisberg 1997). The patient may initially produce movement with co-contraction of agonist and antagonist and, as improvement occurs, there will be sequential contraction, producing an improved quality of movement (Moore & Marteniuk 1986). With improvement, the movement will be carried out more efficiently with less energy used (Sparrow & Irizarry-Lopez 1987), so that there will be less fatigue. This change can be measured by asking patients their rating of perceived effort using the Borg scale, shown in Figure 5.2 (Borg 1982). The clinician can enhance learning in this stage by providing the patient with specific and accurate feedback using mirrors, palpation, verbal feedback, pressure biofeedback unit (PBU, Chattanooga, Australia), ultrasound imaging (Hides et al. 1995) and electromyogram (EMG) biofeedback (Richardson et al. 1999) and encouraging the patient to practise (Moore & Marteniuk 1986; Sparrow & Irizarry-Lopez 1987; McDonald et al. 1989). If the movement is complex, then practice of individual components may help, but, as early as possible, the movement should be practised in its entirety and in its specific context (Carr & Shepherd 1998). This stage may last for several weeks or months.

The patient may then move to the autonomous stage in which a movement can be carried out without the patient having to concentrate on it and there is an increased ability to detect and correct error in performance (McCullagh & Caird 1990). Learning in this stage can continue for months and even years (Crossman 1959). For example, in the manufacture of cigars, workers perform a discrete motor task as quickly as possible. The speed of performance does not appreciably improve until it has been repeated some three million times over a 2-year period (Crossman 1959).

The nervous system is plastic, that is, it adapts and changes as the need arises (Kandel 1991; Niemann et al. 1991; Pascual-Leone et al. 1995; Carr & Shepherd 1998; Kleim & Jones 2008). The trigger for change within the central nervous system is an increased use of a body part or increased sensory feedback from it (Jenkins et al. 1990; Carr & Shepherd 1998). An interesting study controlled the behaviour of the adult owl monkey's hand. The hand was trained to obtain food and repeated the task about 600 times each day for 10 days, equivalent to about 6000 repetitions. This learned motor task was accompanied by an expansion of the area of the brain's cortex concerned with the hand, demonstrating the cortical effects of motor learning (Jenkins et al. 1990). Cortical changes have been found to occur in humans following limb amputation and spinal cord injury (Cohen et al. 1991) and learning a complicated sequence of finger movements (Niemann et al. 1991; Pascual-Leone et al. 1995). Learning alters the pattern of interconnections between the involved sensory and motor systems (Kandel 1991). It appears that Brodmann's area of mapping in the sensory cortex varies between individuals and depends on the dominant pathways in use (Kandel 1991). The underlying mechanisms of these changes have so far been identified as either the development of new neural connections or increased synaptic effectiveness (Kandel 1991; Kidd et al. 1992). PNF, described by a number of workers (Rood 1956; Knott & Voss 1968; Bobath 1990; Carr & Shepherd 1998; Waddington 1999), has provided treatments that encourage and guide normal movement patterns. Treatment aims to facilitate wanted movement and inhibit unwanted movement (Kidd et al. 1992). The basis of these techniques is that, by producing normal movement patterns and repeating them, the central and peripheral nervous system will undergo plastic change such that it learns to initiate and reproduce this normal movement pattern (Carr & Shepherd 1998; Fletcher-Cook 1999).

Continual practice of normal movement patterns over a long period of time is often necessary to produce a change. The Peto Institute in Budapest provides an intensive (13 hours per day) residential teaching programme in motor learning for children and adults with motor disabilities, such as ataxia and hemiplegia (Todd 1990). To alter normal functional movement patterns, treatment needs to use normal functional movement patterns (Carr & Shepherd 1998). This is reinforced by the principle of specificity of learning (Henry 1968), which, when applied to patients, means that the best practice of a movement is that which most closely mimics the functional movement required.

To increase muscle activation

Methods for increasing muscle activation, that is, for facilitating muscle contraction, include active assisted movements, rapid stretch mechanical vibration, PNF, touch, use of overflow, ice and taping (Box 5.4). Electrical stimulation of muscle is also available. With the muscle contracting and in a lengthened position, a rapid stretch is applied to the muscle; this stimulates the muscle spindles to facilitate extrafusal muscle contraction (Newham 2001). Vibration similarly stimulates the muscle spindles. PNF may also prove helpful in facilitating muscle contraction (Knott & Voss 1968; Waddington 1999). Touch can be used to facilitate muscle contraction; stimulation of the skin has been shown to enhance alpha and gamma motor neurone activity in the underlying muscles and cause inhibition of more distal muscles (Eldred & Hagbarth 1954). The principle of overflow may also be helpful in facilitating muscle activation, such that contraction of stronger muscles can lead to increased activation of the weak muscle (Kidd et al. 1992).

Box 5.4

Treatment to increase muscle activation

- Active assisted movements
- Rapid stretch
- Proprioceptive neuromuscular facilitation
- Touch
- Use of overflow
- Mechanical vibration
- Ice
- Taping

Quickly brushing ice over a muscle may facilitate its contraction (Rood 1956). Taping is thought to increase activation of the underlying muscle (Gilleard et al. 1998; Cowan et al. 2002).

Inhibition of an active voluntary contraction was eliminated with a fast-velocity isotonic contraction (Newham et al. 1989). This can be explained by the relationship of force and speed, where increased speed of concentric contraction reduces the force generated (Hill 1938).

The activation of a muscle during functional activities may need to be addressed in treatment. Contraction of the hamstring muscles can increase knee joint stiffness by 100–250% (Louie & Mote 1987) and reduce the strain on the anterior cruciate ligament (ACL) (Renstrom et al. 1986). It may be helpful in treatment to increase the activation of the hamstring muscles to help stabilise the knee joint. It has been found that strengthening the knee flexors over a period of 2–3 weeks results in increased activity of the hamstrings during maximal active knee extension (Baratta et al. 1988). It appears, then, that strengthening a muscle does not just affect its function as an agonist; it also facilitates its recruitment as an antagonist. Thus, hamstring strength training may be beneficial in patients with ACL injury, or after repair, to enhance knee joint stability (Baratta et al. 1988). If this phenomenon occurs with other muscles, then the effect of strengthening a muscle increases its torque as an agonist and also increases its activation as an antagonist.

The plastic nature of muscle activation is highlighted by patients with ACL-deficient knees who have an increased EMG activity of biceps femoris, vastus lateralis and tibialis anterior during a range of functional activities, compared with a control group (Ciccotti et al. 1994). This increased muscle activity is considered to be a protective mechanism which enhances the stability of the knee joint.

Measurement of muscle inhibition varies with joint angle (Suter & Herzog 1997). For this reason, standardisation of the position of the joint is needed on each reassessment. Measurement of quadriceps inhibition, in the presence of a joint effusion, is best carried out at $30°$ knee flexion, as intra-articular pressure is least at this angle (Jayson & Dixon 1970; Levick 1983). Measurement of quadriceps inhibition for patients with ACL reconstruction is best carried out beyond $60°$ (Arms et al. 1984) or $80°$ (Hirokawa et al. 1992) knee flexion because, at this angle, the tibia is translating posteriorly and will thus not strain the ACL.

Increase speed of onset

Using the principles of motor learning, it would seem reasonable to suggest that, to increase the speed of onset of muscle contraction, treatment needs to use normal functional activities that will produce a need for the muscle to contract. With delayed activation of transversus abdominis in patients with low-back pain (Hodges & Richardson 1996), treatment would include functional postures and movements that challenge postural stability and this would need to be continued repetitively over a period of time. The use of a gym ball and sit fit (Sissel UK, Halifax, UK) may help to facilitate speed of onset of muscle contraction (Richardson et al. 1999). In patients with anterior knee pain, a combination of specific muscle exercise with biofeedback, muscle stretches, taping and patellofemoral accessory movements has been shown, over a 6-week period, to increase the timing of muscle onset of vastus medialis, when going up and down stairs (Gilleard et al. 1998; Cowan et al. 2002). The mechanism by which the tape increased the onset of vastus medialis is unclear. Cutaneous stimulation has been shown to alter recruitment threshold and recruitment order of motor units (Garnett & Stephens 1981; Jenner & Stephens 1982).

To reduce muscle activation

This may be needed where the clinician feels there is overactivity of muscles. For example, in the early stages of motor learning there is co-contraction of the agonist and antagonist when carrying out a movement (Moore & Marteniuk 1986). Similarly, there may be unwanted muscle activity as a patient attempts to produce a specific muscle contraction, for example flexion of the lumbar spine, while trying to isolate contraction of the transversus abdominis and lumbar multifidus (Richardson et al. 1999). The patient may have overactivity of muscles because of pain, which may be sufficient to produce muscle spasm. In all of these examples, the clinician may need to reduce the muscle activity. To do this the patient may need to be made aware of the unwanted muscle activity using a mirror, verbal feedback, touch or EMG feedback. Other methods for reducing muscle activation include positioning, PNF, trigger points, deep inhibitory massage, relaxation techniques and taping (Box 5.5). It has been speculated that tape to the posterior thigh inhibits overactive hamstring muscles (McConnell 2002)

Box 5.5

Treatment to reduce muscle activity

- Mirror
- Verbal feedback
- Touch
- Electromyogram feedback
- Positioning
- Proprioceptive neuromuscular facilitation
- Trigger points
- Deep inhibitory massage
- Taping

and some other studies would support this (Tobin & Robinson 2000). Tape across the belly of vastus lateralis in asymptomatic subjects has been found to reduce the EMG activity when coming down stairs (Tobin & Robinson 2000). Tape over the lower fibres of trapezius of asymptomatic subjects was found to inhibit the muscle by as much as 22% when measured using the H reflex (Alexander et al. 2003). The underlying mechanism is not known; it has been postulated that it could be due to an alteration in muscle length and/or stimulation of cutaneous afferents, leading to inhibition of the underlying muscle and/or decrease in descending drive of the motor neurone pool (Alexander et al. 2003).

Altered relative activation of agonist and antagonist

The above sections on increasing and reducing muscle activation address the relative activation of agonist and antagonist.

Altering muscle length

Treatment may aim to decrease or increase length. The reason a muscle may be considered long, and why treatment should be aimed at reducing its length, is likely to be associated with reduced muscle tone. Where the clinician identifies reduced tone, treatment would be directed at increasing the contraction of the muscle, which has been discussed above.

Increasing muscle length

When considering muscle stretching, it can be helpful to categorise muscle into the active contractile

unit and the non-contractile connective tissue, within the muscle belly and tendon. Treatment can be classified according to which effect the clinician is attempting to have on the muscle. Increasing the length of a muscle can be achieved by passively lengthening the connective tissue such that there is a permanent increase in length, or by attempting to produce physiological relaxation of the active contractile unit of the muscle belly using, for example, PNF. Clearly, the contractile and non-contractile elements are inseparable and what is not being stated here is that treatment to lengthen the connective tissue affects the connective tissue alone and has no effect on the contractile unit, or vice versa. The classification of treatment is used simply to aid communication between clinicians and is not attempting to describe the effect of the treatment.

Muscle can be stretched passively, by the clinician or by the patient. The aim of treatment is to produce a permanent (plastic) lengthening of the connective tissue of muscle and tendon with minimal structural weakness.

Passive muscle stretching by the clinician

A passive stretch can be performed in much the same way as a passive stretch to a joint or a nerve, that is, the clinician applies a static or oscillatory force to lengthen the muscle. The dose of passive stretch incorporates a number of factors, and is outlined in Table 5.3.

Position

This includes the general position of the patient, such as lying, sitting or standing, and the specific position of the body part; for example, the hip may be placed in medial rotation and then flexed. The choice of general and specific positioning will depend on a number of factors:

- the comfort and support of the patient
- the comfort of the clinician applying the technique
- accurate application of the technique
- the desired effect of the treatment
- whether weight-bearing or non-weight-bearing is desired
- to what extent the movement is to be functional
- to what extent symptoms are to be produced.

An effective passive stretch is produced when a force moves the proximal and distal muscle attachments further apart; often, this involves fixing the proximal attachment while passively moving the

Table 5.3 Treatment dose for passive stretching by the clinician and active stretching by the patient

Factors	Passive stretching by the clinician	Active stretching by the patient
Patient's position	e.g. supine	e.g. sitting, standing with heel of foot on a stool with knee extended
Direction of movement	e.g. hip flexion	e.g. active knee extension
Magnitude of force applied	Related to therapist's perception of resistance: grades I–V	Related to patient's perception of stretch
Amplitude of oscillation	Static or small or large	Static or small or large
Speed	Slow or fast	Slow or fast (if fast, may be referred to as ballistic)
Rhythm	Smooth or staccato	Smooth or staccato
Time	Of repetitions and number of repetitions	Of repetitions and number of repetitions
Temperature	Room temperature or heat with short-wave diathermy	Room temperature
Symptom response	Short of symptom production Point of onset or increase in resting symptom Partial reproduction of symptom Full reproduction of symptom	Short of symptom production Point of onset or increase in resting symptom Partial reproduction of symptom Full reproduction of symptom

distal attachment. Positioning can often be used to help fix the proximal attachment; for example, supine with one leg flexed on to the chest helps to fix the pelvis as the other hip is moved into extension to lengthen the iliopsoas muscle.

Direction of movement

There is no single direction of movement that will stretch all parts of a muscle; the clinician needs to explore fully and treat all aspects of muscle length by combining movements (Hunter 1998). The muscle attachments, direction of its fibres, position of the muscle and the relationship of the muscle to other structures enable the clinician to decide how to combine movements for any particular muscle. For example, to lengthen biceps femoris fully, a combination of hip flexion, medial rotation and adduction with knee extension and medial tibial rotation needs to be used. Similarly, to lengthen extensor carpi radialis brevis fully, elbow extension with forearm pronation, wrist flexion, ulna deviation and individual finger flexion need to be combined (Hunter 1998).

Magnitude of force

When a muscle is stretched the force is distributed throughout the connective tissue framework of the muscle (Hill 1950). Whenever a permanent lengthening is achieved, there is some degree of mechanical weakening (Rigby et al. 1959; Warren et al. 1971).

Interestingly, the amount of weakening depends on the way the muscle has been lengthened, as well as how much it has been lengthened. A small force for a long duration will induce less weakening than a large force for a short duration (Warren et al. 1971; Sapega et al. 1981; Taylor et al. 1990).

The force applied by the clinician may be described using grades of movement (Magarey 1985, 1986; Maitland et al. 2001). Grades of movement were initially described for forces applied to joint movement, later for lengthening nerve, and in this text for lengthening muscle. As a joint is passively moved to lengthen a muscle, resistance will be felt by the clinician and this can be depicted on a movement diagram (Petty 2011). With physiological movements that lengthen muscle, there is often minimal resistance early in range of movement. For example, hip flexion will have little resistance in the early part of the range and the clinician may mark the onset of resistance (R_1) somewhere towards the end of the movement (Figure 5.5). Grades of movement are then defined according to the resistance curve. The grades of movement defined in this text (Table 5.4) are a modification of Maitland et al. (2001) and Magarey (1985, 1986). The modification allows every possible position in range to be described (Magarey 1985, 1986),

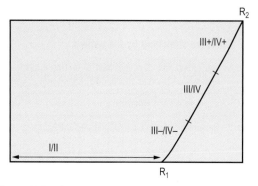

Figure 5.5 • A movement diagram depicting grades of movement for a physiological movement. The onset of resistance (R_1) may be felt by the clinician somewhere towards the end of the movement, with R_2 depicting the end of range.

and each grade to be distinct from the others (Maitland et al. 2001). The choice of magnitude of force, like every other factor of treatment dose, depends on what the clinician is attempting to achieve.

Amplitude of oscillation

The movement can be a sustained or oscillatory force. If the force is oscillated, it is described as having a small or large amplitude. The amplitude is relative to the available range of any movement. The amplitude of oscillatory movement is described within the definition of a grade of movement: grades

Table 5.4 Grades of movement

Grade	Definition
I	Small-amplitude movement short of resistance
II	Large-amplitude movement short of resistance
III−	Large-amplitude movement in the first third of resistance
IV−	Small-amplitude movement in the first third of resistance
III	Large-amplitude movement in the middle third of resistance
IV	Small-amplitude movement in the middle third of resistance
III+	Large-amplitude movement in the last third of resistance
IV+	Small-amplitude movement in the last third of resistance

I and IV are small-amplitude movements, grades II and III are large-amplitude movements. It is impossible for a truly sustained force to be applied: there will always be some variation in the force, albeit very small. For this reason, it is sometimes referred to as a quasistatic force. Where a clinician applies a sustained force, it is suggested that the description would use grades I, IV−, IV, IV+, with the word 'sustained' written prior to the grade; for example, treatment notes would read 'sustained grade IV−'. What is important, however, is not the choice of notation but the full description of the treatment dose.

It can be seen that grades of movement describe the magnitude of the force and the amplitude of oscillation. The choice of grade of movement is determined by the relationship of pain (or other symptom) and resistance through the range of movement. Where resistance limits the range of movement and there is minimal pain, a grade III+ or IV+ would be appropriate (Figure 5.6A). Where pain limits the range of movement, and there is minimal resistance, a grade I or II may be appropriate, so that no pain is produced (Figure 5.6B). A grade III− or IV− may be appropriate if the pain is non-severe and non-irritable and there is no caution related to the nature of the disorder. Where resistance limits the movement and there is a significant amount of pain, or where pain limits the movement and there is a significant amount of resistance, the choice of grade will depend on the degree to which symptoms can be provoked (Figure 5.6C and 5.6D). For example, in Figure 5.6C, if a grade IV is chosen at about 50% of resistance, this would, according to the movement diagram, provoke an intensity of pain of about 3 out of 10 (where A is 0 and C is 10). If a grade IV is chosen for Figure 5.6D, this would provoke about 6 out of 10, which may or may not be acceptable to the patient.

Speed and rhythm of movement

The speed of the movement can be described as slow or fast, and the rhythm as smooth or staccato (jerky); of course, these terms will apply only to oscillatory forces. Speed and rhythm go hand in hand, and movements will tend to be slow and smooth, fast and smooth, or fast and staccato; it would be difficult to apply a slow staccato movement. The connective tissue in muscle is viscoelastic and is therefore sensitive to the speed of the applied force (Norkin & Levangie 1992). A force applied quickly will produce less movement, provoking a greater stiffness; that is, the gradient of the resistance curve will increase; a

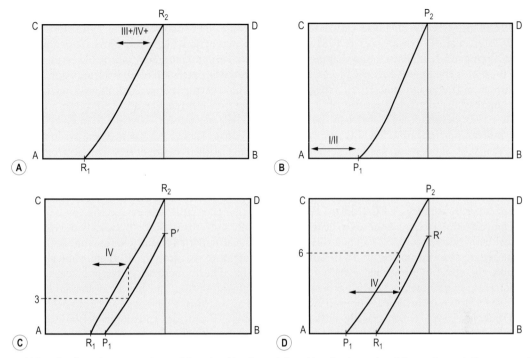

Figure 5.6 • Grades of movement are determined by the relationship of pain and resistance through the range of movement; this is depicted on a movement diagram. **A** Resistance limiting movement. **B** Pain limiting movement. **C** Resistance limiting movement with a significant amount of pain. **D** Pain limiting movement with a significant amount of resistance.

force applied more slowly, on the other hand, will cause more movement as the stiffness is relatively less (Norkin & Levangie 1992). If the intention of treatment is to maximise range of movement by lengthening connective tissue then a slow speed would seem preferable.

Time

In terms of treatment dose, time relates to the amount of time a muscle is placed on a stretch, the number of times this is repeated and the frequency of the appointments.

The required length of time to stretch a muscle is thought to be 6–12 seconds several times a day (Corbin & Noble 1980).

Hamstring muscle length has been found to be as effectively lengthened with daily static stretches using a 30-second stretch as with three repetitions of 1-minute stretches (Bandy et al. 1997). Reassessment after each repetition enables the clinician to determine the effect of treatment on the patient's signs and symptoms. Depending on this change (better, same or worse), the clinician may alter the time and number of repetitions within a treatment session.

When a muscle is placed on a stretch, the time needed to lengthen the connective tissue a certain amount varies inversely with the magnitude of the force; that is, a low force will take longer to lengthen a set amount than a high force (Warren et al. 1971). The proportion of lengthening that remains, once the force is removed, is greater following a long-duration, low force (Warren et al. 1971; Sapega et al. 1981). A permanent (plastic) lengthening of the connective tissue of muscle and tendon with minimal structural weakness is enhanced by a long-duration stretch (Sapega et al. 1981).

Temperature

Temperature influences the mechanical behaviour of connective tissue under tensile load. As temperature rises to about 40–45°C, stiffness decreases and extensibility increases (Rigby et al. 1959; LaBan 1962; Rigby 1964; Lehmann et al. 1970). At about 40°C a change in the microstructure of collagen occurs, which significantly enhances the extensibility and potential for a permanent (plastic) change in length (Rigby et al. 1959; Rigby 1964). The viscoelastic properties can be increased by as much as 170% when muscle temperature is raised to

43°C (Talishev & Fedina 1976). A higher temperature will induce less weakening than a lower temperature (Warren et al. 1971; Sapega et al. 1981). Once the heat is removed, it has been found that maintaining the tension as the tissue cools enhances the plastic deformation (Lehmann et al. 1970; Sapega et al. 1981). Increasing the temperature of a tissue depends on its depth; it will obviously be easier to heat more superficial muscles.

The ability of short-wave diathermy, hot-water baths and ultrasound to increase muscle and tendon temperature has been investigated. Twenty minutes of short-wave diathermy has been shown to raise muscle temperature by as much as 4°C (Millard 1961). If normal muscle temperature is assumed to be the same as normal body temperature, 37°C, then this would raise the temperature of muscle to 41°C, sufficient to enhance the effect of stretching. Twenty minutes of immersion in a water bath at 42.5°C has been found to increase forearm muscle temperature to 39°C (Barcroft & Edholm 1943), which may be sufficient to enhance the effect of a stretch. Ultrasound at a frequency of 1 megacycle with a 12.5 cm² head at an intensity of 1 W/cm² for 7 minutes caused the muscle temperature (3.5 cm below the surface of the skin) to rise to 40°C (Lehmann et al. 1966). This research suggests that heating muscle and tendon with short-wave diathermy, hot water or ultrasound will enhance the effect of muscle stretching.

Symptom response

The clinician decides which symptom, and to what extent, is to be provoked during treatment. Choices include:

- no provocation
- provocation to the point of onset or increase in resting symptoms
- partial reproduction
- total reproduction.

The decision as to what extent symptoms are provoked during treatment depends on the severity and irritability of the symptom(s) and the nature of the condition. If the symptoms are severe, that is, the patient is unable to tolerate the symptom being produced, the clinician would choose not to provoke the symptoms. The clinician may also choose not to provoke symptoms if they are irritable, that is, once symptoms are provoked they take some time to ease. If, however, the symptoms are not severe and not irritable then the clinician is able to reproduce the patient's symptoms during treatment, and the extent to which symptoms are

reproduced will depend on the tolerance of the patient. The nature of the condition may limit the extent to which symptoms are produced, such as a recent traumatic injury. Treatment is progressed or regressed by altering appropriate aspects of the treatment dose: patient position, movement, direction of force, magnitude of force, amplitude of oscillation, speed, rhythm, time or symptom response. Table 5.5 suggests the ways in which each aspect of the treatment dose can be progressed and regressed.

It is suggested that inexperienced clinicians alter only one aspect of treatment dose at an attendance so that they fully understand the value of the alteration; in this way they will quickly develop valuable clinical experience and clinical mileage which will contribute to growth in their clinical reasoning skills. The immediate and more long-term effect of the alteration can then be evaluated by reassessment of the subjective and physical asterisks. Table 5.6 provides an example of how a treatment dose for lengthening the upper fibres of trapezius may be progressed and regressed. An increase in time from 30 seconds to 1 minute provides a progression of the treatment dose, and a reduction in the amount of symptoms accounts for the regression. Other aspects of treatment dose which are

Table 5.5 Progression and regression of treatment dose

Treatment dose	Progression	Regression
Position	Muscle towards end of available range	Muscle towards beginning of available range
Direction of force	More provocative	Less provocative
Magnitude of force	Increased	Decreased
Amplitude of oscillation	Decreased	Increased
Rhythm	Staccato	Smoother
Time	Longer	Shorter
Speed	Slower or faster	Slower
Symptom response	Allowing more symptoms to be provoked	Allowing fewer symptoms to be provoked

Table 5.6 Example of how a treatment dose for increasing the passive length of the upper fibres of trapezius can be progressed and regressed

Regression	Dose	Progression
In full cervical flexion and 1/2 range contralateral flexion, static hold for 30 seconds to partial reproduction of patient's neck pain	In full cervical flexion and 1/2 range contralateral flexion, static hold for 30 seconds to full reproduction of patient's neck pain	In full cervical flexion and 1/2 range contralateral flexion, static hold for 1 minute to full reproduction of patient's neck pain

closely linked are the length of time for each repetition and the number of repetitions; these, together, provide a dose of time and so each can be altered at the same time.

Passive muscle stretching by the patient

The patient can actively stretch a muscle. The factors defining the treatment dose are exactly the same as passive muscle stretching carried out by the clinician (Table 5.3). The only difference is that, with passive stretching by the patient, the patient is in total control of the stretching movement and relies on his or her own perception of stretch and symptom production to determine the way the stretch is carried out. The patient needs to be fully informed as to how to carry out the stretch, that is, how forceful to be and to what extent to reproduce the symptoms. The clinician in this case takes on a more educational and advisory role.

In sports medicine, two types of stretching are advocated: ballistic and static stretching. Ballistic stretching involves the person performing bouncing, rhythmic end-range movements. Static stretching involves a simple hold at the end of range. Controversy exists over the effectiveness of each type of stretching in producing an increase in muscle length. One study found that both methods were ineffective; only hold–relax produced an increase in muscle length (Sady et al. 1982). The best method of stretching to cause a permanent increase in muscle length remains unclear (Corbin & Noble 1980).

Summary of increasing muscle length

The important factors that affect a permanent increase in length of muscle following a passive stretch include the magnitude of force, time of force application and temperature of the muscle (Sapega et al. 1981). From research to date, it appears that a permanent (plastic) lengthening of the connective tissue of muscle and tendon with minimal structural weakness will be enhanced by a relatively low force for a long-duration stretch (Warren et al. 1971; Sapega et al. 1981) at high temperatures (Rigby et al. 1959; Rigby 1964; Talishev & Fedina 1976; Sapega et al. 1981).

Increasing length via the contractile unit of muscle

The aim of this type of treatment is to cause a relaxation of the contractile unit of muscle in order to increase muscle length. Muscle energy techniques and positional release techniques can also be used to cause muscle relaxation (Chaitow 2001a, b). PNF is advocated to achieve this muscle relaxation (Knott & Voss 1968; Waddington 1999). These are rotational movement patterns through full range of movement, hold–relax, contract–relax and agonist–contract.

Rotational movement patterns
These patterns of movement take muscles from full outer range, where they are fully lengthened, to a fully shortened position. Specific patterns of movement for the head and neck, trunk and limbs have been described (Knott & Voss 1968).

Hold–relax
The muscle is positioned in its stretched position, either actively or passively. A strong isometric contraction of the muscle is achieved by the clinician providing manual resistance. The muscle contraction needs to be carefully controlled by the clinician. This is achieved by saying to the patient 'don't let me move you' or 'hold' and by slowly and smoothly increasing the manual resistance to maximum contraction. Following contraction the patient is asked to relax, the clinician gradually reduces the resistance and time is allowed for muscle relaxation to occur. The clinician then moves further into range to increase the length of the muscle. The procedure of

contraction followed by relaxation is then repeated until no further increase in muscle length can be achieved.

Contract–relax

This is the same as hold–relax except that, following the isometric contraction, the patient actively contracts to lengthen the antagonistic muscle further, rather than the clinician passively lengthening the muscle. For example, to lengthen quadriceps the patient isometrically contracts the quadriceps at, for example, 60° flexion for 3–6 seconds. The patient is then asked to relax and actively to contract the hamstrings in an attempt to increase knee flexion and stretch the quadriceps muscle group. As in hold–relax, the procedure is repeated in the new range of movement and repeated until no further increase in muscle length is achieved.

Agonist–contract

The muscle is put in a position of stretch and a contraction of the agonist attempts to increase movement and thus increase stretch of the muscle. The clinician facilitates this movement by carefully applying a passive force. For example, to lengthen quadriceps the knee is positioned in 60° flexion. The patient actively contracts the hamstrings in an attempt to increase knee flexion and stretch the quadriceps muscle group. The clinician applies a force to the lower leg to enhance this movement.

Soft-tissue mobilisation of muscle

Hunter (1998) has coined the phrase 'specific soft-tissue mobilisation' (SSTM). It is essentially the application of manual force to soft tissue, which can be considered to include muscle and tendon as well as skin, fascia, ligament and nerve.

There are essentially three types of treatment techniques: physiological SSTM, accessory SSTM and combined SSTM (physiological and accessory).

1. Physiological SSTM involves full exploration of all anatomical regions of the muscle and tendon by a combination of physiological movements – in other words, putting a stretch on a muscle with a combination of movements. For example, to explore biceps femoris fully, hip flexion and knee extension need to be combined with medial rotation and adduction of the hip with medial rotation of the tibia (Hunter 1998).

2. Accessory SSTM involves applying manual force to muscle and tendon. For example, a horizontal force across the fibres of the tendocalcaneus could be applied. It is recommended that the force be applied

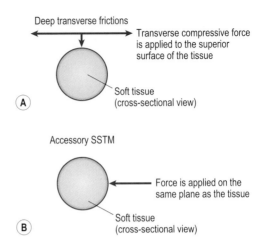

Figure 5.7 • Direction of force and position of force for A deep transverse frictions and B accessory specific soft-tissue mobilisation (SSTM) (from Hunter 1998, with permission).

in the plane of the muscle or tendon and at right angles to the site of dysfunction (Hunter 1998). In this regard it differs from transverse frictions (Figure 5.7). Manual force can be applied with the muscle or tendon relaxed or with an isometric, concentric or eccentric muscle contraction.

3. Combined accessory and physiological SSTM involves the muscle and tendon in a lengthened position while an accessory force is applied. For example, the transverse glide across the tendocalcaneus could be carried out with the knee extended and the foot in dorsiflexion. It could also involve applying accessory movement with isometric, concentric or eccentric muscle contraction.

Treatment dose

The decisions to be made by the clinician, in terms of treatment dose, include the patient's position, movement, direction, magnitude of force applied, amplitude of oscillation, speed and rhythm of movement, time and symptom response. Table 5.7 provides a summary of the treatment options and is identical to the treatment dose for joint and nerve in Chapters 3 and 7 respectively.

The underlying effect of soft-tissue mobilisation is not yet known. Soft-tissue mobilisation is considered to be appropriate following soft-tissue injury during the regeneration and remodelling phase of healing (Hunter 1998), details of which are given below with muscle injury. During the regeneration and remodelling phases soft-tissue mobilisation is thought to enhance collagen synthesis and cross-linkage development,

Table 5.7 Treatment dose for soft-tissue mobilisation

Factors	Variables
Patient's position	e.g. prone, side lie, sitting
Movement	Physiological movement Accessory movement or a mixture of accessory and physiological
Direction of force applied	e.g. medial transverse, lateral transverse, anteroposterior, posteroanterior, caudad, cephalad
Magnitude of force applied	Related to therapist's perception of resistance: grades I–V
Amplitude of oscillation	None: sustained (quasistatic) Small: grades I and IV Large: grades II and III
Speed	Slow or fast
Rhythm	Smooth or staccato
Time	Of repetition and number of repetitions
Symptom response	Short of symptom production Point of onset or increase in resting symptom Partial reproduction of symptom Full reproduction of symptom

promote the orientation of collagen fibres along functional lines of stress, and promote 'normal' viscoelastic behaviour (Hunter 1998). SSTM is also proposed to be beneficial for degenerative lesions by stimulating an inflammatory response that initiates healing (Hunter 1998).

Reducing symptoms

A useful premise for the clinician is to consider that the symptom is whatever patients say it is, existing whenever they say it is (McCaffery 1979). This was originally used for pain, but can be widened to any symptom the patient feels.

The assumption in this text is that the cause of the muscle pain is some sort of injury to the muscle and/or tendon. In this situation, the pain will be a result of mechanical and/or chemical irritation of the muscle nociceptors. The subjective information from the patient, particularly the behaviour of symptoms

and mechanism of injury, may enable the clinician to identify whether it is the contractile unit of muscle and/or connective tissue of muscle that is involved in the pain (Vicenzino et al. 2002). For example, an overstretch injury may affect the connective tissue of muscle and require treatment to increase the muscle length and, by so doing, reduce pain.

Various palpatory techniques can be used to reduce symptoms emanating from muscle, including SSTM massage, connective tissue massage trigger points and frictions. Joint mobilisations, taping and electrotherapy can also be used. SSTM has been described above. Electrotherapy is beyond the scope of this text; the reader is referred to other texts such as Low & Reed (1990) and an excellent review by Watson (2000).

Massage can be applied to muscle to reduce pain, using stroking, effleurage, kneading, picking up, wringing and skin rolling (Thomson et al. 1991). Additional effects are thought to include an increase in the flow of the circulation, muscle relaxation, lengthening of tissues and an increased tissue drainage and pain relief (Thomson et al. 1991). For further details see Thomson et al. (1991).

Connective tissue massage involves applying specific strokes to the skin and subcutaneous tissues from the lumbar spine to the upper limbs or from the lumbar spine to the lower limbs. It has been suggested that it affects the autonomic nervous system and, via this system, increases circulation which aids healing and eases pain (Thomson et al. 1991). For further details see Thomson et al. (1991).

A trigger point is defined as a focus of hyper-irritability of a muscle and is thought to contribute to muscle tightness. On palpation of the muscle, an area of local tightness with tenderness, possible muscle twitch and referral of pain in a typical pattern is found. Having identified this, treatment involves applying manual pressure over the area. The reader is referred to the textbook by Travell & Simons (1983, 1992) for further information. The underlying cause of the phenomenon of trigger points has been proposed as secondary hyperalgesia originating from peripheral nerves (Quintner & Cohen 1994).

Frictions are small-amplitude deep pressures applied to tissue such as muscle and tendon. The clinician's finger or thumb moves with the patient's skin across the tissue. The tissue is often positioned such that it is in a lengthened position. It has been proposed that frictions cause hyperaemia, break down adhesions and stimulate mechanoreceptors (Cyriax

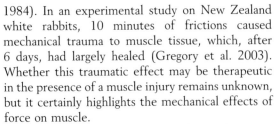

1984). In an experimental study on New Zealand white rabbits, 10 minutes of frictions caused mechanical trauma to muscle tissue, which, after 6 days, had largely healed (Gregory et al. 2003). Whether this traumatic effect may be therapeutic in the presence of a muscle injury remains unknown, but it certainly highlights the mechanical effects of force on muscle.

Joint mobilisations may be used to reduce pain and change muscle. For example, anterior knee pain often involves the dysfunction of the quadriceps muscle group and the patellofemoral joint. Treatment to the muscle will affect the joint, and, similarly, treatment to the joint will affect the muscle. Accessory movements applied to the patellofemoral joint, with or without concentric, eccentric or isometric quadriceps contraction, may be useful. Similarly, with lateral elbow pain there may be dysfunction of the extensor muscles of the forearm as well as a radiohumeral joint dysfunction. Again, accessory movements may be applied to the joint with or without concentric, eccentric or isometric contraction of the wrist and finger extensor muscles. For example, a lateral glide combined with the patient performing an isometric grip with the hand has been found in a randomised double-blind placebo-controlled study to increase by approximately 10% the pressure pain threshold and increase by almost 60% the painfree grip strength (Vicenzino et al. 2001). In another study, spinal accessory movements have been found to reduce pain and improve muscle activation in the cervical spine (Sterling et al. 2001). Further information on accessory movements combined with active muscle contractions can be found elsewhere (Mulligan 1995; Vicenzino 2003). The mechanism by which joint accessory movements reduce pain and cause a change in muscle activity is discussed in Chapter 3.

Tape may be used to relieve muscle pain. A useful principle is to apply the tape in such a way that it replicates the direction of the pain-relieving force applied by the clinician during treatment. For details of methods of taping the reader is referred to other texts (Macdonald 1994; Vicenzino 2003).

The mechanism by which pain is relieved with each of these manual techniques is still unclear. Large-diameter type III afferents are distributed throughout muscle tissue and are stimulated by pressure, mechanical force caused by lengthening

muscle or by muscle contraction (Mense & Meyer 1985). It is possible that the manual techniques described above may stimulate the type III afferents and cause a reflex inhibition of the type IV muscle nociceptors according to the pain gate theory (Melzack & Wall 1965). Clearly, large-diameter afferents in the skin and joint may also contribute to this pain inhibition. The pain may also be reduced via a descending inhibitory system explained below and expanded rather more in Chapter 7 on nerve treatment.

Descending inhibition of pain

The periaqueductal grey (PAG) area has been found to be important in the control of nociception. PAG projects to the dorsal horn and has a descending control of nociception (Figure 5.8). It also projects upwards to the medial thalamus and orbital frontal cortex, and so may have an ascending control of nociception (Fields & Basbaum 1999). The PAG has two distinct regions, the dorsolateral PAG (dPAG) and the ventrolateral PAG (vPAG).

dPAG

The dPAG runs to the dorsolateral pons and ventrolateral medulla, which is involved in autonomic control (Fields & Basbaum 1999). In the rat, stimulation of the dPAG causes analgesia, increased blood pressure, increased heart rate, vasodilation of the hindlimb muscles, increased rate and depth of respiration and coordinated hind-limb, jaw and tail movements, suggesting increased activity of the sympathetic nervous system, and alpha motor neurones (Lovick 1991). The neurotransmitter from dPAG is noradrenaline (norepinephrine), and the analgesic effect appears to mediate morphine analgesia of mechanical nociceptor stimuli (Kuraishi et al. 1983). At the spinal cord level, dPAG causes inhibition of substance P from peripheral noxious mechanical stimulation (Kuraishi 1990).

vPAG

The vPAG runs mainly to the nucleus raphe magnus. In the rat, stimulation of vPAG causes analgesia with decreased blood pressure, decreased heart rate, vasodilation of the hind-limb muscles and reduced hind-limb, jaw and tail movements, suggesting inhibition of the sympathetic nervous system

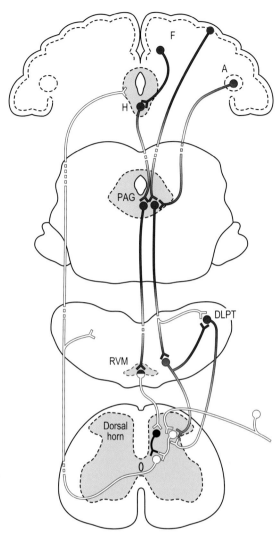

Figure 5.8 • Pain-modulating pathway. Periaqueductal grey (PAG) receives input from the frontal lobe (F), the amygdala (A) and the hypothalamus (H). Afferents from PAG travel to the rostral ventromedial medulla (RVM) and the dorsolateral pontomesencephalic tegmentum (DLPT) and on to the dorsal horn. The RVM has bidirectional control of nociceptive transmission. There are inhibitory (filled) and excitatory (unfilled) interneurones. (From Fields & Basbaum 1999, with permission.)

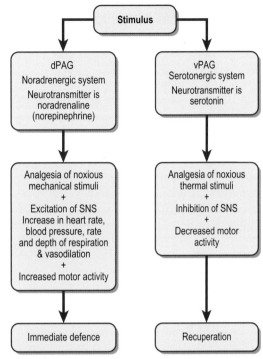

Figure 5.9 • Descending inhibition of mechanical nociception from the dorsolateral periqueductal grey (dPAG: noradrenergic system) and thermal nociception from the ventrolateral periaqueductal grey (vPAG: serotonergic system). SNS, sympathetic nervous system.

and inhibition of alpha motor neurones (Lovick 1991). The neurotransmitter used in vPAG is serotonin, and the analgesic effect appears to mediate morphine analgesia of thermal nociceptive stimuli (Kuraishi et al. 1983). At the dorsal horn vPAG inhibits the release of somatostatin, produced by

peripheral noxious thermal stimulation (Kuraishi 1990). These mechanisms have been linked to the behaviour of an animal under threat, which initially acts with a defensive flight-or-fight response, followed by recuperation (Fanselow 1991; Lovick 1991); this is summarised in Figure 5.9.

Noxious stimuli can cause activation of the descending control system (Yaksh & Elde 1981; Fields & Basbaum 1999), which may reduce nociceptive transmission. Noxious stimulation has been found to cause release of enkephalins at the supraspinal and spinal levels (Yaksh & Elde 1981). It has also been found that stimulation of the spinothalamic tract, transmitting nociceptive information from one foot, can be inhibited by noxious input from the contralateral foot, hand, face or trunk (Gerhart et al. 1981). It has been suggested that this may explain the relief of pain with acupuncture, and pain behaviours such as 'biting your lip and banging your head against a wall' (!) (Melzack 1975). Painful treatment of muscle may also activate the descending control system.

Addressing the biopsychosocial aspects of symptoms

Injury, or the perception of injury, produces anxiety and fear (Craig 1999). Who has ever injured themselves, however minimally, and not experienced an emotional reaction? The psychological aspects of pain sometimes focus on 'emotional individuals', or on chronic pain patients. However, all of us will have a cognitive and emotional response to injury, because injury interrupts our lives. There is never a right time for an injury: it will always be, to a greater or lesser degree, a nuisance to us. That 'nuisance' will drive our emotional reactions. It seems reasonable to suggest, therefore, that all patients with neuromusculoskeletal dysfunction will have thoughts and feelings about their problem, and it would be an oversight on the part of the clinician not to enquire about these. This enquiry involves the clinician understanding the patient's thoughts and feelings. This is no easy task, and to do it well requires a high level of skill in active listening. Active listening involves putting our own thoughts, beliefs and feelings to one side and choosing, instead, to hear what the patient has to say. It involves trying to understand patients and their world, through their eyes, and avoiding the all-too-easy error of reinterpreting through our eyes. It requires the clinician to listen with compassion and patience and without judgement. It involves the clinician using words carefully and meaningfully and using open-ended questions to search for information, until understanding is reached. It involves sensitive verbal and non-verbal communication, encouraging safe and open communication. This is a tall order, but the benefits of truly being able to come alongside the patient will far outweigh the effort of developing these skills.

The use of 'yellow flags' was devised specifically for acute low-back pain to identify beliefs, emotions and behaviours that may contribute to long-term disability (Watson & Kendall 2000). Screening questionnaires (Main & Waddell 1999) have been devised; these, like all questionnaires, have major limitations. Questions provide a superficial, and sometimes false, understanding of the problem – as anyone who has filled in any questionnaire knows only too well. For example, when a question asks: 'How much have you been bothered by feeling depressed in the last week?' and the recipient answers on a 0–10 scale from 'not at all' to 'extremely', little information is gleaned from this – there may be a wide variety of factors underlying the given score. For this reason, if a questionnaire is used, a discussion with the patient will also be necessary to understand the problems the patient faces (Watson & Kendall 2000). The questionnaire can be useful for providing the clinician with aspects to discuss with the patient; however, there is a danger that it becomes a mechanistic form-filling exercise. It is worth remembering that the clinical management of patients is fundamentally based on human relationships which are not normally enriched by form-filling!

Following the enquiry of patients as to their thoughts and feelings, two further steps are recommended: education and exposure (Vlaeyen & Crombez 1999). Education involves the clinician carefully facilitating the patient's understanding of his or her problem. How this is carried out with patients will vary according to a number of factors, including their prior knowledge, thoughts and beliefs, and how they feel about the problem. All the listening skills discussed above will be essential in this process. The ability of the clinician to be honest is important. The clinician needs to explain the problem to the patient in a careful way. There is a world of difference between 'The pain in your back is from the disc' and 'I think the pain in your back could be coming from the disc'. The former explanation suggests that you know that the pain is coming from the disc, and yet there is overwhelming evidence that you cannot make such claims; it has been estimated that a definite diagnosis of pathology can be made in about only 15% of cases (Waddell 1999). Furthermore, there is a long-term problem with being so confident as the patient may, in the future, have a recurrence of the same pain and may see another clinician who may say 'The pain in your back is from your sacroiliac joint'. The patient is aware that this is a repeat episode and now, quite rightly, begins to have doubts about the ability of these two clinicians. This will be a familiar story to experienced clinicians, who will have come across patients who may have received three, four or even more confident 'diagnoses' of the same problem, and who come to you depressed, cynical and disillusioned with the medical profession.

The final aspect is exposure, which involves careful and graded exposure to the movements or postures that provoke pain (Vlaeyen & Crombez 1999). While this is designed for chronic pain patients who learn to avoid movements and posture through fear (Waddell & Main 1999), it may also be an important part of the treatment of acute tissue damage. Using movements and postures in a careful, controlled and graded way may help to avoid long-term movement dysfunctions.

Muscle injury and repair

Muscle can be damaged by a direct injury, such as a laceration or contusion, or indirectly by a sudden forceful contraction causing a muscle or tendon tear; damage may also be due to a chronic overuse injury (Kellett 1986). Whatever the mechanism of injury, the effect on muscle tissue is similar (Hurme et al. 1991) and can be considered in three phases: inflammatory or lag phase, regeneration phase and remodelling phase (Jarvinen & Lehto 1993).

The inflammatory or lag phase is characterised by haematoma formation, tissue necrosis and an inflammatory reaction. Necrosis of muscle tissue occurs with retraction of the muscle fibres on either side of the necrotic zone. It is generally accepted that treatment for the first 48–72 hours of a muscle injury is summarised by RICE: rest, ice, compression and elevation (Evans 1980; Kellett 1986).

During the regeneration phase there is phagocytosis of damaged tissue, and production of connective scar tissue. Capillary growth satellite cells migrate into the necrotic area. Muscle fibres regenerate by differentiation into myoblasts and then into myotubes, which link the two stumps on either side of the necrotic region (McComas 1996). The connective tissue within muscle is also damaged and undergoes healing with subsequent scar formation (Jarvinen & Lehto 1993). Following a short period of immobilisation – more than 3–5 days for rats (Jarvinen & Lehto 1993) – it is considered beneficial to mobilise the muscle, within the limits of symptoms. Early mobilisation is thought to enhance tensile strength, orientation of the regenerating muscle fibres, resorption of connective scar tissue and blood flow to the damaged area and to avoid atrophy brought about by immobilisation (Jarvinen & Lehto 1993). The tensile strength of a tendon has been found to increase as a result of 60 repetitions per day of manual wrist and finger flexion/extension following a primary repair (Takai et al. 1991).

The remodelling phase is characterised by the maturation of regenerated muscle (Jarvinen & Lehto 1993). There is contraction and reorganisation of scar tissue and a gradual recovery of the functional capacity of the muscle.

An experimental crush injury of the semitendinosus muscle of the rat reveals necrosis of muscle tissue in the first 2 days, with new myotubes within the damaged area at 5 days and regeneration of muscle fibres bridging the necrotic area by 10 days, with full regeneration at 30 days (Stuart et al. 1981). A controlled strain injury of the musculotendinous junction of tibialis anterior muscle was carried out on New Zealand white rabbits (Nikolaou et al. 1987). Necrosis and infiltration of inflammatory cells, oedema and haemorrhage occurred after 1 day. After 2 days the damaged fibres had been broken down with proliferation of inflammatory cells, macrophages and fibroblasts. After 7 days inflammation was reduced and fibrocytes were evident (Nikolaou et al. 1987). Clear evidence of muscle regeneration was evident after 4 days following an experimental strain injury of a rat tendon (Almekinders & Gilbert 1986).

Treatment of a muscle injury may include soft-tissue mobilisation, frictions, controlled exercises, lengthening, tape and electrotherapy. The reader is directed to relevant texts for further information.

It is worth mentioning here that a patient presenting with classical signs of a hamstring tear may, in fact, have a neurodynamic component to the problem. In Australian Rules football, players with signs of a hamstring tear had a positive slump test and when this was addressed in treatment there was a better result than with more traditional muscle treatment techniques (Kornberg & Lew 1989). This highlights the need for a full and comprehensive examination of a patient.

Delayed muscle soreness

Muscle strain injury occurs with eccentric exercise, producing delayed muscle soreness (Friden et al. 1983; Jones et al. 1986). Pain, weakness and muscle stiffness are felt after unaccustomed eccentric exercise. There is breakdown of collagen (Brown et al. 1997) and disruption of the Z band, predominantly in type II fibres, with repair largely completed by 6 days (Friden et al. 1983; Jones et al. 1986). The reason for the delayed muscle soreness following eccentric contraction may be that eccentric contraction produces more force within the muscle than other types of muscle contraction (Katz 1939).

Tendon injury and repair

Tendons can tear in the middle region, by avulsion of bone and, more rarely, at the insertion site (Woo et al. 1988). The myotendinous region is the weakest part of the tendon–muscle unit and is the region most susceptible to strain injuries (Nikolaou et al. 1987; Garrett et al. 1989; Garrett 1990; Tidball 1991). Healing of tendon is similar to that of other soft tissues and consists of three phases: lag or inflammation phase (1–7 days), regeneration or proliferation phase (7–21 days) and remodelling or maturation phase (21 days to 1 year) (Jozsa & Kannus 1997).

Repetitive strain may alter the collagenous structure of tendon with resultant inflammation, oedema and pain (Jozsa & Kannus 1997). Overuse injury occurs where this repetitive strain causing tissue damage is greater than the natural repair and healing process (Archambault et al. 1995; Jozsa & Kannus 1997). Conditions including tendinopathies may lead, with further strain, to partial or complete rupture of the tendon. Eccentric exercises have been advocated for chronic Achilles tendinopathy (Alfredson et al. 1998).

In work-related upper-limb tendon injuries, the repetitive nature of the task may be sufficient to cause change in the tissue. It is proposed that, initially, in the first 5 days, there is ischaemia, metabolic disturbance and cell membrane damage leading to inflammation (Jozsa & Kannus 1997). The increase in tissue pressure further impairs the circulation and enhances the ischaemic changes. In the proliferation phase (5–21 days) there is fibrin clotting, and fibroblast, synovial cell and capillary proliferation followed by the maturation phase (<21 days) in which adhesions and thickening of the tenosynovium and paratenon occur (Kvist & Kvist 1980; Jozsa & Kannus 1997).

Treatment of a tendon injury may include soft-tissue mobilisation, frictions, controlled exercises, lengthening, tape and electrotherapy. The reader is directed to relevant texts for further information.

Choice of muscle treatment

The choice of treatment depends on the assessment of the patient, whether the patient has a dysfunction of muscle and, if so, what that dysfunction is. Treatment may be to increase muscle strength, power and/or endurance, increase muscle length, alter motor control (increase muscle activation, reduce muscle activation, increase time of onset) and reduce symptoms. The overall aim of treatment is to normalise a dysfunction, that is, to eradicate the abnormal signs and symptoms.

There is a wide variety of treatment techniques, and it is not the intention of this textbook to reproduce what is already well described in other texts.

Rather, this text aims to provide a broad overview of the principles behind the broad range of treatments to enable clinicians to solve the problem of what might be best for a particular patient at a particular time.

The best treatment is the one that improves the patient's signs and symptoms in the shortest period of time. The clinician monitors the patient's signs and symptoms within and between treatment sessions in order to identify the effectiveness of the treatment choice. Any change in signs and symptoms is considered in the light of the prognosis and treatment goals, following the examination and assessment on day 1. In this way, the clinician can be creative and imaginative in considering all the possible treatment choices, while constantly monitoring the effectiveness of treatment. If the treatment is proved to be ineffective, then the clinician can alter the treatment; if it proves to be effective, and the patient is improving at the expected rate, then the treatment can be continued or progressed.

Any physical test which reproduces or eases the patient's symptoms can be converted to a treatment technique by applying the components of a treatment dose. Converting positive physical testing procedures to treatment techniques would seem the most logical approach to choosing treatment, as the clinician can be confident that the treatment is somehow or other affecting the structure at fault. Reproduction of the patient's symptoms is a vital anchor from which to decide aspects of treatment dose. Only when symptoms are produced can the clinician be sure that they are affecting, somehow or other, the structure(s) at fault. For example, the classic test of the length of the upper fibres of trapezius is contralateral lateral flexion and flexion of the cervical spine with the shoulder girdle depressed. If a patient's symptoms are brought on only when this test is accompanied by slight ipsilateral rotation, then it seems reasonable to ignore the classical test and follow the movement that reproduces the patient's symptoms. It may be that this particular patient has some sort of anatomical variation that requires the rotation movement.

Modification, progression and regression of treatment

The continuous monitoring of the patient's subjective and physical asterisks guides the entire treatment and management programme of the patient. The clinician judges the degree of change with treatment and relates this to the expected rate of change from the prognosis, and decides whether or not a treatment needs to be altered in some way. The nature of this alteration can be to modify the technique in some way, to progress or regress the treatment. Regardless of which alteration is made, the clinician makes every effort to determine what effect this alteration has on the patient's subjective and physical asterisks. In order to do this, the clinician alters one aspect of treatment at a time, and reassesses immediately to determine the value of the alteration.

Modification of treatment

The clinician may modify the treatment given to a patient by altering an existing treatment, adding a new treatment or stopping a treatment. At all times the treatment should have the functional goals of the patient in mind. Altering an existing treatment involves altering some aspect of the treatment dose (outlined earlier). The immediate and more long-term effect of the alteration is then evaluated by re-assessment of the subjective and physical asterisks; this process is outlined in Figure 5.10. The clinician then decides whether, overall, the patient is better, the same or worse, relating this to the prognosis. For instance, if a quick improvement was expected but only some improvement occurred, the clinician may progress treatment. If the patient is worse after treatment, the dose may be regressed in some way,

and if the treatment made no difference at all then a more substantial modification may be made. Before discarding a treatment it is worth making sure that it has been fully utilised, as it may be that a much stronger or much weaker treatment dose may be effective.

Progression and regression of treatment

A treatment is progressed or regressed by altering appropriate aspects of the treatment dose in such a way that more treatment, or less treatment, is applied to the tissues.

Prognosis

A full discussion on muscle and tendon injuries and their prognosis is beyond the scope of this text. Muscle rehabilitation following an ACL tear is briefly outlined to highlight the difficulties in obtaining a restoration of muscle function. There is often incomplete recovery of muscle function following joint injury, despite a rehabilitation programme (Ciccotti et al. 1994; Suter & Herzog 2000). A deficit in motor performance (Pfeifer & Banzer 1999), altered EMG activity (Ciccotti et al. 1994), quadriceps strength (Hurley et al. 1994) and muscle power (DeVita et al. 1998) have been found during the first year following an injury or reconstruction of the ACL

Figure 5.10 • Modification, progression and regression of treatment.

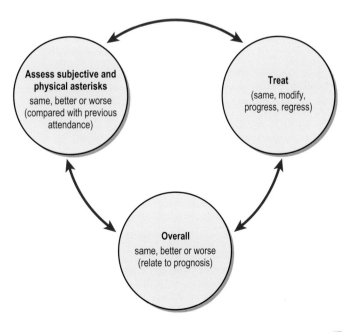

of the knee. Patients who had greater muscle inhibition at the beginning of treatment had a poorer outcome by the end of the year (Hurley et al. 1994). A deficit in muscle strength of up to 20% may continue for 4–9 years (Seto et al. 1988; Natri et al. 1996; Arangio et al. 1997) owing to muscle atrophy (Arangio et al. 1997) and incomplete muscle activation (Suter & Herzog 2000). The consequences of these deficits is unclear; it has been suggested that alterations in muscle activity may alter joint loading and this may, in the long term, lead to osteoarthritis in the joint (Brandt 1997; Felson & Zhang 1998). This is partly supported by the prediction that 50–70% of patients with a rupture of the ACL will develop radiographical signs of osteoarthritis 15–20 years postinjury (Gillquist & Messner 1999). Osteoarthritic changes have been found 14 years (McDaniel & Dameron 1983) and between 2 and 27 years (Walla et al. 1985) after an untreated ACL rupture and were found to be associated with varus deformity and medial meniscectomy (McDaniel & Dameron 1983). This evidence suggests that joint injury will have profound effects on muscles, and restoration of muscle function may take a considerable length of time, and, even then, may be incomplete.

Summary

This chapter has outlined the principles of muscle treatment. Treatment is only a part of the overall management of a patient; the reader is therefore encouraged to go now to Chapter 9, where the principles of management are discussed.

References

Alexander, C.M., Stynes, S., Thomas, A., et al., 2003. Does tape facilitate or inhibit the lower fibres of trapezius? Man. Ther. 8 (1), 37–41.

Alfredson, H., Pietila, T., Jonsson, P., et al., 1998. Heavy load eccentric calf muscle training for the treatment of chronic achilles tendinosis. Am. J. Sports Med. 26, 360–366.

Almekinders, L.C., Gilbert, J.A., 1986. Healing of experimental muscle strains and the effects of nonsteroidal antiinflammatory medication. Am. J. Sports Med. 14 (4), 303–308.

American College of Sports Medicine (ACSM), 1998. Resource manual for guidelines for exercise testing and prescription, third ed. Williams & Wilkins, Baltimore.

Andersen, J.L., Aagaard, P., 2000. Myosin heavy chain IIX overshoot in human skeletal muscle. Muscle Nerve 23 (7), 1095–1104.

Arangio, G.A., Chen, C., Kalady, M., et al., 1997. Thigh muscle size and strength after anterior cruciate ligament reconstruction and rehabilitation. J. Orthop. Sports Phys. Ther. 26 (5), 238–243.

Archambault, J.M., Wiley, J.P., Bray, R.C., 1995. Exercise loading of tendons and the development of overuse injuries, a review of current literature. Sports Med. 20 (2), 77–89.

Arms, S.W., Pope, M.H., Johnson, R.J., et al., 1984. The biomechanics of anterior cruciate ligament rehabilitation and reconstruction. Am. J. Sports Med. 12 (1), 8–18.

Bandy, W.D., Irion, J.M., Briggler, M., 1997. The effect of time and frequency of static stretching on flexibility of the hamstring muscles. Phys. Ther. 77 (10), 1090–1096.

Baratta, R., Solomonow, M., Zhou, B.H., et al., 1988. Muscular coactivation: the role of the antagonist musculature in maintaining knee stability. Am. J. Sports Med. 16 (2), 113–122.

Barcroft, H., Edholm, O.G., 1943. The effect of temperature on blood flow and deep temperature in the human forearm. J. Physiol. 102, 5–20.

Berger, R., 1962. Effect of varied weight training programs on strength. Res. Q. 33 (2), 168–181.

Berger, R.A., 1982. Applied exercise physiology. Lea & Febiger, Philadelphia.

Bobath, B., 1990. Adult hemiplegia: evaluation and treatment, third ed. Butterworth-Heinemann, Oxford.

Borg, G.A.V., 1982. Psychophysical bases of perceived exertion. Med. Sci. Sports Exerc. 14 (5), 377–381.

Braith, R.W., Graves, J.E., Pollock, M.L., et al., 1989. Comparison of 2 vs 3 days/week of variable resistance training during 10- and 18-week programs. Int. J. Sports Med. 10, 450–454.

Brandt, K.D., 1997. Putting some muscle into osteoarthritis. Ann. Intern. Med. 127 (2), 154–156.

Brosseau, L., Pelland, L., Wells, G., et al., 2004. Efficacy of aerobic exercises for osteoarthritis (part II): a meta-analysis. Phys. Ther. Rev. 9, 125–145.

Brown, S.J., Child, R.B., Day, S.H., et al., 1997. Indices of skeletal muscle damage and connective tissue breakdown following eccentric muscle contractions. Eur. J. Appl. Physiol. 75, 369–374.

Bruton, A., 2002. Muscle plasticity: response to training and detraining. Physiotherapy 88 (7), 398–408.

Carr, J.H., Shepherd, R.B., 1998. Neurological rehabilitation, optimizing motor function. Butterworth-Heinemann, Oxford.

Chaitow, L., 2001a. Muscle energy techniques, second ed. Churchill Livingstone, Edinburgh.

Chaitow, L., 2001b. Positional release techniques, second ed. Churchill Livingstone, Edinburgh.

Ciccotti, M.G., Kerlan, R.K., Perry, J., et al., 1994. An electromyographic analysis of the knee during functional activities. II. The anterior cruciate ligament-deficient and -reconstructed profiles. Am. J. Sports Med. 22 (5), 651–658.

Cohen, L.G., Roth, B.J., Wassermann, E.M., et al., 1991.

Magnetic stimulation of the human cerebral cortex, an indicator of reorganization in motor pathways in certain pathological conditions. J. Clin. Neurophysiol. 8 (1), 56–65.

Corbin, C.B., Noble, L., 1980. Flexibility: a major component of physical fitness. J. Phys. Educ. Recreation Dance 51 (6), 23–24, 57–60.

Cowan, S.M., Bennell, K.L., Crossley, K.M., et al., 2002. Physical therapy alters recruitment of the vasti in patellofemoral pain syndrome. Med. Sci. Sports Exerc. 34 (12), 1879–1885.

Craig, K.D., 1999. Emotions and psychobiology. In: Wall, P.D., Melzack, R. (Eds.), Textbook of pain. fourth ed. Churchill Livingstone, Edinburgh, pp. 331–343.

Crossman, E.R.F.W., 1959. A theory of the acquisition of speed-skill. Ergonomics 2, 153–166.

Cyriax, J., 1984. Textbook of orthopaedic medicine, vol. 2. Baillière Tindall, London.

Danneels, L.A., Vanderstraeten, G.G., Cambier, D.C., et al., 2001. Effects of three different training modalities on the cross sectional area of the lumbar multifidus muscle in patients with chronic low back pain. Br. J. Sports Med. 35, 186–191.

DeLateur, B., Lehmann, J.F., Warren, C. G., et al., 1972a. Comparison of effectiveness of isokinetic and isotonic exercise in quadriceps strengthening. Arch. Phys. Med. Rehabil. 53, 60–64.

DeLateur, B., Lehmann, J., Stonebridge, J., et al., 1972b. Isotonic versus isometric exercise: a double-shift transfer-of-training study. Arch. Phys. Med. Rehabil. 53, 212–216.

DeMichele, P.L., Pollock, M.L., Graves, J.E., et al., 1997. Isometric torso rotation strength: effect of training frequency on its development. Arch. Phys. Med. Rehabil. 78, 64–69.

Demirel, H.A., Powers, S.K., Naito, H., et al., 1999. Exercise-induced alterations in skeletal muscle myosin heavy chain phenotype: dose–response relationship. J. Appl. Physiol. 86, 1002–1008.

DeVita, P., Hortobagyi, T., Barrier, J., 1998. Gait biomechanics are not normal after anterior cruciate ligament reconstruction and accelerated rehabilitation. Med. Sci. Sports Exerc. 30 (10), 1481–1488.

deVries, H.A., Housh, T.J., 1994. Physiology of exercise for physical education, athletics and exercise science, fifth ed. Brown & Benchmark, Madison, Wisconsin.

DiNubile, N.A., 1991. Strength training. Clin. Sports Med. 10 (1), 33–62.

Eldred, E., Hagbarth, K.E., 1954. Facilitation and inhibition of gamma efferents by stimulation of certain skin areas. J. Neurophysiol. 17, 59–65.

Enoka, R.M., 1988. Muscle strength and its development: new perspectives. Sports Med. 6, 146–168.

Evans, P., 1980. The healing process at cellular level: a review. Physiotherapy 66 (8), 256–259.

Fanselow, M.S., 1991. The midbrain periaqueductal gray as a coordinator of action in response to fear and anxiety. In: Depaulis, A., Bandler, R. (Eds.), The midbrain periaqueductal gray matter. Plenum Press, New York, pp. 151–173.

Feigenbaum, M.S., Pollock, M.L., 1999. Prescription of resistance training for health and disease. Med. Sci. Sports Exerc. 31 (1), 38–45.

Felson, D.T., Zhang, Y., 1998. An update on the epidemiology of knee and hip osteoarthritis with a view to prevention. Arthritis. Rheum. 41 (8), 1343–1355.

Fields, H.L., Basbaum, A.I., 1999. Central nervous system mechanisms of pain modulation. In: Wall, P.D., Melzack, R. (Eds.), Textbook of pain. fourth ed. Churchill Livingstone, Edinburgh, pp. 309–329.

Fitts, R.H., Widrick, J.J., 1996. Muscle mechanics: adaptations with exercise-training. Exerc. Sport Sci. Rev. 24, 427–473.

Fletcher-Cook, P., 1999. Neurophysiology of movement. In: Hollis, M., Fletcher-Cook, P. (Eds.), Practical exercise therapy. fourth ed. Blackwell Science, Oxford, pp. 189–201.

Friden, J., Sjostrom, M., Ekblom, B., 1983. Myofibrillar damage following intense eccentric exercise in man. Int. J. Sports Med. 4, 170–176.

Garnett, R., Stephens, J.A., 1981. Changes in the recruitment threshold of motor units produced by cutaneous stimulation in man. J. Physiol. (Lond) 311, 463–473.

Garrett, W.E., 1990. Muscle strain injuries: clinical and basic aspects. Med. Sci. Sports Exerc. 22 (4), 436–443.

Garrett, W.E., Rich, F.R., Nikolaou, P.K., et al., 1989. Computed tomography of hamstring muscle strains. Med. Sci. Sports Exerc. 21 (5), 506–514.

Gea, J.G., 1997. Myosin gene expression in the respiratory muscles. Eur. Respir. J. 10, 2404–2410.

Gerhart, K.D., Yezierski, R.P., Giesler, G.J., et al., 1981. Inhibitory receptive fields of primate spinothalamic tract cells. J. Neurophysiol. 46 (6), 1309–1325.

Gillam, G.M., 1981. Effects of frequency of weight training on muscle strength enhancement. J. Sports Med. 21, 432–436.

Gilleard, W., McConnell, J., Parsons, D., 1998. The effect of patellar taping on the onset of vastus medialis obliquus and vastus lateralis muscle activity in persons with patellofemoral pain. Phys. Ther. 78 (1), 25–32.

Gillquist, J., Messner, K., 1999. Anterior cruciate ligament reconstruction and the long term incidence of gonarthrosis. Sports Med. 27 (3), 143–156.

Graves, J.E., Pollock, M.L., Foster, D., et al., 1990. Effect of training frequency and specificity on isometric lumbar extension strength. Spine 15 (6), 504–509.

Gregory, M.A., Deane, M.N., Mars, M., 2003. Ultrastructural changes in untraumatised rabbit skeletal muscle treated with deep transverse friction. Physiotherapy 89 (7), 408–416.

Grimby, G., 1995. Muscle performance and structure in the elderly as studied cross-sectionally and longitudinally. J. Gerontol. 50A (special issue), 17–22.

Hakkinen, K., Newton, R.U., Gordon, S.E., et al., 1998. Changes in muscle morphology, electromyographic activity, and force production characteristics during progressive strength training in young and older men. J. Gerontol. 53A (6), B415–B423.

Haskell, W.L., Lee, I.M., Pate, R.R., et al., 2007. Physical activity and public health: updated recommendation for adults from the American College of Sports Medicine and the American Heart Association.

Med. Sci. Sports Exerc. 39 (8), 1423–1434.

Henry, F.M., 1968. Specificity vs. generality in learning motor skill. In: Brown, R.C., Kenyon, G.S. (Eds.), Classical studies on physical activity. Prentice Hall, New Jersey, pp. 328–331.

Hermansen, L., Wachtlova, M., 1971. Capillary density of skeletal muscle in well-trained and untrained men. J. Appl. Physiol. 30 (6), 860–863.

Hides, J., Richardson, C., Jull, G., et al., 1995. Ultrasound imaging in rehabilitation. Aust. J. Physiother. 41 (3), 187–193.

Hill, A.V., 1938. The heat of shortening and the dynamic constants of muscle. Proc. R. Soc. Lond. (Biology) 126, 136–195.

Hill, A.V., 1950. The series elastic component of muscle. Proc. R. Soc. B137, 273–280.

Hirokawa, S., Solomonow, M., Lu, Y., et al., 1992. Anterior-posterior and rotational displacement of the tibia elicited by quadriceps contraction. Am. J. Sports Med. 20 (3), 299–306.

Hodges, P.W., Richardson, C.A., 1996. Inefficient muscular stabilization of the lumbar spine associated with low back pain. A motor control evaluation of transversus abdominis. Spine 21 (22), 2640–2650.

Holloszy, J.O., 1976. Adaptations of muscular tissue to training. Prog. Cardiovasc. Dis. 18 (6), 445–458.

Honey, P., Mumford, A., 1986. The manual of learning styles. Printique, London.

Hortobagyi, T., Hill, J.P., Houmard, J.A., et al., 1996. Adaptive responses to muscle lengthening and shortening in humans. J. Appl. Physiol. 80 (3), 765–772.

Hortobagyi, T., Dempsey, L., Fraser, D., et al., 2000. Changes in muscle strength, muscle fibre size and myofibrillar gene expression after immobilization and retraining in humans. J. Physiol. 524 (1), 293–304.

Housh, D.J., Housh, T.J., Johnson, G.O., et al., 1992. Hypertrophic response to unilateral concentric isokinetic resistance training. J. Appl. Physiol. 73, 65–70.

Hunter, G., 1998. Specific soft tissue mobilization in the management of soft tissue dysfunction. Man. Ther. 3 (1), 2–11.

Hurley, M.V., Jones, D.W., Newham, D.J., 1994. Arthrogenic quadriceps inhibition and rehabilitation of patients with extensive traumatic knee injuries. Clin. Sci. 86, 305–310.

Hurley, M.V., Walsh, N.E., Mitchell, H.L., et al., 2007. Clinical effectiveness of a rehabilitation program integrating exercise, self-management, and active coping strategies for chronic knee pain: a cluster randomized trial. Arthritis. Rheum. 57 (7), 1211–1219.

Hurme, T., Kalimo, H., Lehto, M., et al., 1991. Healing of skeletal muscle injury: an ultrastructural and immunohistochemical study. Med. Sci. Sports Exerc. 23 (7), 801–810.

Ingjer, F., 1979. Capillary supply and mitochondrial content of different skeletal muscle fiber types in untrained and endurance-trained men. A histochemical and ultrastructural study. Eur. J. Appl. Physiol. Occup. Physiol. 40, 197–209.

Jarvinen, M.J., Lehto, M.U.K., 1993. The effects of early mobilisation and immobilisation on the healing process following muscle injuries. Sports Med. 15 (2), 78–89.

Jayson, M.I.V., Dixon St, A.J., 1970. Intra-articular pressure in rheumatoid arthritis of the knee. III. Pressure changes during joint use. Ann. Rheum. Dis. 29, 401–408.

Jenkins, W.M., Merzenich, M.M., Ochs, M.T., et al., 1990. Functional reorganization of primary somatosensory cortex in adult owl monkeys after behaviorally controlled tactile stimulation. J. Neurophysiol. 63 (1), 82–104.

Jenner, J.R., Stephens, J.A., 1982. Cutaneous reflex responses and their central nervous system pathways studied in man. J. Physiol. (Lond) 333, 405–419.

Jones, D.A., Newham, D.J., Round, J.M., et al., 1986. Experimental human muscle damage: morphological changes in relation to other indices of damage. J. Physiol. 375, 435–448.

Jozsa, L., Kannus, P., 1997. Human tendons: anatomy, physiology and pathology. Human Kinetics, Champaign, Illinois.

Kandel, E.R., 1991. Cellular mechanisms of learning and the biological basis of individuality. In: Kandel, E.R., Schwartz, J.H., Jessell, T.M. (Eds.), Principles of neural science. third ed. Elsevier, New York.

Kanehisa, H., Miyashita, M., 1983. Specificity of velocity in strength training. Eur. J. Appl. Physiol. 52, 104–106.

Kaser, L., Mannion, A.F., Rhyner, A., et al., 2001. Active therapy for chronic low back pain part 2. Effects on paraspinal muscle cross-sectional area, fiber type size, and distribution. Spine 26 (8), 909–919.

Katz, B., 1939. The relation between force and speed in muscular contraction. J. Physiol. 96, 45–64.

Kawakami, Y., Abe, T., Fukunaga, T., 1993. Muscle-fiber pennation angles are greater in hypertrophied than in normal muscles. J. Appl. Physiol. 74 (6), 2740–2744.

Kawakami, Y., Abe, T., Kuno, S.-Y., et al., 1995. Training-induced changes in muscle architecture and specific tension. Eur. J. Appl. Physiol. 72, 37–43.

Kellett, J., 1986. Acute soft tissue injuries – a review of the literature. Med. Sci. Sports Exerc. 18 (5), 489–500.

Kerr, K., 1998. Exercise in rehabilitation. In: Pitt-Brooke, J., Reid, H., Lockwood, J. et al., (Eds.), Rehabilitation of movement, theoretical basis of clinical practice. W B Saunders, London, pp. 423–457.

Kidd, G., Lawes, N., Musa, I., 1992. Understanding neuromuscular plasticity a basis for clinical rehabilitation. Edward Arnold, London.

Kleim, J.A., Jones, T.A., 2008. Principles of experience-dependent neural plasticity: implications for rehabilitation after brain damage. J. Speech Hear. Res. 51, S225–S239.

Knott, M., Voss, D.E., 1968. Proprioceptive neuromuscular facilitation. Harper Row, New York.

Komi, P.V., 1986. Training of muscle strength and power: interaction of neuromotoric, hypertrophic, and mechanical factors. Int. J. Sports Med. 7 (Suppl.), 10–15.

Kornberg, C., Lew, P., 1989. The effect of stretching neural structures on grade one hamstring injuries. J. Orthop. Sports Phys. Ther. 6, 481–487.

Kuraishi, Y., 1990. Neuropeptide-mediated transmission of nociceptive information and its regulation. Novel mechanisms of analgesics. Yakugaku Zasshi 110 (10), 711–726.

Kuraishi, Y., Harada, Y., Aratani, S., et al., 1983. Separate involvement of the spinal noradrenergic and serotonergic systems in morphine analgesia: the differences in mechanical and thermal algesic tests. Brain Res. 273, 245–252.

Kvist, H., Kvist, M., 1980. The operative treatment of chronic calcaneal paratenonitis. J. Bone Joint Surg. 62B (3), 353–357.

LaBan, M.M., 1962. Collagen tissue: implications of its response to stress in vitro. Arch. Phys. Med. Rehabil. 43 (9), 461–466.

Labarque, V.L., Eijnde, B., Van Leemputte, M., 2002. Effect of immobilization and retraining on torque–velocity relationship of human knee flexor and extensor muscles. Eur. J. Appl. Physiol. 86, 251–257.

Leggett, S.H., Graves, J.E., Pollock, M. L., et al., 1991. Quantitative assessment and training of isometric cervical extension strength. Am. J. Sports Med. 19 (6), 653–659.

Lehmann, J.F., DeLateur, B.J., Silverman, D.R., 1966. Selective heating effects of ultrasound in human beings. Arch. Phys. Med. Rehabil. 47, 331–339.

Lehmann, J.F., Masock, A.J., Warren, C.G., et al., 1970. Effect of therapeutic temperature on tendon extensibility. Arch. Phys. Med. Rehabil. 51 (8), 481–487.

Levick, J.R., 1983. Joint pressure–volume studies: their importance, design and interpretation. J. Rheumatol. 10, 353–357.

Liu, J., Wrisberg, C.A., 1997. The effect of knowledge of results delay and the subjective estimation of movement form on the acquisition and retention of a motor skill. Res. Q. Exerc. Sport 68 (2), 145–151.

Louie, J.K., Mote, C.D., 1987. Contribution of the musculature to rotatory laxity and torsional stiffness at the knee. J. Biomech. 20 (3), 281–300.

Lovick, T., 1991. Interactions between descending pathways from the dorsal and ventrolateral periaqueductal gray matter in the rat. In: Depaulis, A.,

Bandler, R. (Eds.), The midbrain periaqueductal gray matter. Plenum Press, New York, pp. 101–120.

Low, J., Reed, A., 1990. Electrotherapy explained, principles and practice. Butterworth-Heinemann, London.

Macdonald, R., 1994. Taping techniques. Butterworth-Heinemann, Oxford.

MacDougall, J.D., 1986. Morphological changes in human skeletal muscle following strength training and immobilization. In: Jones, N.L., McCartney, N., McComas, A.J. (Eds.), Human muscle power. Human Kinetics, Champaign, Illinois, pp. 269–288.

MacDougall, J.D., Elder, G.C.B., Sale, D.G., et al., 1980. Effects of strength training and immobilization on human muscle fibres. Eur. J. Appl. Physiol. 43, 25–34.

Magarey, M.E., 1985. Selection of passive treatment techniques. In: Proceedings of 4th Biennial conference of the Manipulative Therapists' Association of Australia. Brisbane, pp. 298–320.

Magarey, M.E., 1986. Examination and assessment in spinal joint dysfunction. In: Grieve, G.P. (Ed.), Modern manual therapy of the vertebral column. Churchill Livingstone, Edinburgh, pp. 481–497.

Main, C.J., Waddell, G., 1999. Psychological distress. In: Waddell, G. (Ed.), The back pain revolution. Churchill Livingstone, Edinburgh, pp. 173–186.

Maitland, G.D., Banks, K., English, K., et al., 2001. Maitland's vertebral manipulation, sixth ed. Butterworth-Heinemann, Oxford.

Mannion, A.F., Taimela, S., Muntener, M., et al., 2001. Active therapy for chronic low back pain. Part I. Effects on back muscle activation, fatigability, and strength. Spine 26 (8), 897–908.

McArdle, W.D., Katch, F.I., Katch, V.L., 1996. Exercise physiology: energy, nutrition and human performance, fourth ed. Williams & Wilkins, Baltimore.

McCaffery, M., 1979. Nursing the patient in pain. Harper & Row, London.

McComas, A.J., 1996. Skeletal muscle: form and function. Human Kinetics, Champaign, Illinois.

McConnell, J., 2002. Recalcitrant chronic low back and leg pain – a new theory and different approach to management. Man. Ther. 7 (4), 183–192.

McCullagh, P., Caird, J.K., 1990. Correct and learning models and the use of model knowledge of results in the acquisition and retention of a motor skill. J. Hum. Mov. Stud. 18, 107–116.

McDaniel, W.J., Dameron, T.B., 1983. The untreated anterior cruciate ligament rupture. Clin. Orthop. Relat. Res. 172, 158–163.

McDonald, P.V., van Emmerick, R.E.A., Newell, K.M., 1989. The effects of practice on limb kinematics in a throwing task. J. Mot. Behav. 21 (3), 245–264.

Melissa, L., MacDougall, J.D., Tarnopolsky, M.A., et al., 1997. Skeletal muscle adaptations to training under normobaric hypoxic versus normoxic conditions. Med. Sci. Sports Exerc. 29 (2), 238–243.

Melzack, R., 1975. Prolonged relief of pain by brief, intense transcutaneous somatic stimulation. Pain 1, 357–373.

Melzack, R., Wall, P.D., 1965. Pain mechanisms: a new theory. Science 150, 971–979.

Mense, S., Meyer, H., 1985. Different types of slowly conducting afferent units in cat skeletal muscle and tendon. J. Physiol. 363, 403–417.

Millard, J.B., 1961. Effect of high-frequency currents and infra-red rays on the circulation of the lower limb in man. Ann. Phys. Med. 6 (2), 45–66.

Montgomery, H.E., Marshall, R., Hemingway, H., et al., 1998. Human gene for physical performance. Nature 393, 221–222.

Moore, S.P., Marteniuk, R.G., 1986. Kinematic and electromyographic changes that occur as a function of learning a time-constrained aiming task. J. Mot. Behav. 18 (4), 397–426.

Moritani, T., DeVries, H.A., 1979. Neural factors versus hypertrophy in the time course of muscle strength gain. Am. J. Phys. Med. 58 (3), 115–130.

Morrissey, M.C., Harman, E.A., Johnson, M.J., 1995. Resistance training modes: specificity and effectiveness. Med. Sci. Sports Exerc. 27 (5), 648–660.

Mulligan, B.R., 1995. Manual therapy 'nags', 'snags', 'MWM' etc, third ed. Plane View Services, New Zealand.

Narici, M.V., Hoppeler, H., Kayser, B., et al., 1996. Human quadriceps cross-sectional area, torque and neural activation during 6 months strength training. Acta. Physiol. Scand. 157, 175–186.

Natri, A., Jarvinen, M., Latvala, K., et al., 1996. Isokinetic muscle performance after anterior cruciate ligament surgery. Int. J. Sports Med. 17, 223–228.

Nelson, M.E., Rejeski, W.J., Blair, S.N., et al., 2007. Physical activity and public health in older adults: recommendation from the American College of Sports Medicine and the American Heart Association. Med. Sci. Sports Exerc. 39 (8), 1435–1445.

Newham, D.J., 2001. Strength, power and endurance. In: Trew, M., Everett, T. (Eds.), Human movement, fourth ed. Churchill Livingstone, Edinburgh, pp. 105–128.

Newham, D.J., Hurley, M.V., Jones, D.W., 1989. Ligamentous knee injuries and muscle inhibition. J. Orthop. Rheumatol. 2, 163–173.

Niemann, J., Winker, T., Gerling, J., et al., 1991. Changes of slow cortical negative DC-potentials during the acquisition of a complex finger motor task. Exp. Brain Res. 85, 417–422.

Nikolaou, P.K., MacDonald, B.L., Glisson, R.R., et al., 1987. Biomechanical and histological evaluation of muscle after controlled strain injury. Am. J. Sports Med. 15 (1), 9–14.

Norkin, C.C., Levangie, P.K., 1992. Joint structure and function, a comprehensive analysis, second ed. F A Davis, Philadelphia.

O'Neill, D.S., Zheng, D., Anderson, W.K., et al., 1999. Effect of endurance exercise on myosin heavy chain gene regulation in human skeletal muscle. Am. J. Physiol. 276, R414–R419.

Parkkola, R., Kujala, U., Rytokoski, U., 1992. Response of the trunk muscles to training assessed by magnetic resonance imaging and muscle strength. Eur. J. Appl. Physiol. Occup. Physiol. 65, 383–387.

Pascual-Leone, A., Dang, N., Cohen, L.G., et al., 1995. Modulation of muscle responses evoked by transcranial magnetic stimulation during the acquisition of new fine motor skills. J. Neurophysiol. 74 (3), 1037–1045.

Petty, N.J., 2011. Neuromusculoskeletal examination and assessment: a handbook for therapists, fourth ed. Elsevier, Edinburgh.

Pfeifer, K., Banzer, W., 1999. Motor performance in different dynamic tests in knee rehabilitation. Scand. J. Med. Sci. Sports 9, 19–27.

Pollock, M.L., Graves, J.E., Bamman, M.M., et al., 1993. Frequency and volume of resistance training: effect on cervical extension strength. Arch. Phys. Med. Rehabil. 74, 1080–1086.

Quintner, J.L., Cohen, M.L., 1994. Referred pain of peripheral nerve origin: an alternative to the 'myofascial pain' construct. Clin. J. Pain 10 (3), 243–251.

Renstrom, P., Arms, S.W., Stanwyck, T.S., 1986. Strain within the anterior cruciate ligament during hamstring and quadriceps activity. Am. J. Sports Med. 14 (1), 83–87.

Richardson, C., Jull, G., Hodges, P., et al., 1999. Therapeutic exercise for spinal segmental stabilization in low back pain, scientific basis and clinical approach. Churchill Livingstone, Edinburgh.

Rigby, B.J., 1964. The effect of mechanical extension upon the thermal stability of collagen. Biochim. Biophys. Acta. 79 (SC 43008), 634–636.

Rigby, B.J., Hirai, N., Spikes, J.D., et al., 1959. The mechanical properties of rat tail tendon. J. Gen. Physiol. 43, 265–283.

Rohter, F.D., Rochelle, R.H., Hyman, C., 1963. Exercise blood flow changes in the human forearm during physical training. J. Appl. Physiol. 18 (4), 789–793.

Rood, M.S., 1956. Neurophysiological mechanisms utilized in the treatment of neuromuscular dysfunction. Am. J. Occup. Ther. 10 (4), 220–224.

Sady, S.P., Wortman, M., Blanke, D., 1982. Flexibility training: ballistic, static or proprioceptive neuromuscular facilitation? Arch. Phys. Med. Rehabil. 63 (6), 261–263.

Sale, D.G., 1988. Neural adaptation to resistance training. Med. Sci. Sports Exerc. 20 (5), S135–S145.

Sale, D.G., MacDougall, J.D., Upton, A. R.M., et al., 1983. Effect of strength training upon motor neurone excitability in man. Med. Sci. Sports Exerc. 15 (1), 57–62.

Sapega, A.A., Quedenfield, T.C., Moyer, R.A., et al., 1981. Biophysical factors in range-of-motion exercise. Phys. Sportsmed. 9 (12), 57–65.

Schmidt, R.A., Wrisberg, C.A., 2000. Motor learning and performance, a problem-based learning approach, second ed. Human Kinetics, Champaign, Illinois.

Scott, W., Stevens, J., Binder-Macleod, S.A., 2001. Human skeletal muscle fiber type classifications. Phys. Ther. 81 (11), 1810–1816.

Seto, J.L., Orofino, A.S., Morrissey, M.C., et al., 1988. Assessment of quadriceps/hamstring strength, knee ligament stability, functional and sports activity levels five years after anterior cruciate ligament reconstruction. Am. J. Sports Med. 16 (2), 170–180.

Simoneau, J.A., Lortie, G., Boulay, M.R., et al., 1986. Inheritance of human skeletal muscle and anaerobic capacity adaptation to high-intensity intermittent training. Int. J. Sports Med. 7, 167–171.

Sparrow, W.A., Irizarry-Lopez, V.M., 1987. Mechanical efficiency and metabolic cost as measures of learning a novel gross motor task. J. Mot. Behav. 19 (2), 240–264.

Starkey, D.B., Pollock, M.L., Ishida, Y., et al., 1996. Effect of resistance training volume on strength and muscle thickness. Med. Sci. Sports Exerc. 28, 1311–1320.

Staron, R.S., Karapondo, D.L., Kraemer, W.J., et al., 1994. Skeletal muscle adaptations during early phase of heavy-resistance training in men and women. J. Appl. Physiol. 76, 1247–1255.

Sterling, M., Jull, F., Wright, A., 2001. Cervical mobilisation: concurrent effects on pain, sympathetic nervous system activity and motor activity. Man. Ther. 6 (2), 72–81.

Stuart, A., McComas, A.J., Goldspink, G., et al., 1981. Electrophysiologic features of muscle regeneration. Exp. Neurol. 74, 148–159.

Suter, E., Herzog, W., 1997. Extent of muscle inhibition as a function of knee angle. J. Electromyogr. Kinesiol. 7 (2), 123–130.

Suter, E., Herzog, W., 2000. Muscle inhibition and functional deficiencies associated with knee pathologies. In: Herzog, W. (Ed.), Skeletal muscle mechanics, from mechanisms to function. John Wiley, Chichester, pp. 365–376.

Takai, S., Woo, S.L.-Y., Horibe, S., et al., 1991. The effects of frequency and duration of controlled passive mobilization on tendon healing. J. Orthop. Res. 9, 705–713.

Talishev, F.M., Fedina, T.I., 1976. Influence of muscle viscoelastic characteristics on the accuracy of movement control. In: Komi, P.V. (Ed.), Biomechanics V-A. University Park, Baltimore, pp. 124–128.

Taylor, D.C., Dalton, J.D., Seaber, A.V., et al., 1990. Viscoelastic properties of muscle–tendon units the biomechanical effects of stretching. Am. J. Sports Med. 18 (3), 300–309.

Taylor, N.F., Dodd, K.J., Shields, N., et al., 2007. Therapeutic exercise in physiotherapy practice is beneficial: a summary of systematic reviews 2002–2005. Aust. J. Physiother. 53, 7–16.

Terrados, N., Jansson, E., Sylven, C., et al., 1990. Is hypoxia a stimulus for synthesis of oxidative enzymes and myoglobin? J. Appl. Physiol. 68, 2369–2372.

Thomson, A., Skinner, A., Piercy, J., 1991. Tidy's physiotherapy, twelveth ed. Butterworth-Heinemann, Oxford.

Tidball, J.G., 1991. Myotendinous junction injury in relation to junction structure and molecular composition. Exerc. Sport Sci. Rev. 19, 419–445.

Tobin, S., Robinson, G., 2000. The effect of McConnell's vastus lateralis inhibition taping technique on vastus lateralis and vastus medialis obliquus activity. Physiotherapy 86 (4), 173–183.

Todd, J.E., 1990. Conductive education: the continuing challenge. Physiotherapy 76 (1), 13–16.

Tonkonogi, M., Walsh, B., Svensson, M., et al., 2000. Mitochondrial function and antioxidative defence in human muscle: effects of endurance training and oxidative stress. J. Physiol. 528 (2), 379–388.

Travell, J.G., Simons, D.G., 1983. Myofascial pain and dysfunction: the trigger point manual, the upper extremities, vol. 1. Williams & Wilkins, Baltimore.

Travell, J.G., Simons, D.G., 1992. Myofascial pain and dysfunction: the trigger point manual, the lower extremities, vol. 1. Williams & Wilkins, Baltimore.

Vanderhoof, E.R., Imig, C.J., Hines, H. M., 1961. Effect of muscle strength and endurance development on blood flow. J. Appl. Physiol. 16 (5), 873–877.

Vicenzino, B., 2003. Lateral epicondylalgia: a musculoskeletal physiotherapy perspective. Man. Ther. 8 (2), 66–79.

Vicenzino, B., Paungmali, A., Buratowski, S., et al., 2001. Specific manipulative therapy treatment for chronic lateral epicondylalgia produces uniquely characteristic hypoalgesia. Man. Ther. 6 (4), 205–212.

Vicenzino, B., Souvlis, T., Wright, A., 2002. Musculoskeletal pain. In: Strong, J., Unruh, A.M., Wright, A. et al. (Eds.), Pain: a textbook for therapists. Churchill Livingstone, Edinburgh, pp. 327–349.

Vlaeyen, J.W.S., Crombez, G., 1999. Fear of movement/(re)injury, avoidance and pain disability in chronic low back pain patients. Man. Ther. 4 (4), 187–195.

Waddell, G., 1999. Diagnostic triage. In: Waddell, G. (Ed.), The back pain revolution. Churchill Livingstone, Edinburgh, p. 9.

Waddell, G., Main, C.J., 1999. Beliefs about back pain. In: Waddell, G. (Ed.), The back pain revolution. Churchill Livingstone, Edinburgh, pp. 187–202.

Waddington, P.J., 1999. Hollis, M., Fletcher-Cook, P. (Eds.), Practical exercise therapy. Blackwell Scientific, Oxford.

Walla, D.J., Albright, J.P., McAuley, E., et al., 1985. Hamstring control and the unstable anterior cruciate ligament-deficient knee. Am. J. Sports Med. 13 (1), 34–39.

Warren, C.G., Lehmann, J.F., Koblanski, J.N., 1971. Elongation of rat tail tendon: effect of load and temperature. Arch. Phys. Med. Rehabil. 52, 465–474.

Watson, T., 2000. The role of electrotherapy in contemporary physiotherapy practice. Man. Ther. 5 (3), 132–141.

Watson, P., Kendall, N., 2000. Assessing psychological yellow flags. In: Gifford, L. (Ed.), Topical issues in pain. 2. Biopsychosocial assessment and management relationships and pain. CNS, Kestral, pp. 111–129.

Westcott, W.L., 1986. Four key factors in building a strength program. Scholastic Coach 55 (104–105), 123.

Westcott, W.L., Greenberger, K., Milius, D., 1989. Strength-training research: sets and repetitions. Scholastic Coach 58 (98), 100.

Wilmore, J.H., Costill, D.L., 1999. Physiology of sport and exercise, second ed. Human Kinetics, Illinois.

Woo, S., Maynard, J., Butler, D., et al., 1988. Ligament, tendon, and joint capsule insertions to bone. In: Woo, S.L.-Y., Buckwalter, J. (Eds.), Injury and repair of the musculoskeletal soft tissues. American Academy of Orthopaedic Surgeons, Park Ridge, Illinois, pp. 133–166.

Yaksh, T.L., Elde, R.P., 1981. Factors governing release of methionine enkephalin-like immunoreactivity from mesencephalon and spinal cord of the cat in vivo. J. Neurophysiol. 46 (5), 1056–1075.

Young, A., Stokes, M., Round, J.M., et al., 1983. The effect of high-resistance training on the strength and cross-sectional area of the human quadriceps. Eur. J. Clin. Invest. 13, 411–417.

Function and dysfunction of nerve

6

Kieran Barnard   Colette Ridehalgh

CHAPTER CONTENTS

Whilst joint and muscle allow movement through range, in multiple planes and with varying degrees of subtlety, it is nerve which provides the physiological means by which movement can occur. It is important to stress however that nerves do not act in isolation; the function of nerve, joint and muscle is highly interdependent. For a nerve to function optimally, there must be normal functioning of the relevant joints and muscles. Some examples of how nerves, joints and muscles function together may help to highlight this close relationship. Anatomically, nerve tissues are clearly related to joint and

muscle. Sensory nerve endings lie within ligamentous tissue, in extrafusal muscle fibres and in musculotendinous junctions. Peripheral nerves also lie close to muscle and joint; for example, the median nerve at the elbow runs under a fibrous arch of flexor digitorum superficialis, the sciatic nerve sometimes pierces through piriformis and the common peroneal nerve runs around the superior tibiofibular joint.

As well as there being a close anatomical relationship between nerve, joint and muscle, there is a complex physiological relationship. Indeed the true complexity of neural systems in the control and modulation of motor function is yet to be completely understood. Clearly, movement is initiated as a result of the innervation of a muscle by a given motor nerve. This is not the whole story however as the complexity of human movement requires the central nervous system to take advantage of diverse neural pathways, including the exploitation of muscle, cutaneous and joint afferent activity to modulate muscle contraction (Grey et al. 2001).

The stretch reflex, discussed in Chapter 4, is the simplest example of a reflex arc; however, it is now known that group II afferent activity can induce muscle contraction in different muscle groups. For example, in humans, reflexes have been observed from the tibial flexors to the quadriceps (Marchand-Pauvert & Nielsen 2002; Marchand-Pauvert et al. 2005) and from gastrocnemius to the hamstrings (Simonetta-Moreau et al. 1999; Marchand-Pauvert et al. 2005). Furthermore, it is thought that such pathways may also receive significant modulation via descending control systems from the cortex (Chaix et al. 1997;

Marchand-Pauvert et al. 1998, 1999). Similar reflex activity has also been demonstrated when stimulating cutaneous afferents around the foot both electrically (Zehr et al. 1997, 1998) and with von Frey hairs (Fallon et al. 2005). It is thought that these reflex pathways may play an important role in the gait cycle by ensuring appropriate sequential activation of the muscles involved (Zehr & Duysens 2004).

Stimulation of mechanoreceptors around a joint can also elicit a reflex muscular response. Freeman & Wyke (1967) have demonstrated in cats that passive ankle joint movement leads to reflex activation of tibialis anterior and gastrocnemius motor neurones, whilst later studies around the knee reveal that this reflex response may be due to afferent discharge both from the joint capsule (Johansson et al. 1986) and from ligaments (Dyhre-Poulsen & Krogsgaard 2000). It is thought that such reflexes may enhance joint stability via dynamic muscle splinting. Further examples of such reflexes have been observed in the lumbar spine; the supraspinous ligament (Solomonow et al. 1998), facet joint capsule and intervertebral disc (Indahl et al. 1995, 1997) contain mechanoreceptors which, when stimulated, cause a reflex contraction of the multifidus muscle which is thought to improve spinal stability (Solomonow et al. 1998).

These examples clearly illustrate the complexity of the neural systems involved in human movement. To highlight this complexity further, proprioception would suggest that the approach of these systems is coordinated and evidence suggests that the brain uses information collectively from joint, muscle and skin afferents and that isolated information from one of these tissues provides limited information (Gandevia et al. 1983; Moberg 1983; McCloskey et al. 1987; Macefield et al. 1990). Clearly, the nerves are the means by which this information is relayed to the central nervous system. Normal control of movement occurs as a result of incoming sensory information and is integrated at all levels of the nervous system. Automatic and simple reflex movements occur in the spinal cord, postural and balance reactions occur at the level of the brainstem and basal ganglia and more complicated movements are initiated and controlled at the motor/sensory cortices, while the cerebellum controls and coordinates movement (Crow & Haas 2001).

These examples have sought to highlight the complex interdependent nature of nerve with joint and muscle. It seems clear that normal joint and muscle functions are prerequisites for normal nerve function.

Nerve function

This chapter is limited to aspects of nerve function that underpin nerve examination and treatment in patients with neuromusculoskeletal dysfunction. It is anticipated that readers will need to refer to anatomy and physiology textbooks for further information.

The nervous system can be broadly divided into the central nervous system (brain and spinal cord), autonomic nervous system (which will be discussed under nerve movement) and peripheral nervous system (cranial nerves and spinal nerves with their branches).

The following aspects of nerve function will be considered:

- anatomy and physiology of the spinal cord and nerve roots
- tracts of the spinal cord
- anatomy and physiology of peripheral nerves
- biomechanics of peripheral nerves
- movement of the nervous system

Anatomy and physiology of the spinal cord

The human spinal cord extends from the foramen magnum to the conus medullaris around the level of the first lumbar vertebra. From the conus medullaris, the roots of the cauda equina (horse's tail) project inferiorly (Figure 6.1). Three layers of connective tissue, collectively known as the meninges, surround and protect the delicate brain and the spinal cord; they are the dura mater, arachnoid mater and pia mater (Figure 6.2). The pia mater, the innermost meningeal layer, is a thin, highly vascular structure that blends and intimately follows the contours of the underlying brain and spinal cord. Cerebrospinal fluid and larger blood vessels fill the subarachnoid space which lies between the pia mater and the overlying arachnoid mater. The outermost meningeal layer, the dura mater, is a tough fibrous stucture. The subdural space between the arachnoid mater and the dura mater contains no cerebrospinal fluid and few blood vessels. In the cranium the dura mater is continuous with the periosteum. The space between the dura mater of the spinal cord and the vertebral periosteum is known as the epidural space. The epidural space extends to the level of the second

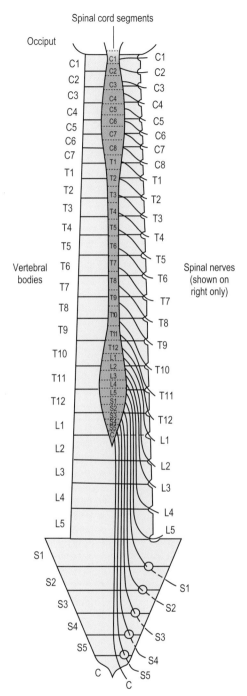

Figure 6.1 • The human spinal cord extending from the occiput to the conus medullaris, from where the roots of the cauda equina project inferiorly (from Oliver & Middleditch 1991, with permission).

sacral vertebra and contains the spinal nerve roots, fat and the epidural venous plexus. The epidural space may be injected with anaesthetic for pain relief or with steroid to reduce inflammation, for example in the conservative treatment of a lumbar disc herniation (Buttermann 2004).

Blood is supplied to the spinal cord segmentally from the aorta and other adjacent arteries, including the vertebral, cervical, intercostal, lumbar and sacral arteries. As a consequence, spinal cord ischaemia may occur in 5–15% of patients undergoing extensive aortic aneurysm surgery (Morishita et al. 2003). Each segmental artery passes through the inteverterbal foramina and divides into the dorsal (posterior) and ventral (anterior) radicular arteries. The ventral radicular arteries supply the anterior spinal artery, which runs in the midline down the ventral aspect of the cord. The anterior artery provides 75% of the cord's vascularity. The dorsal radicular arteries feed the two posterior spinal arteries, which supply the remainder of the cord (Figure 6.3). As well as the arterial system, which envelops the spinal cord from the anterior and posterior arteries, venous drainage occurs via an extensive venous plexus.

Spinal rootlets project from the spinal cord both dorsally and ventrally. These rootlets unite to form the dorsal and ventral roots. The dorsal roots contain sensory fibres whilst the ventral roots contain motor fibres (Figure 6.4). The cell bodies of the ventral nerve axons lie in the grey matter of the ventral horn within the spinal cord whilst the cell bodies of the dorsal axons lie outside the spinal cord in the dorsal root ganglion. The dorsal and ventral roots are enveloped by an extension of the dura mater known as the dural sleeve. The dorsal and ventral roots soon converge to form the roots of the spinal nerves, which contain the sensory and motor nerve fibres responsible for the innervation of a segment of the body. The dural sleeve becomes the epineurium.

The spinal nerve roots descend within the spinal canal by varying amounts and then exit the intervertebral foramina, as shown in Figure 6.1. The nerve roots are named according to the level of the spine from which they emerge. There are eight pairs of cervical roots (the first of which emerges above the level of C1), 12 pairs of thoracic roots, five pairs of lumbar roots, five pairs of sacral roots and one pair of coccygeal roots. The sensory nerve fibres within each nerve root supply a specific segment of skin known as a dermatome (shown in Figure 2.38). Similarly, the motor fibres within each nerve root supply a given muscle (shown in Figure 4.39). Although

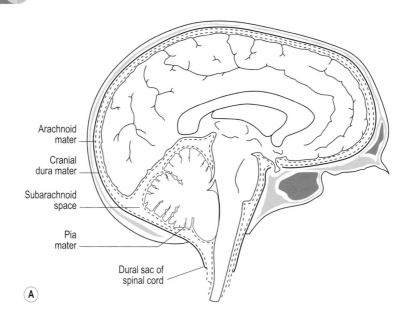

Arachnoid mater

Cranial dura mater

Subarachnoid space

Pia mater

Dural sac of spinal cord

(A)

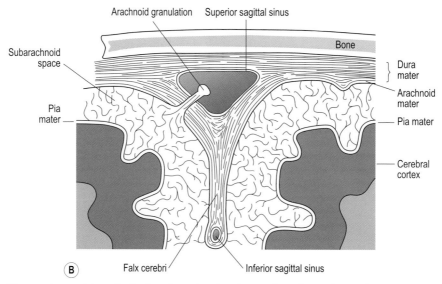

Arachnoid granulation   Superior sagittal sinus

Bone

Subarachnoid space

Dura mater

Arachnoid mater

Pia mater

Pia mater

Cerebral cortex

(B)   Falx cerebri   Inferior sagittal sinus

Figure 6.2 • The meninges. A Longitudinal section, showing the meningeal covering of the brain. B The meningeal covering at the falx cerebri. (From Palastanga et al. 2002, with permission.)

dermatomal and myotomal innervation is not exact as there is some cross-over in the dermatomal fields and muscles are typically supplied by more than one nerve root; clinically, this arrangement can be very useful in determining the site of a lesion. For example, if a patient has some numbness across the anterior aspect of the thigh with some weakness to the quadriceps, a lesion affecting the L3 or L4 nerve roots

is suspected. In addition, an impaired patellar tendon reflex will further implicate these nerve roots as this reflex is supplied by the same segmental levels.

On exiting the intervertebral foramina, the spinal nerve divides into two branches: the dorsal and ventral rami. The dorsal rami supply the zygapophyseal joints, muscles and skin overlying the head, neck and spine. The ventral rami supply the anterior

Figure 6.3 • Arterial blood supply to the spinal cord (from Middleditch & Oliver 2005, with permission).

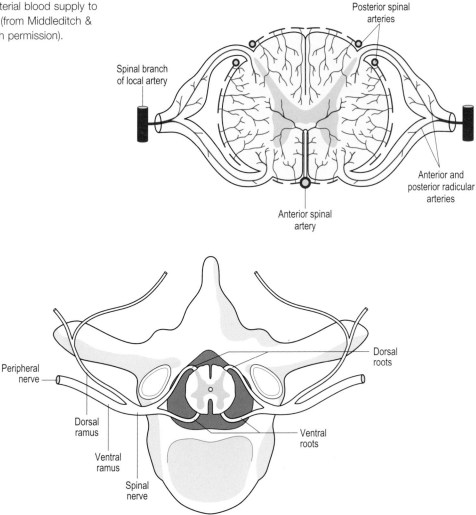

Posterior spinal arteries

Spinal branch of local artery

Anterior and posterior radicular arteries

Anterior spinal artery

Dorsal roots

Peripheral nerve

Dorsal ramus

Ventral ramus

Spinal nerve

Ventral roots

Figure 6.4 • A horizontal cross-section of the spinal cord demonstrating the dorsal and ventral roots (after Palastanga et al. 2002, with permission).

and lateral trunk, and the upper and lower limbs. The ventral rami, which become the peripheral nerves, join in the cervical region to form the cervical and brachial plexi and in the lumbar and sacral regions to form the lumbar, lumbosacral and sacral plexi (Figure 6.5). A branch from the ventral rami together with an autonomic branch from the grey ramus communicans forms the sinuvertebral nerve, which passes into the intervertebral foramen. On entering the canal, the sinuvertebral nerve branches to form a complex neural network that innervates the outer third of the annulus fibrosus, the posterior longitudinal ligament and the dura mater (Adams et al. 2006).

Tracts of the spinal cord

Information is continually relayed to and from the peripheries along a series of well-organised tracts within the white matter of the spinal cord. An ascending nerve signal must however first enter the spinal cord. This occurs via a given axon that enters the dorsal horn and terminates in the grey matter. In cross-section, the grey matter conforms to a pattern of lamination know as Rexed's laminae (Figure 6.6). Anatomically there are 10 identifiable laminae. Aα fibres from muscle spindles and Golgi tendon organs terminate in laminae VI, VII and IX. Aβ fibres from cutaneous mechanoreceptors terminate

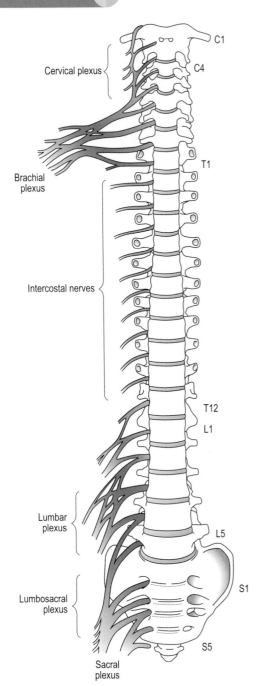

Figure 6.5 • Spinal nerves exit the intervertebral foramina to form the cervical, brachial, lumbar, lumbosacral and sacral plexi (from Palastanga et al. 2002, with permission).

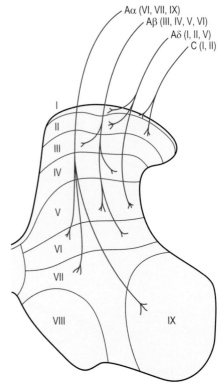

Figure 6.6 • Laminae of Rexed and the termination of afferent fibres (after Todd & Koerber 2006).

one or more synapses to pass into the appropriate ascending tract within the white matter. The ascending signal eventually reaches the thalamus, from where it is projected to the cortex. For a descending nerve signal the converse is true. The signal travels down a descending tract within the white matter before synapsing, passing into the grey matter and exiting the spinal cord via the ventral horn.

Ascending tracts

The distinct tracts which convey ascending and descending information are represented in Figure 6.7. The tracts conveying general sensory and proprioceptive information can be broadly catogorised into three systems: the dorsal column medial lemniscus pathway, the spinothalamic tracts and the spinocerebellar tracts.

- **Dorsal column medial lemniscus pathway** (Figure 6.8A): this pathway comprises a sequence of three orders of neurones which convey light touch, pressure and vibration sensation, and limb and joint position sense to the sensory cortex. The first-order neurone enters the dorsal horn and

in laminae III–VI, Aδ nociceptive fibres terminate in laminae I, II and V, whilst C nociceptive fibres terminate in laminae I and II (Noback et al. 2005). The ascending nerve signal must therefore cross

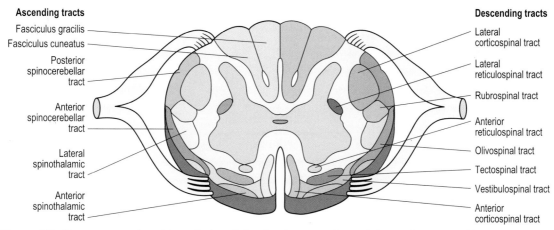

Ascending tracts
- Fasciculus gracilis
- Fasciculus cuneatus
- Posterior spinocerebellar tract
- Anterior spinocerebellar tract
- Lateral spinothalamic tract
- Anterior spinothalamic tract

Descending tracts
- Lateral corticospinal tract
- Lateral reticulospinal tract
- Rubrospinal tract
- Anterior reticulospinal tract
- Olivospinal tract
- Tectospinal tract
- Vestibulospinal tract
- Anterior corticospinal tract

Figure 6.7 • Transverse section of the spinal cord showing the ascending and descending tracts. (From Marieb 1995. Copyright © 1995 by The Benjamin/Cummings Publishing Company, Inc. Reprinted by permission of Pearson Education, Inc.)

terminates in laminae III and IV. The signal then synapses and travels up the second-order neurone in the ipsilateral fasciculus gracilis or cuneatus bundles of the dorsal columns as far as the medulla oblongata. A few nociceptor fibres run in these columns. Fasciculus cuneatus runs as far as the mid-thoracic region and conveys sensation from the upper limb, trunk and neck whilst fasciculus gracilis conveys sensation from the lower limb and lower trunk. At the medulla, the signal passes contralaterally to join the medial lemniscal tract before synapsing in the thalamus. The third-order neurone projects to the cortex.

- **Spinothalamic tracts:** there are two spinothalamic tracts, the lateral and anterior. The lateral spinothalamic tract (Figure 6.8B) conveys pain and temperature, whilst the anterior spinothalamic tract transmits crude touch and pressure information to the sensory cortex. Both tracts again comprise a sequence of three orders of neurones. Approximately half of first-order neurones of the spinothalamic tracts terminate in lamina I whilst the remainder terminate in laminae II–IV and VII–VIII (Noback et al. 2005). Once the signal has passed from the dorsal horn to the contralateral lateral or anterior spinothalamic tract it continues upwards to the thalamus to synapse and onwards to the sensory cortex.
- **Spinocerebellar tracts** (Figure 6.8A): tracts conveying information relating to muscle or tendon stretch to the cerebellum include the anterior and posterior spinocerebellar tracts, although there are a number of other direct

and indirect pathways. First-order neurones destined for the cerebellum via the posterior spinocerebellar tract terminate in laminae VII of the grey matter before synapsing, passing ipsilaterally into the aforementioned tracts and continuing unimpeded to the cerebellum.

The five principal tracts conveying nociceptive information from the spinal cord to the brain include the lateral spinothalamic, spinoreticular, spino-mesencephalic, spinocervical and the dorsal columns. These tracts are described briefly below:

- **Dorsal column medial lemniscus pathway** (Figure 6.8A): this pathway, described above, transmits nociceptive information to the cortex from lamina III and IV.
- **Lateral spinothalamic tract** (Figure 6.8B): this pathway, described above, transmits nociceptive information from laminae I, V, VI and VII. It contains both nociceptive-specific neurones as well as wide-dynamic neurones.
- **Spinoreticular tract** (Figure 6.9): this tract transmits nociceptive information from laminae VII and VIII where the first-order neurones terminate, via the contralateral spinoreticular tract, to the reticular formation; second-order neurones then synapse and the signal continues onwards towards the thalamus and sensory cortex as the spinoreticulothalamic pathway.
- **Spinomesencephalic tract** (Figure 6.9): this tract transmits nociceptive information from lamina I and lamina V where the first-order neurones

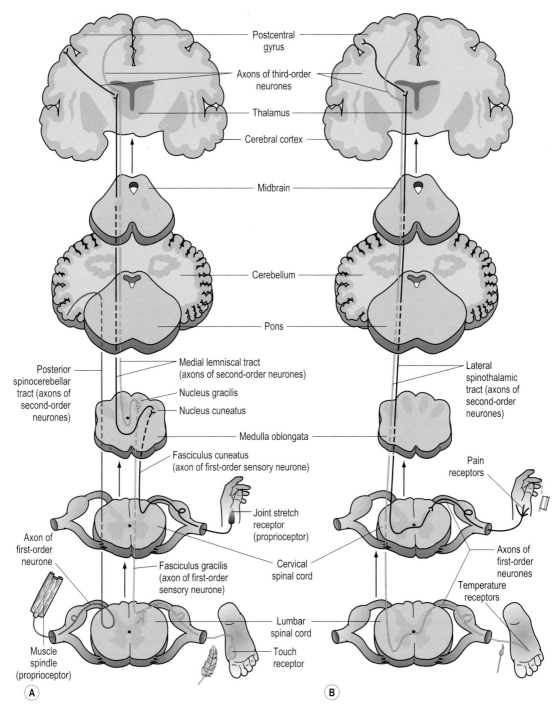

Figure 6.8 • Ascending tracts in the spinal cord. A Dorsal column medial lemniscus pathway and spinocerebellar tract for touch, pressure and proprioception. B Lateral spinothalamic tract for pain, temperature, deep pressure and crude touch. (From Marieb 1995. Copyright © 1995 by The Benjamin/Cummings Publishing Company, Inc. Reprinted by permission of Pearson Education, Inc.)

Figure 6.9 • Ascending pathways transmitting nociceptor information from the dorsal horn via the spinoreticular and spinomesencephalic pathways (from Jessell & Kelly 1991).

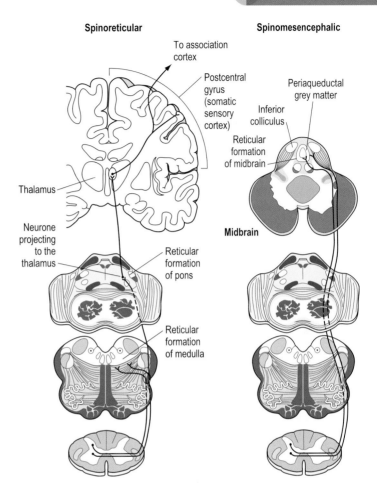

terminate, via the spinomesencephalic tract, the mesencephalic reticular formation, the lateral part of the periaqueductal grey (PAG) region and parts of the midbrain. The PAG is linked to the limbic system via the hypothalamus.

- **Spinocervical tract:** this final ascending tract lies in the upper cervical spine and transmits nociceptive information from laminae III and IV, via the lateral cervical nucleus, to the midbrain and thalamus.

Descending tracts

The descending pathways of the spinal cord which facilitate motor function include the following:

- **Corticospinal (pyramidal) tracts** (Figure 6.10): these are the largest of the descending pathways and comprise the anterior and lateral corticospinal tracts. These tracts originate in the pyramidal cells of the motor cortex and form pyramidal-shaped

enlargements in the medulla. In all, 85% of the nerve fibres cross-over (decussate) at this point. The motor nerve impulses synapse in laminae IV–VII and IX before leaving the anterior horn via a motor neurone to activate the appropriate skeletal muscle. The corticospinal tracts have a specific role in the control of precise and skilled movements. Owing to decussation of the pyramids, damage to one cerebral hemisphere, for example from a cardiovascular accident, leads to paralysis of the contralateral half of the body. Furthermore, disruption to the corticospinal tract leads to hyperreflexia and a positive Babinski sign in which the hallux extends and the toes splay when a sharp object is drawn up the outer border of the foot. A positive Babinski sign is normal in newborn babies but is otherwise a sign of upper motor neurone pathology.

- **Rubrospinal tract** (Figure 6.10): this tract runs from the red nucleus in the midbrain and decends

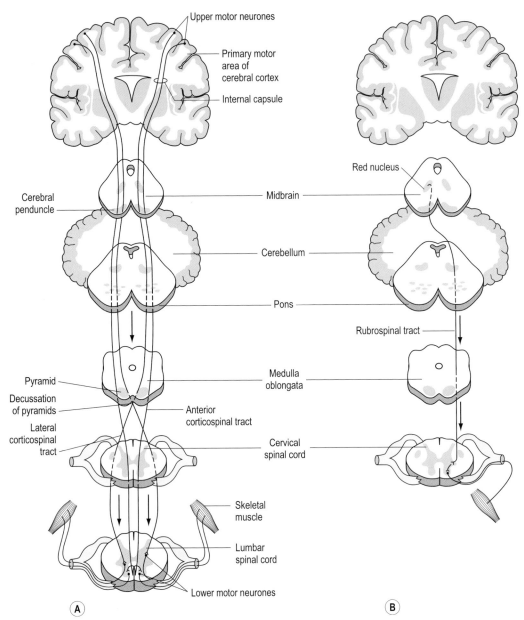

Figure 6.10 • Descending tracts. **A** Lateral and anterior corticospinal tracts activate skeletal muscle, and **B** rubrospinal tract involved in maintaining muscle tone. (From Marieb 1995. Copyright © 1995 by The Benjamin/Cummings Publishing Company, Inc. Reprinted by permission of Pearson Education, Inc.)

contralaterally to the anterior horn where it terminates in laminae V–VII. It maintains muscle tone of mostly distal flexor muscles in the limbs. Interestingly, ablation studies caried out on monkeys during the 1960s by Lawrence and Kuypers (cited in Bear et al. 2006) in which lesions were experimentally induced in both the corticospinal and rubrospinal tracts produced similar results. The monkeys were able to sit upright and stand with normal posture but had lost the ability to activate individual muscles of the arm and hand in a coordinated fashion. It thus seems that these laterally lying tracts are primarily responsible for fine motor control.

• **Vestibulospinal tract:** the vestibulospinal tract originates in the vestibular nuclei of the brainstem and decends mainly ipsilaterally to terminate in laminae VII–IX. It maintains muscle tone and activates limb and trunk extensor muscles, thus aiding posture and balance. This tract receives some modulation from the vestibular nuclei of the cerebellum.

- **Reticulospinal tract:** this tract decends from the reticular formation in the brainstem both ipsilaterally and contralaterally to terminate in laminae VII–IX. It maintains muscle tone and visceral motor function.

- **Tectospinal tract:** the tectospinal tract decends both contralaterally and ipsilaterally from the midbrain to terminate in laminae VII and VIII. This tract transmits motor impulses for coordinated movement of the head and eyes.

Anatomy and physiology of peripheral nerves

Sensory and motor fibres

Peripheral nerves typically consist of sensory and motor nerve fibres surrounded by connective tissue. A typical sensory nerve fibre consists of dendrites at its distal end (peripheral axon), a cell body lying in the dorsal root ganglion in the intervertebral foramen, and a central axon to the dorsal horn in the spinal cord (Figure 6.11A). A typical motor nerve fibre consists of dendrites, a cell body in the ventral horn of the spinal cord and an axon (Figure 6.11B). Each sensory or motor nerve fibre is a single, extremely elongated cell which may run from the spinal cord as far as the toe or finger.

The fascicles (nerve fibres enclosed by the endoneurium; see later in this chapter) do not have a straight course along a nerve; rather, they repeatedly join and divide to form a complex plexus (Figure 6.12). The number of fascicles seen on cross-section of a nerve increases where a nerve crosses a joint, increasing its tensile strength (Sunderland 1990).

Most axons are myelinated, that is, they are surrounded by a myelin sheath; some, however, do not have this covering and are said to be unmyelinated. The myelin sheath is formed by Schwann cells wrapped a number of times around part of an axon (Figure 6.13A). Longitudinally along the axon, gaps occur between the Schwann cells, and these are known as nodes of Ranvier. Impulses travel along the nerve and 'jump' from one node of Ranvier to the next, a process known as saltatory conduction,

which increases the speed of nerve conduction (Rydevik et al. 1989). Unmyelinated nerve fibres are also covered in Schwann cells but they have no myelin sheath (Figure 6.13B). Impulses travel in a continuous manner along an unmyelinated nerve fibre; there is no 'jumping', which reduces the speed of conduction. Large myelinated nerve fibres conduct the sense of touch, pressure, sense of position, temperature and sharp pain, while the small unmyelinated nerve fibres conduct dull diffuse pain (Rydevik et al. 1989).

Peripheral nerve fibres (sensory, motor and autonomic) are classified according to their conduction velocities (Table 6.1). Afferent fibres can be classified in a variety of ways (Palastanga et al. 2002). In this text the following terms only are used:

- $A\alpha$, which is the same as group I afferent
- $A\beta$, which is the same as group II afferent
- $A\delta$, which is the same as group III afferent
- C fibres, which are the same as group IV fibres.

Efferent fibres, that is, motor fibres supplying muscle, can be broadly classified as $A\alpha$ and $A\gamma$ (or fusimotor) fibres, both of which are fast-conducting myelinated fibres (Palastanga et al. 2002).

The sensory nerves end distally in various types of receptor in almost all the tissues of the body. The sensory receptors in joint and muscle have been covered in the relevant chapters on joint and muscle. What remains to be clarified here are the receptors found in skin, which will clearly have relevance for all types of nerve, muscle and joint treatments.

Cutaneous sensory receptors

There is a variety of sensory receptors in the skin (Figure 6.14); these are briefly outlined below:

1. Free nerve endings. These lie in the dermis and at the root of hair follicles. They respond to low-threshold mechanical stimuli such as touch, pressure and temperature, and high-threshold noxious mechanical stimuli; they thus act as nociceptors.

2. Merkel's discs. These lie in the epidermis in hairless skin, particularly the fingertips, and are low-threshold mechanical receptors providing the sense of touch.

3. Meissner's corpuscles. These are surrounded by a fibrous capsule and lie in the dermis. They respond to touch.

4. Krause end bulbs. These are also surrounded by a fibrous capsule and lie in the dermis. They are

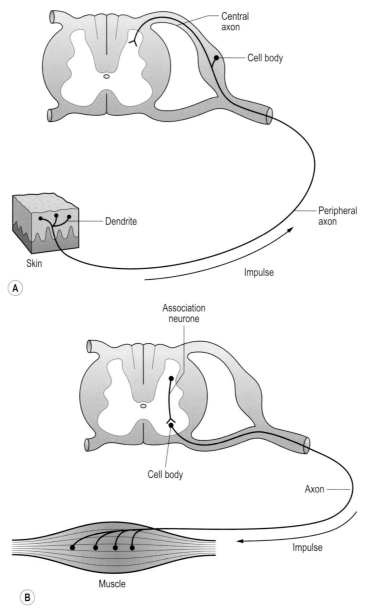

Figure 6.11 • Typical **A** sensory and **B** motor nerve fibres. (After Marieb 1995. Copyright © 1995 by The Benjamin/ Cummings Publishing Company, Inc. Reprinted by permission of Pearson Education, Inc.)

low-threshold mechanical receptors, and so respond to touch.

5. Ruffini corpuscles. These lie within a covering of collagen fibres and lie in the dermis. They respond to pressure.

6. Pacinian corpuscles. These are covered in layers of modified Schwann cells encased in a fibrous capsule. They lie in the dermis and respond to pressure.

Free nerve endings responding to noxious mechanical and thermal stimuli are supplied by fast myelinated Aδ and slow unmyelinated C fibres (Palastanga et al. 2002). All the other skin receptors are supplied by fast-conducting myelinated Aβ fibres (Palastanga et al. 2002).

Normal, age-related change in nerve function occurs by approximately the seventh decade (Schaumburg et al. 1983). The clinical tests manifesting reduced

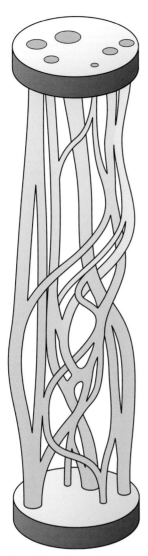

Figure 6.12 • Fascicular plexus within a nerve (from Sunderland 1990, with permission).

nerve function reflect both anatomical and physiological changes. There are degenerative changes in both myelinated and unmyelinated afferent fibres and their receptors, and efferent fibres and their motor endings, as well as a thickening of the connective tissue in the perineurium and endoneurium (Schaumburg et al. 1983). These alterations are reflected in a reduction in sensitivity to touch, two-point discrimination and vibration in the lower limbs, and a slightly elevated pain threshold (Schaumburg et al. 1983). Motor changes include a reduction in tendon reflexes and a reduction in nerve conduction velocity (Kimura 1983). There is also a reduced function of the autonomic nervous system with increasing age (Schaumburg et al. 1983).

Axoplasmic flow

Nerve cells contain axoplasm (synonymous with cytoplasm) which, as in all cells, plays a vital role in cell function. Nerve cells (cell body and axon) can be extremely elongated structures, running, for example, from the lumbar spine to the toe, or from the cervical spine to the finger. Because of these long distances, a special method is required to transport substances from the cell body to the end of the axon and back. This method of transportation is known as axoplasmic flow (Schwartz 1991). Substances transported include proteins, membranous vesicles, neurotransmitters, lipids, mitochondria and RNA (Grafstein & Forman 1980). There are three methods of axonal transport: fast anterograde (forward-moving to the end of the axon, to the periphery), fast retrograde (backward-moving towards the cell body) and slow anterograde axoplasmic flow (Schwartz 1991).

1. Fast anterograde axoplasmic flow transports synaptic vesicles to the terminal of the nerve where they take part in the release of transmitter substances. Axoplasmic flow occurs at a rate of approximately 400 mm/day (Dahlin & Lundborg 1990).

2. Fast retrograde axoplasmic flow transports materials from the end of the axon to the cell body. These materials can be degraded or recycled, or inform the cell body about events at the end of the axon (Bisby 1982; Dahlin & Lundborg 1990). For example, where nerve growth factor is released to stimulate growth of neurones, this is transported back to inform the cell body (Schwartz 1991). The rate of flow is about 200–260 mm/day.

3. Slow anterograde axoplasmic flow is the method by which the majority of axoplasm moves. Fibrous and soluble proteins and enzymes are transported slowly along the axon either at a rate of 0.2–2.5 mm/day or at a slightly faster rate of 0.4–5 mm/day.

Connective tissue covering of peripheral nerves

Nerve fibres are organised into a bundle (or fascicle) by a layer of connective tissue called the endoneurium; this makes up the functional unit of a nerve. The endoneurium surrounding individual nerve fibres is made up of collagen and fibroblasts. The pressure within the endoneurium is slightly more than in the tissues surrounding a nerve (Rydevik et al. 1989). A number of fascicles are surrounded by another

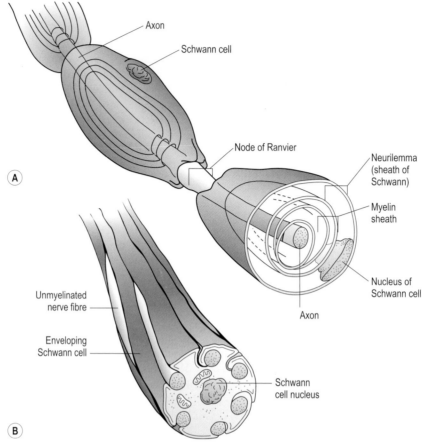

Figure 6.13 • Nerve fibres: A myelinated and B unmyelinated. (From Marieb 1995. Copyright © 1995 by The Benjamin/ Cummings Publishing Company, Inc. Reprinted by permission of Pearson Education, Inc.)

layer of connective tissue called the perineurium. The perineurium acts as a diffusion barrier between the adjacent tissues (Rydevik & Lundborg 1977; Sunderland 1990) and is considered by Sunderland (1990) to be mostly responsible for providing nerve with tensile strength and elasticity. The outermost layer of connective tissue of a peripheral nerve is called the epineurium (Figure 6.15). The epineurium consists of loose connective tissue which helps to protect the nerve during movement. The epineurium rather than the perineurium is considered by Haftek (1970) to be mostly responsible for providing nerve with tensile strength and elasticity.

Blood supply of peripheral nerves

Peripheral nerves are well vascularised (Figure 6.16). Blood vessels running alongside nerves send regional feeding vessels to the epineurium which then divide and supply the deep and superficial layers of the

epineurium, perineurium and endoneurium (Lundborg et al. 1987). The blood vessels are coiled, which allows a certain amount of lengthening to occur without affecting blood flow (Figure 6.17). Vessels lie obliquely in the perineurium, and it is thought that increased endoneurial pressure will therefore close these vessels (Lundborg 1975). This is supported by the fact that a small increase in endoneurial pressure results in a reduction in blood flow within the endoneurium (Lundborg et al. 1983). For example, if a nerve is elongated by more than 8%, the intraneural blood flow is reduced, and at 15% the vessels are completely occluded, causing nerve ischaemia (Lundborg & Rydevik 1973).

Nerve supply of peripheral nerves

The connective tissue sheaths surrounding peripheral nerves are innervated by the nervi nervorum (Figure 6.18) (Hromada 1963; Bove & Light 1995).

Table 6.1 Classification of peripheral nerve fibres (Williams & Warwick 1980)

Characteristics of fibre Type of sheath	Myelinated					Non-myelinated
Fibre diameter	22 μm				1.5 μm	2.0–0.1 μm
Conduction speed (metres/second)	120 60		50 30		4 0.5	
Classification 1. Erlanger and Gasser All fibres	A			B		C
Subclasses: Efferent	Aα Skeletomotor	Aβ Fusimotor collaterals of A fibres	Aγ Fusimotor	B Preganglionic autonomic		C Postganglionic autonomic
Afferent	Aα and smaller. Muscle and tendon; cutaneous			Aβ Cutaneous muscle, visceral, etc.		C Cutaneous muscle, visceral, etc.
2. Lloyd Afferent – skeletal muscle and articular	I (a) Primary spindle ending (b) Tendon ending		II Secondary spindle ending	III Free ending (nociceptor etc.), paciniform ending?		IV Free ending (nociceptor, etc.)

It should be noted that the scale for conduction velocities is not arithmetical.

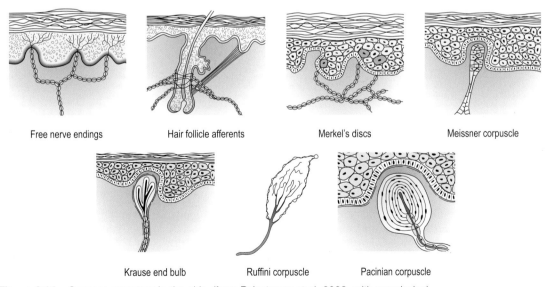

Free nerve endings   Hair follicle afferents   Merkel's discs   Meissner corpuscle

Krause end bulb   Ruffini corpuscle   Pacinian corpuscle

Figure 6.14 • Sensory receptors in the skin (from Palastanga et al. 2002, with permission).

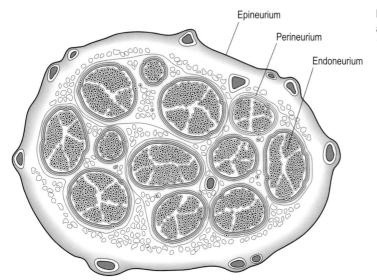

Figure 6.15 • Layers of connective tissue around nerve fibres (after Lundborg et al. 1987, with permission).

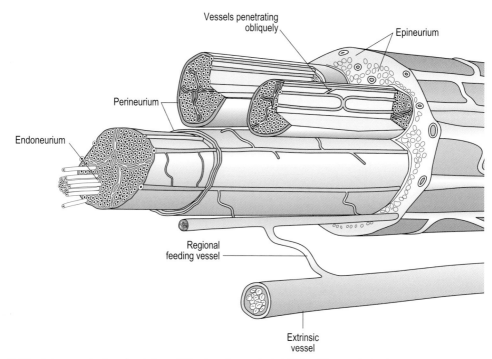

Figure 6.16 • Intraneural microcirculation. (After Lundborg et al. 1987, with permission.)

The epineurium, perineurium and endoneurium contain both free nerve endings and encapsulated endings, and the afferent fibres are mostly unmyelinated C fibres with some thinly myelinated fibres (Hromada 1963). The nerve supply originates from the axons within the sheath and from the blood vessels that supply the nerve (Hromada 1963; Bahns et al. 1986; Bove & Light 1995). The nerve endings respond to high-threshold mechanical stimuli as well as chemical stimuli (capsaicin, bradykinin, hypertonic sodium chloride or potassium chloride) and thermal stimuli, and are therefore considered to have a

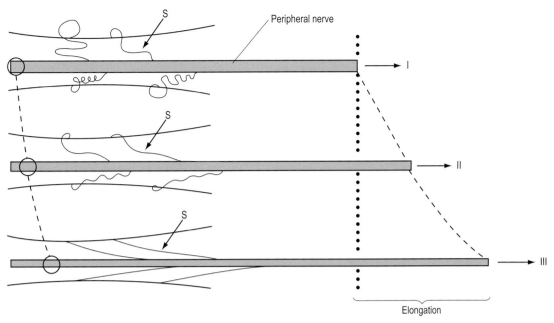

Figure 6.17 • Effect of stretching on the blood supply to the rabbit tibial nerve. Stage I is where the coiled segmental (S) blood vessels are unaffected by nerve lengthening. Stage II is where further increase in nerve lengthening begins to stretch the blood vessels and impair flow. Stage III is where the cross-sectional area of the nerve (circled) is reduced, which further impairs blood flow. (From Rydevik et al. 1989, with permission.)

nociceptive function (Bahns et al. 1986; Bove & Light 1995). The connective tissue of nerve can therefore be a direct source of pain, by mechanical deformation or chemicals released with inflammation.

The epineurium covering the ventral and dorsal roots is also innervated, as are the spinal and sympathetic ganglia (Hromada 1963).

Biomechanics of peripheral nerves

Because peripheral nerves lie on either side of joints they must shorten and lengthen with movement. The connective tissue surrounding nerves contains elastin. This therefore enables nerves to return to a shortened position following lengthening; for example, the median nerve has to shorten by about 15% on elbow flexion (Zoech et al. 1991).

When lengthening occurs, tensile (longitudinal) force is transmitted along the length of a nerve. Nerves have considerable tensile strength to withstand this tensile force. For example, the maximum load that can be sustained by the median nerve ranges from 71 to 218 N, by the ulnar nerve from 63 to 152 N, the medial popliteal nerve from 202 to 329 N, and the lateral popliteal nerve from 116

to 210 N (Sunderland & Bradley 1961). The tensile properties of nerve roots, compared with bone, cartilage, ligament, muscle and tendon, are given in Table 6.2 (Panjabi & White 2001).

Peripheral nerve is viscoelastic and, as such, has a force–displacement (or stress–strain) curve similar to that of other tissues (Sunderland & Bradley 1961). The load–displacement curve is dependent on the rate of lengthening (Sunderland 1990): the faster the lengthening, the greater the resistance. A typical force–displacement curve of a rabbit tibial nerve demonstrates an early toe region (Figure 6.19) where a small force causes a relatively large displacement (Haftek 1970). During the toe region, the undulation of the nerve is straightened out (Haftek 1970), accounting for about 75% of the total change in length (Zoech et al. 1991). Resistance then increases to produce the linear part of the curve until the limit of elasticity is reached. During this phase, all of the nerve, but particularly the epineurium and perineurium, resists the movement until, at the limit of elasticity, the epineurium ruptures (Haftek 1970). Generally this occurs at about 20% elongation, although it can occur as low as 8% (Sunderland & Bradley 1961). Resistance then decreases as elongation continues. Complete

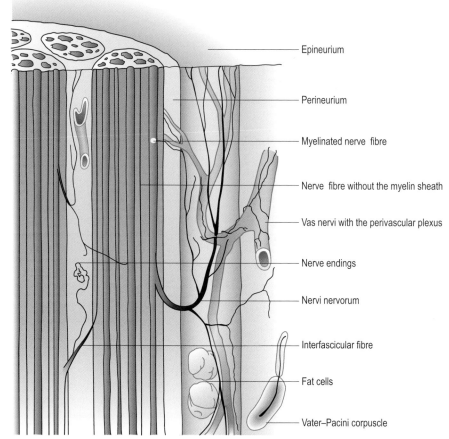

Epineurium

Perineurium

Myelinated nerve fibre

Nerve fibre without the myelin sheath

Vas nervi with the perivascular plexus

Nerve endings

Nervi nervorum

Interfascicular fibre

Fat cells

Vater–Pacini corpuscle

Figure 6.18 • A longitudinal schematic drawing demonstrating the nervi nervorum and nerve endings within the connective tissue sheath of a peripheral nerve. (After Hromada 1963, with permission from the publisher, S. Karger AG, Basel.)

Table 6.2 Tensile properties of nerve roots compared with bone, cartilage, ligament, muscle and tendon (Panjabi & White 2001)

Tissue	Stress at failure (MPa)	Strain at failure (%)
Nerve roots	15	19
Cortical bone	100–200	1–3
Cancellous bone	10	5–7
Cartilage	10–15	80–120
Ligament	10–40	30–45
Muscle (passive)	0.17	60
Tendon	55	9–10

rupture generally occurs at about 30% of elongation, although there is a wide variation between nerves (Sunderland & Bradley 1961).

A stress–strain graph of human median nerve from cadavers is shown in Figure 6.20 (Zoech et al. 1991). It can be seen that there is an increase in stress at quite low strain values. On the graph, the stress is not sufficient to identify the limit of elasticity.

Like all viscoelastic materials, nerve undergoes stress relaxation. A 6% strain held for 1 hour causes a 57% reduction in tension (Wall et al. 1992), an 8% strain held for 30 minutes causes a 50% reduction in tension (Clark et al. 1992) while a 12% strain held for 1 hour causes a 50% reduction in tension (Wall et al. 1992) and a 15% strain held for 30 minutes causes a 40% reduction in tension (Clark et al. 1992). There is no structural damage to the nerve after a 12% strain

Figure 6.19 • Force–displacement curve of the tibial nerve of the albino rabbit (after Haftek 1970, with permission).

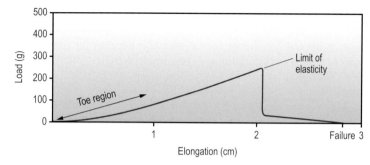

Figure 6.20 • Stress–strain curve of the median nerve at the cubital fossa during elbow extension (after Zoech et al. 1991, with permission).

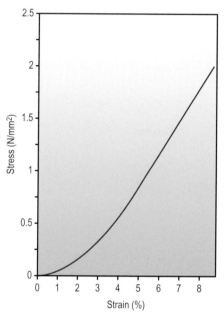

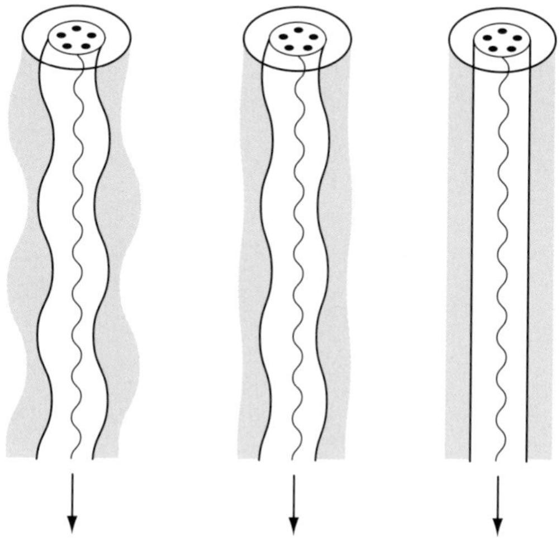

Figure 6.21 • Changes to nerve when it is lengthened (from Sunderland 1990, with permission).

held for 1 hour (Wall et al. 1992), although there could be a change in function if the blood supply to the nerve is affected.

Lengthening a nerve will cause a number of changes: there will be a reduction in the cross-sectional area, increased tension within the nerve, compression of the nerve fibres and a reduction in the microcirculation of nerve (Sunderland 1990).

Whether the resistance to lengthening a nerve is provided mainly by the perineurium (Sunderland 1990) or by the epineurium (Haftek 1970), it seems clear that it is the connective tissue in nerve that resists the lengthening, and not the nerve fibres (Figure 6.21). It can be seen that, under normal physiological lengthening, the nerve fibres remain undulated and thus protected (Sunderland 1990).

The thickness of the epineurium varies between different nerves, and at different parts of the same nerve. Where a nerve requires greater protection there is an increase in the thickness of the epineurium (Sunderland 1978). So, for example, the cross-sectional area of the epineurium of the median nerve in the forearm is about 39% but at the elbow and wrist it is about 60% (Sunderland 1978). The epineurium around the sciatic nerve in the gluteal region is as much as 70–80% (Sunderland 1990). The percentage of epineurium that makes up the cross-sectional area of a nerve varies between 30 and 70% (Sunderland 1990). Nerve roots, on the other hand, exiting from the spinal cord, lack an epineurium and perineurium and are less protected from a traction or compression injury (Sunderland 1990).

Movement of the nervous system

During normal functional movements the nervous system moves as a continuum, as one whole system. For descriptive purposes here, movement of the brain, spinal cord and peripheral nerves will be considered separately.

Movement of the brain

As mentioned previously, three layers of connective tissue, collectively known as the meninges, surround the brain and spinal cord; they are the dura mater, arachnoid mater and pia mater. The dura mater covering the brain is referred to as cerebral dura mater, and that around the spinal cord as spinal dura mater.

The cerebral dura mater is the outermost layer and is attached to the inner aspect of the cranium. Large folds are reflected into the centre of the cranial cavity (Figure 6.22), the largest being the falx cerebri and the tentorium cerebelli (Palastanga et al. 2002). The arachnoid layer contains the subarachnoid space filled with cerebrospinal fluid, which absorbs forces. The pia mater is adherent to the outside of the brain. The dura mater, arachnoid and pia mater in the cranium are all innervated and therefore can be a source of symptoms.

The cranial nerves are covered in connective tissue and lie close to the cerebral dura mater (Williams et al. 1995). Movements of the head are thought to cause sliding, elongation and compression of the dura mater, falx cerebri, tentorium cerebelli and the cranial nerves (Breig 1978; von Piekartz & Bryden 2001). Upper

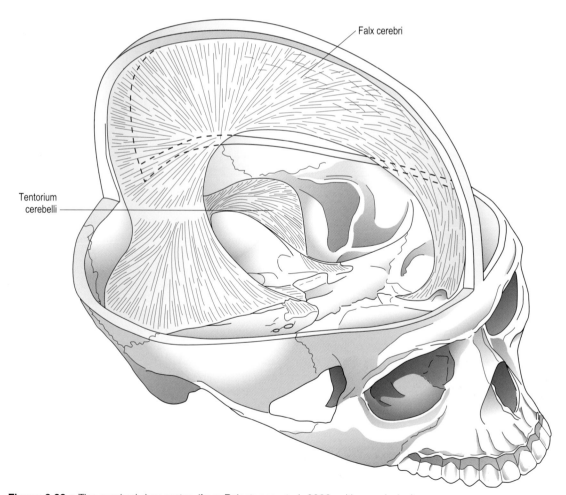

Figure 6.22 • The cerebral dura mater (from Palastanga et al. 2002, with permission).

Figure 6.23 • Effect of cervical flexion on the spinal cord and branches of the mandibular nerve (from von Piekartz & Bryden 2001, with permission).

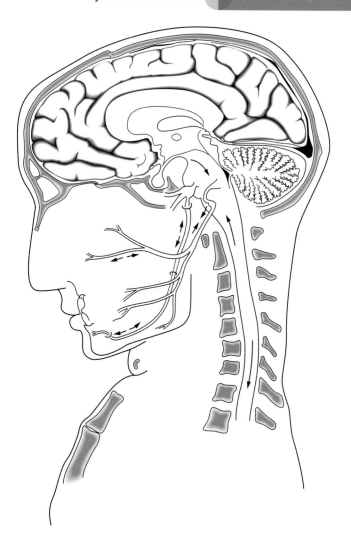

cervical flexion and contralateral lateral flexion have been found to cause 5–7 mm of movement in the trigeminal, hypoglossal, facial and accessory cranial nerves (Breig 1978). Figure 6.23 demonstrates the effect of cervical flexion on the spinal cord and branches of the mandibular nerve.

Movement of the spinal cord

The spinal cord is covered in dura mater, arachnoid mater and pia mater (Figure 6.24). The pia mater is a thin transparent membrane covering the spinal cord; caudally it attaches to the coccyx. The arachnoid contains the subarachnoid space, which is filled with cerebrospinal fluid. Dorsal ligaments link the inner surface of the arachnoid with the spinal cord. The outermost layer of spinal dura mater forms a tube known as the dural theca, which contains the spinal cord. Twenty-one pairs of fibrous denticulate ligaments (or ligamentum denticulatum) lie between the level of the foramen magnum and the T12/L1 level and attach to the pia mater and the dural sac (Figure 6.25). They keep the spinal cord central in the dural theca, and they deform and move during spinal movements (Epstein 1966).

The dura mater is made up of longitudinally arranged collagen and a few elastic fibres, and has great tensile strength. The dura mater is innervated anteriorly by the sinuvertebral nerve, but not posteriorly. The anterior innervation of the dura seems a useful defence mechanism. It lies adjacent to the posterior longitudinal ligament of the spine, which is also innervated, and these two structures form a protective wall between the intervertebral disc and

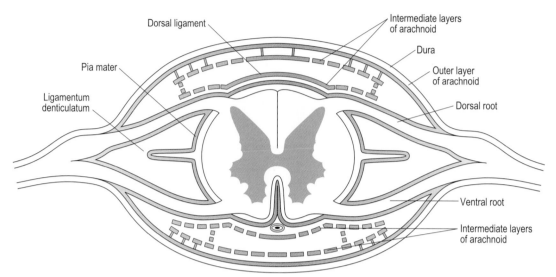

Figure 6.24 • Horizontal cross-section of the spinal cord with the connective tissue layers, dura mater, arachnoid and pia mater (from Williams et al. 1995).

the spinal cord (Figure 6.26). The pia mater and arachnoid are also innervated (Williams et al. 1995). Thus the dura mater, arachnoid and pia mater may transmit nociception and thus be a source of pain.

The autonomic nervous system must also adapt with movement, and of particular interest is the sympathetic trunk that is closely related to the vertebral column (Figure 6.27). It can be seen that the trunk lies anterior to the axis of movement in the cervical region and posterior to the axis in the thoracic and lumbar regions. Consequently, the trunk will be lengthened when the cervical spine is extended and when the thoracic and lumbar regions are flexed. From the anterior view of the vertebral column it can be seen that the trunk lies to one side and will therefore be lengthened on contralateral lateral flexion, that is, the left side of the trunk will be lengthened when the spine laterally flexes to the right. It is perhaps also worth highlighting the close position of the sympathetic trunk to the costotransverse joints; movement at this joint will cause movement of the trunk. The close anatomical arrangement of the pre- and postganglionic axons of the grey and white rami communicans (Figure 6.28) also demonstrates that movements that affect the spinal nerve roots will also affect the sympathetic nervous system.

Cervical flexion in isolation has also been shown to move and tension the spinal dura in the cervical spine in particular, but also in the thoracic and lumbar regions (Breig & Marions 1963; Tencer et al. 1985).

With whole-spine movements, from full extension to full flexion, the spinal canal lengthens by about 5–9 cm (Inman & Saunders 1942; Breig 1978; Louis 1981). The axis of flexion and extension movements lies in the vertebral bodies, which are anterior to the spinal canal. For this reason, during flexion, the posterior wall lengthens more than the anterior wall. During flexion the neuroaxis (all the nervous tissue and meninges in the skull and vertebral canal) elongates and moves anteriorly in the spinal canal (Breig 1978). The movement, however, is not even throughout: little movement occurs at C6, T6 and L4 (Louis 1981). Butler (1991) refers to these regions as 'tension points' (Figure 6.29). Accompanying the increase in length will be an increase in tissue tension (Butler 1991). It should be noted that the neuroaxis moves relative to its meningeal covering: they do not move as one (Louis 1981).

With the reverse movement, from full flexion to full extension, the spinal canal reduces its length and the contents shorten and lie more posteriorly in the spinal canal (Breig 1978). Lateral flexion movements will lengthen the spinal canal on the contralateral side and shorten it on the ipsilateral side; the neuraxis and meningeal coverings will mirror these movements.

Movements of the spine also affect the size of the intervertebral foramen, where the nerve root lies. In the lumbar spine, from a neutral start position, lumbar spine flexion has been found to increase the size

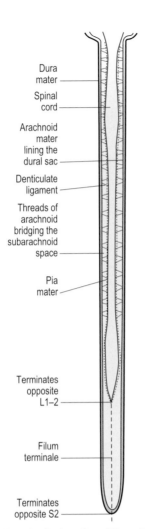

Dura mater

Spinal cord

Arachnoid mater lining the dural sac

Denticulate ligament

Threads of arachnoid bridging the subarachnoid space

Pia mater

Terminates opposite L1–2

Filum terminale

Terminates opposite S2

Figure 6.25 • Longitudinal section of the spinal cord (from Palastanga et al. 2002, with permission).

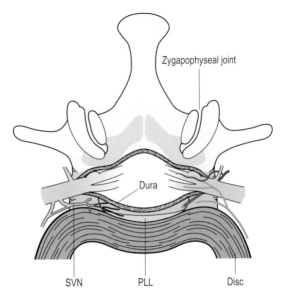

Zygapophyseal joint

Dura

SVN   PLL   Disc

Figure 6.26 • Transverse section of the lumbar spine demonstrating the relationship of the dura mater, posterior longitudinal ligament (PLL) and the intervertebral disc, with sinuvertebral nerve (SVN) (after Bogduk 1997, with permission).

Movement of peripheral nerves

Peripheral nerves are covered with a conjunctiva-like adventitia that allows extraneural gliding with adjacent tissues; there is also gliding between the fascicles (intraneural gliding) (Rempel et al. 1999). There is much data available on peripheral nerve movement. What is provided here are a few examples of the median and ulnar nerve movement. The effects of neurodynamic test movements, as a whole, on peripheral nerve movement are addressed in Chapter 7.

Nerve movement can be measured using magnetic resonance imaging (Greening et al. 1999) and by ultrasound imaging (Hough et al. 2000a, b; Dilley et al. 2001; Greening et al. 2001). Both longitudinal and transverse movements have been measured.

Movement of the fingers causes movement of the median nerve in the forearm and wrist. From full flexion of the index finger to 30° extension at the interphalangeal joints, the median nerve in the forearm moves longitudinally between 1.6 and 4.5 mm (Dilley et al. 2001). Under the flexor retinaculum at the wrist joint, index finger extension causes the median nerve to glide up to 2 mm in an ulnar direction (Nakamichi & Tachibana 1995).

Movement of the wrist also causes movement of the median nerve at the wrist and at the elbow. Wrist

of the intervertebral foramen by 12%, and extension decreases it by 15% (Inufusa et al. 1996). Flexion would therefore reduce compression on the exiting nervous tissue, but would increase its tension, while extension would increase compression, but reduce tension (Adams et al. 2006).

The spinal arachnoid and pia mater are continuous with the perineurium of a peripheral nerve, and the spinal dura mater is continuous with the epineurium of a peripheral nerve (Williams et al. 1995). Thus, the cerebral meninges, spinal meninges, and perineurium and epineurium of peripheral nerves are one continuous structure.

distal movement of the median nerve at the wrist with a reduction in tension and proximal movement of the nerve at the elbow. Shoulder abduction to 110° caused proximal movement and increased tension of the median nerve at both the wrist and elbow. Supination caused proximal movement at both the wrist and elbow, with increased tension at the wrist and reduced tension at the elbow; all changes in movement and tension were small. Pronation caused the median nerve to move distally, with reduced tension at the wrist, and to move proximally with increased tension at the elbow; again, all the changes in movement and tension were small. It should be remembered that these values are based on five cadavers, and greater variation may have been found if a larger number had been used. In addition, cadaveric measurements may be rather different from in vivo measurements. Nevertheless, the study provides useful information about nerve movement and provides support for some of the movements used in the upper-limb neurodynamic tests (ULNT1 and 2a) to increase tension in the median nerve (Butler 2000). Shoulder abduction, wrist extension and finger hyperextension all caused an increased tension in the median nerve, at both the elbow and wrist, and supination caused an increased tension at the wrist.

Summary of nerve function

The central and peripheral nervous systems are anatomically, biomechanically and physiologically linked as part of one whole system. This highly complex system not only produces movement of the body, through the coordinated activation of numerous muscles, but is also adapted to cope with the physical stresses applied to it during these very movements.

Nerve dysfunction

As highlighted at the beginning of this chapter, nerves do not act in isolation as the function of nerve, joint and muscle is highly interdependent. For a nerve to function optimally, there must be normal functioning of the relevant joints and muscles. Conversely, dysfunction of nerve can lead to dysfunction of joints and muscles. Some specific examples which follow may help to highlight how nerve dysfunction will often be accompanied by joint and/or muscle dysfunction.

Nerve dysfunction appears to accelerate joint degeneration. An experimental study on dogs found

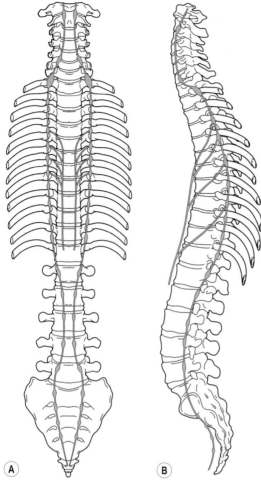

Figure 6.27 • Relationship of the sympathetic trunk and the vertebral column: **A** anterior view and **B** lateral view (from Butler 1991, with permission).

movement from 30° flexion to 30° extension causes the median nerve at the wrist to move approximately 3–5 mm in an ulnar direction (Greening et al. 1999, 2001) and 2 mm in an anterior direction (Greening et al. 2001). With rather more wrist movement, from 55° flexion to 55° extension, the median nerve at the elbow has been found to move distally between 10 and 21 mm (Hough et al. 2000a).

Median nerve movement and tension have been measured in the upper limb in five cadavers (Wright et al. 1996). As might be expected, finger hyperextension and wrist extension caused distal movement and increased tension at the wrist and, to a lesser degree, movement at the elbow (tension at the elbow was not measured). Elbow flexion caused

Figure 6.28 • Cross-section of the spinal cord demonstrating the pre- and postganglionic axons of the white and grey rami communicans (from Palastanga et al. 2002, with permission).

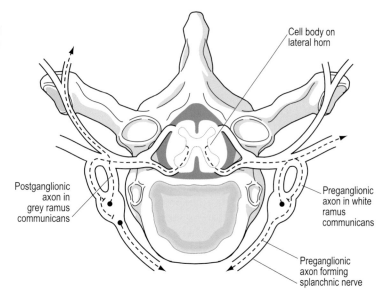

Cell body on lateral horn

Postganglionic axon in grey ramus communicans

Preganglionic axon in white ramus communicans

Preganglionic axon forming splanchnic nerve

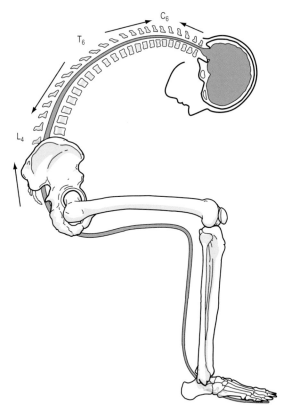

Figure 6.29 • Tension points in the neuroaxis where little movement occurs (from Butler 1991, with permission).

that cutting the joint nerve supply around the knee, combined with rupturing the anterior cruciate ligament, caused severe knee joint degeneration within 3 weeks, while the dogs with only the anterior cruciate ligament cut had no such degeneration (O'Connor et al. 1985; Vilensky et al. 1997).

Compression of nerves, for example the median nerve in the carpal tunnel, can lead to a condition known as carpal tunnel syndrome (CTS), characterised by tingling or numbness in the median nerve distribution of the hand, a perception of swelling of the hand or fingers and possible weakness and atrophy to the muscles of the thenar eminence (Bland 2007). As well as muscle dysfunction, end-of-range wrist movements may be avoided by the patient as these positions increase the carpal tunnel pressure, thus provoking symptoms. Therefore nerve dysfunction in the form of CTS may also lead to joint and muscle dysfunction.

The following aspects of nerve dysfunction will be considered in this section:

- classification of nerve injury
- effect of nerve compression
- reduced nerve movement
- CTS – a clinical example
- effect of nerve stretching
- nerve regeneration and repair
- production of symptoms
- summary of nerve dysfunction.

Classification of nerve injury

As peripheral nerves are made up of sensory, motor and autonomic fibres, any disruption of nerve conduction will produce alterations in sensation, muscle activation and autonomic control. The sensory and motor alterations are tested clinically by the neurological integrity tests of sensation, isometric muscle strength and reflex testing, described in detail in the companion text (Petty 2011). Where there are changes in all three aspects of nerve function, a nerve lesion is suspected (Magee 2002). Where the findings relate to dermatome and myotome patterns, with or without reflex changes, nerve root dysfunction would be suspected. Where the findings implicate a peripheral nerve, this is termed a mononeuropathy; where more than one peripheral nerve is involved, a polyneuropathy.

Altered nerve conduction may be due to structural damage of the nerve, and can be classified into:

- neuropraxia, where there is a temporary interruption of conduction, with or without segmental demyelination, and no structural damage to the axon
- axonotmesis, where there is structural damage to the axon and myelin sheath, but intact connective tissue
- neurotmesis, where there is structural damage to the axon, the myelin sheath and the surrounding connective tissue.

Clinical findings of a neuropraxia, at the level of the nerve root, are most commonly seen in patients with neuromusculoskeletal dysfunction. The signs and symptoms include altered sensation in the relevant dermatome, muscle weakness in the relevant myotomes and diminished reflexes (where relevant).

Clinical findings for an axonotmesis and neurotmesis (Magee 2002) are:

- sensory changes, which include loss or abnormal sensation; the skin may be warm, flushed, scaly (early nerve lesions) or cold, white, thin and shiny (later signs of nerve lesion); loss of skin creases and alterations to nails (Magee 2002)
- motor changes, which include muscle weakness, muscle atrophy, reduced muscle length, reduced joint range of movement and increased stiffness to movement (Magee 2002)
- autonomic function is suggested by abnormalities of temperature, colour and sweating (Scadding 2003).

Effect of nerve compression

Large compressive force may result in major disruption to nerve function. Smaller levels of pressure can however cause ischaemic or mechanical changes to the nerve. Lundborg (2004) suggested that acute compression to nerve can lead to chronic changes due to microenvironmental and fibrotic changes (Figure 6.30). Compression of a normal nerve root or peripheral nerve will initially not cause pain, but may cause numbness, due to nerve ischaemia (Lundborg et al. 1982).

Nerves are susceptible to compression predominantly because of their superficial arrangement, location close to nerve interfaces (e.g. bone or passing through tight tunnels, for example the carpal tunnel), and their response to changes in circulation and alterations in intraneural pressure (Sunderland 1978; Rempel et al. 1999). The effects of such compression will depend on the magnitude and duration of the compression (Rydevik & Lundborg 1977; Dahlin & McLean 1986) and to some extent the make-up of the nerve. For example, a nerve which has fewer, larger fascicles, embedded therefore in less connective tissue, will be more vulnerable to compression than a nerve which has numerous fascicles and therefore more connective tissue (Figure 6.31; Sunderland 1978; Lundborg 2004). In addition certain sections of the same nerve are more vulnerable to compression than others, depending on their location; nerve fibres located on the periphery of the nerve are more susceptible to compressive forces than those in the middle of the nerve (Lundborg 2004).

Nerve can be broadly compressed in one of two ways, either a circumferential pressure or a lateral pressure. As the name suggests, a circumferential pressure is where the compression is applied circumferentially around the nerve, for example with CTS or spinal stenosis. The forces applied to the nerve and the alteration in shape of the nerve are demonstrated in Figure 6.32. The main effect is at the edge of the compressed segment and is referred to as the 'edge effect' (Ochoa et al. 1972).

A lateral pressure is where something presses on the side of a nerve, causing deformation of the nerve – such as a posterolateral disc protrusion compressing an exiting nerve root (Figure 6.33). It can be seen that the site of compression causes the nerve to be lengthened, and will increase nerve tension, if its ends are fixed (Rydevik et al. 1984). It has been speculated that this lengthening of the nerve fibre membrane

Acute effects   Chronic effects

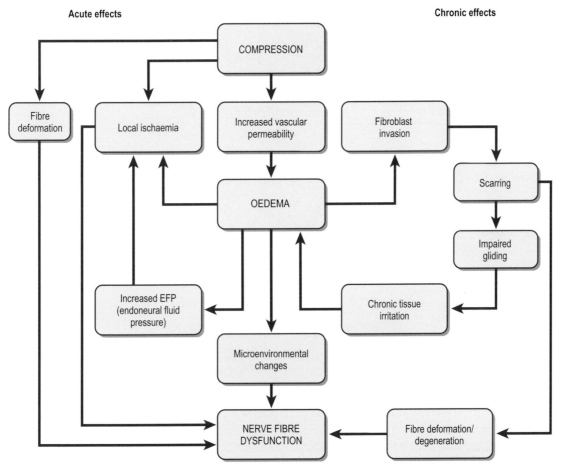

Figure 6.30 • Acute compression of nerve can lead to chronic changes due to microenvironmental and fibrotic change (from Lundborg 2004, with permission).

may alter its permeability and conductivity, which could trigger nociception (Rydevik et al. 1989).

Experimental studies have investigated the effects of compression on animal peripheral nerves. The effects include ischaemia due to mechanical injury to the blood vessels and endoneurial oedema (Lundborg et al. 1983), and direct injury to the nerve fibres (Dyck et al. 1990; Rempel et al. 1999; Rempel & Diao 2004; Topp & Boyd 2006).

The blood vessels within the epineurium of the nerve are the parts most sensitive to compression injuries (Rydevik & Lundborg 1977; Lundborg et al. 1983). Compression injury of the blood vessels results in increased permeability of the vessel walls, with oedema formation within the epineural space (Rydevik & Lundborg 1977). The perineurium provides an important barrier to oedema, protecting the endoneurial space and therefore the nerve fibres

themselves; however, more severe compression can lead to damage of the endoneurial vessels, resulting in oedema within the endoneurium (Rydevik & Lundborg 1977; Rydevik et al. 1981). Interestingly, it appears that the failure of the blood–nerve barrier function of the perineurium is more susceptible to direct trauma from the compression itself rather than ischaemia (Lundborg 1970). It is of importance to note that much higher pressures (above 200 mmHg) are necessary for endoneurial oedema to be present (Rydevijk & Lundborg 1977) compared with 50 mmHg for epineurial oedema, and the authors suggest that this is more to do with endoneurial vessel leakage than failure of the perineurial barrier. Another important response to compression of the vessels is a reduction in blood flow (Ogata & Naito 1986). Pressures as low as 20–30 mmHg can reduce the blood flow to the epineurium (Rydevik et al. 1981); pressures of 80

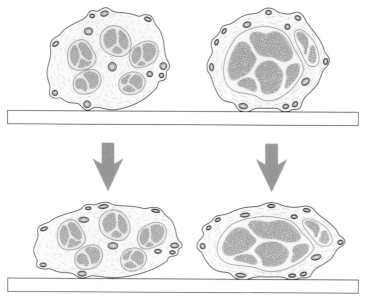

Figure 6.31 • Smaller fascicles within larger amounts of epineurium are less vulnerable than large fascicles in less epineurium (from Lundborg 2004, with permission).

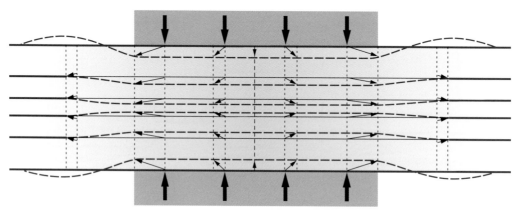

Figure 6.32 • The 'edge effect' whereby a circumferential pressure is applied to a nerve with maximal effect at the edge of the compression (from Rydevik et al. 1984, with permission).

mmHg for over 4 hours are needed to cause endoneurial oedema (Lundborg et al. 1983).

Mechanical injury of nerve fibres reduces the axonal transport (Dahlin & McLean 1986) and causes nerve degeneration and demyelination (Lundborg et al. 1983; Powell & Myers 1986).

Pressure of about 30 mmHg held for 8 hours can cause a reduction in the slow and fast axonal transport systems (Dahlin & McLean 1986). Such changes to the axonal transport systems could result in the distal axon being depleted of certain structures essential for repair and maintenace of the cell structure and transmitter substances needed to allow synaptic function (Lundborg 2004). In addition, retrograde axonal transport is inhibited at pressures as low as 20 mmHg (Lundborg & Dahlin 1992) and this results in the suspension in provision of specific neurotrophic factors to the cell body. A depletion of these factors at the cell body has been suggested to activate the cell death programme in nerve cells (Kandel et al. 2000).

Pressures of 50 mmHg held for 2 minutes (Dyck et al. 1990), 30 mmHg for 2 hours (Powell & Myers 1986) and 80 mmHg for 4 hours (Lundborg et al. 1983) have been shown to cause demyelination of nerve fibres and axonal damage. Fibrosis between the epineurium and adjacent muscles has been observed following a compression injury (Powell &

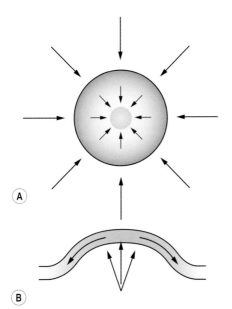

Figure 6.33 • A Circumference pressure, such as spinal stenosis. B Lateral pressure on a nerve – from a prolapsed intervertebral disc, for example – causing nerve deformation. (From Rydevik et al. 1984, with permission.)

Myers 1986); such fibrosis is likely to disrupt the normal movement of nerve through the interface.

Certain nerve fibres appear to be more susceptible to ischaemia and compression. In rabbit common peroneal nerve, C fibres (transmitting pain) were found to be the most resistant to compression, while the large myelinated fibres, Aβ, were found to be the most resistant to ischaemia (Dahlin et al. 1989). However, in contrast to this, Fink & Cairns (1982) found that C fibres showed more resistance to anoxia than Aβ fibres. It is difficult to compare these studies directly due to differences in methodology.

Nerve compression of above 20 mmHg thus causes widespread mechanical and ischaemic changes in nerves, which will alter nerve conduction, nerve movement and normal reparative processes. Such alterations to repair processes and the restriction of neurotrophic factors which in turn appear to be responsible for causing cell death are thought to lead to a condition termed double-crush phenomenon and reversed double-crush phenomenon (Lundborg 1988).

The changes to nerve function described have all been carried out in animal studies in order to establish the levels of pressure and duration of time needed to cause such damage. In vivo, several clinical conditions exist which result in nerve compression and the most commonly found is CTS (Rempel & Diao 2004).

Reduced nerve movement

As previously mentioned, neural mobility in response to limb movement appears to be a normal and desirable phenomenon. Upper-limb neural mobility in response to movement is particularly well documented. Studies examining the median nerve have shown that not only does the nerve move longitudinally in asymptomatic subjects (McLellan & Swash 1976; Hough et al. 2000c; Dilley et al. 2003), but there is also a small amount of transverse gliding of the median nerve beneath the flexor retinaculum during flexion/extension of the wrist (Nakamichi & Tachibana 1995; Greening et al. 1999).

It has been suggested that injury or pathology affecting peripheral neural tissue may lead to a reduced neural compliance (Elvey 1986) and thereby an alteration in the patterns of normal nerve movement. Reduced neural mobility may include an impaired ability of a nerve to lengthen and move relative to adjacent tissues (referred to as the interface). It seems reasonable to suggest that, if there is a restriction in the longitudinal movement, there will be a restriction in interface movements, and vice versa.

CTS provides a useful example of how nerve compression relative to an interface can directly and adversely affect a nerve's physiological and mechanical function.

Carpal tunnel syndrome – a clinical example

The development of signs and symptoms of CTS has been linked to the effects of circumferential nerve compression of the median nerve. Early signs are intermittent paraesthesia and alteration in sensation, particularly at night; this may be due to changes in the intraneural circulation with some oedema accumulating at night and disappearing during the day (Lundborg et al. 1983). Later in the progression of nerve compression there is increased numbness and paraesthesia, impaired dexterity and muscle weakness. These symptoms may be present during the day as well as at night and may be related to altered circulation and the presence of oedema (Fuchs et al. 1991) along with demyelination. Minor mechanical irritation can cause radiating pain (Smyth & Wright 1958; MacNab 1972; Howe et al. 1977; Rydevik et al. 1984). Finally, there is constant pain, atrophy of the thenar muscles and permanent sensory changes; this may be due to a neuropraxia caused by lesions of the myelin sheath of the nerve fibres (Lundborg & Dahlin 1996). Clinical measurement of nerve conduction velocity and latency can be carried out objectively; however, there is a 20% false-negative response in patients with CTS (Spindler & Dellon 1982).

The pressure within the carpal tunnel is generally increased in patients with CTS. Indeed, in a study of intracanal pressure utilising a wick catheter, the carpal tunnels of 15 subjects with CTS were found to be subject to significantly greater mean pressure in neutral (32 mmHg) compared with an asymptomatic population of 12 (2 mmHg: Gelberman et al. 1981). Although the samples studied were small, these differences were statistically significant.

It appears that pressures increase substantially in the carpal tunnel during maximal wrist flexion and extension in both asymptomatic and symptomatic subjects. The aforementioned study by Gelberman et al. (1981) recorded mean flexion pressures of 94 mmHg in symptomatics, compared with 42 mmHg in asymptomatics, and extension pressures of 110 mmHg in symptomatics, compared with 33 mmHg in asymptomatics. Another study has recorded flexion pressures in symptomatics as high as 192 mmHg in flexion and 222.8 mmHg in extension (Okutsu et al. 1989); however, it must be noted that these figures are substantially higher than other similar studies (Szabo & Chidgey 1989; Seradge et al. 1995). Research examining more functional tasks has also demonstrated significant rises in carpal tunnel pressure. Making a fist with the hand, for example, has been shown to increase carpal tunnel pressure from 24 to 234 mmHg (Seradge et al. 1995); this is almost a 10-fold increase. Furthermore, finger and thumb pinch grip has been shown to increase carpal tunnel pressure from 5 to about 50 mmHg (Keir et al. 1998).

Environmental factors may also play a role in the development of CTS. The increasing use of computer keyboards, for example, has been postulated for a rise in CTS (Keir et al. 1999). Keir et al. (1999) found that a marked rise in carpal tunnel pressure occurred during dragging and pointing tasks using a mouse.

Furthermore, patients with CTS who are regularly exposed to hand-held vibration tools have been found to have demyelination and incomplete regeneration of the dorsal interosseous nerve at the wrist (Stromberg et al. 1997). This suggests that, in some patients, CTS may be caused by two mechanisms: nerve compression and nerve vibration (Stromberg et al. 1997).

Experimental compression of nerves in normal subjects provides valuable information on the effect of nerve compression on clinical neurological testing. A catheter inserted into the carpal tunnel allows for controlled and accurate increases in carpal pressure to 30, 40, 50, 60, 70 and 90 mmHg (Lundborg et al. 1982; Gelberman et al. 1983; Szabo et al. 1983). The earliest signs of nerve impairment are the subjective reporting of numbness, tingling or paraesthesia in the distribution of the median nerve (Gelberman et al. 1983; Szabo et al. 1983). At 40–50 mmHg sensation is completely blocked (Gelberman et al. 1983), and in hypertensive subjects with a higher neural arteriole pressure, sensory block occurs at 60–70 mmHg (Szabo et al. 1983). This suggests that patients with raised or lowered blood pressure may respond differently to a given amount of nerve compression (Szabo et al. 1983). At 90 mmHg paraesthesia in the hand was felt after 20 minutes, after 30–50 minutes there was a complete sensory block and after a further 10–30 minutes there was a complete motor block (Lundborg et al. 1982).

Clinically it is useful to be able to test the function of the peripheral nerves in individuals with suspected minor nerve pathology. The most sensitive physical tests of nerve impairment are vibration sensibility (Gelberman et al. 1983; Szabo et al. 1983) using a 256 cycles-per-second tuning fork (Dellon 1980, 1981) or vibrameter (Goldberg & Lindblom 1979; Martina et al. 1998) and pressure testing (Gelberman et al. 1983; Szabo et al. 1983) using von Fry monofilaments (Levin et al. 1978). These sensory changes occurred before any motor changes (Gelberman et al. 1983; Szabo et al. 1983). Conversely another sensory test, two-point discrimination, has been found to be an extremely insensitive measure of nerve compression (Lundborg et al. 1982; Gelberman et al. 1983; Szabo et al. 1983). The sensitivity of vibration sensibility is supported by earlier research which found 72% of patients with symptoms of CTS had abnormal vibration sensibility (Dellon 1978). Vibration sense is more pronounced in the upper limbs than in the lower limbs and there is a decrease in vibration threshold with increasing age (Martina et al. 1998). Because of these variations the comparison of the left and right sides of a patient would seem the most reliable method of determining a difference.

As well as the physiological changes described, reduced median nerve mobility in CTS may further compromise nerve function. Reduced transverse mobility of the median nerve has certainly been observed in subjects with CTS (Nakamichi & Tachibana 1995; Allmann et al. 1997; Erel et al. 2003). Interestingly, however, there is some discrepancy in the literature with reference to longitudinal movement of the median nerve in CTS. Erel et al. (2003) studied the longitudinal excursion of the median nerve using ultrasound imaging in 17 patients with CTS and compared the data with a matched control group. Longitudinal excursion was measured 5–15 cm proximal to the distal wrist crease with the metacarpophalangeal joints extended from 90° of flexion to neutral. There was found to be no significant difference in longitudinal excursion between the control and CTS groups. In contrast, a more recent ultrasound study by Hough et al. (2007) measured longitudinal excursion in 19 patients with CTS and 37 healthy control subjects during elbow extension and flexion. Mean excursion was found to be significantly greater in the control group during elbow extension ($P = 0.013$) but not elbow flexion ($P = 0.089$). Methodological differences are thought to explain the differing results of these two similar studies: Erel et al. (2003) measured nerve excursion during metacarpophalangeal flexion/extension, whereas Hough et al. (2007) measured nerve excursion during elbow flexion/extension. Also, as Erel et al. (2003) collected data proximal to the wrist and Hough et al. (2007) collected data directly at the carpal tunnel, it could be argued that the study by Hough et al. (2007) may represent more accurately what is occurring at the carpal tunnel.

Effect of nerve stretching

Lengthening a nerve beyond its normal resting length can also cause dysfunction of the nerve by both mechanical and ischaemic means. In animal studies increasing strain by as little as 5–10% can reduce the blood flow in a nerve and alter nerve function (Lundborg & Rydevik 1973; Clark et al. 1992). In rats, it has been found that an 8% strain of the sciatic nerve results in a 50% reduction in blood flow to the nerve, which recovers on release of the strain; a 15% strain results in an 80% reduction in blood flow which does not recover on release of the strain (Clark et al.

1992). A similar study found that a stretch of about 16% resulted in complete occlusion of the blood flow in the sciatic nerve (Ogata & Naito 1986).

The nerve injury at the limit of elasticity (Figure 6.19) would correspond to a neuropraxia (temporary interruption of conduction, with or without segmental demyelination, but no structural damage to the axon) or an axonotmesis (structural damage to axon and myelin sheath but intact connective tissue) (Haftek 1970). Beyond the limit of elasticity the injury would correspond to a neurotmesis (structural damage to axon, myelin sheath and surrounding connective tissue) (Haftek 1970). The effects of excessive nerve stretch on one fasciculus are depicted in Figure 6.34.

Clinically it is difficult to consider conditions where excessive nerve lengthening changes occur. During some surgical procedures such as leg-lengthening procedures, care must be taken not to strain excessively the nerve adjacent to the bone that is being lengthened. It has been suggested that neurodynamic tests and techniques could lengthen the nerve beyond normal resting length and therefore

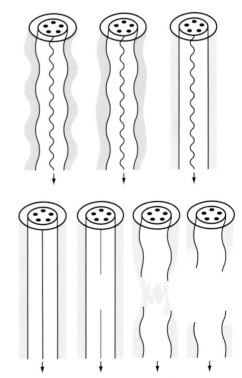

Figure 6.34 • Changes to one fasciculus in a nerve as it is stretched to structural failure (from Sunderland 1990, with permission).

be responsible for changes in nerve function, particularly in individuals with an already-present neuropathy. However there is very little evidence to support this theory. Ridehalgh et al. (2005) found no change to vibration thresholds after the application of the straight-leg raise (SLR) test and treatment using ankle movements in the SLR position thought to load the common peroneal nerve. The subjects used were asymptomatic runners and non-runners. It has been postulated that runners may be more susceptible to changes in nerve function due to the repetitive nature of running (Colak et al. 2005), and therefore this study suggests that SLR does not alter function even in potentially susceptible individuals.

Nerve regeneration and repair

Following nerve injury the distal portion of the nerve undergoes wallerian degeneration. Distal to the site of injury, the Schwann cells proliferate and the myelin and axoplasm disintegrate and are reabsorbed by macrophagic activity. Proximal to the site of injury axons grow a large number of sprouts, which grow at approximately 1 mm/day towards the distal segment. If the Schwann cell columns remain intact the sprouting axons will be guided to reinnervate the target organ. If the Schwann cell columns have been destroyed by the injury then sprouting axons may grow and innervate inappropriate areas, giving a poorer clinical result.

The reinnervation and sensory restoration following a myocutaneous skin flap have been investigated and highlight the clinical outcome of nerve regeneration. Some axons were found to sprout into Schwann cell columns, whereas a number of axons were found to be unmyelinated and associated with blood vessels (Turkof et al. 1993; Terenghi 1995). The degree of sensory restoration varied widely between individuals; some flaps were totally numb while others had moderate sensation (Turkof et al. 1993). From this research it seems that there is a wide variation in the functional regeneration of sensory nerves, from very poor to moderately good.

An additional effect in regeneration of nerve axons occurs at the dorsal horn within 2 weeks of a nerve injury (Doubell & Woolf 1997). C fibres, which synapse in lamina II of the dorsal horn, atrophy and leave vacant synaptic spaces (Figure 6.35). Large myelinated A fibres sprout into these spaces, altering the processing of mechanoreceptor input from A fibres (Woolf et al. 1992; Doubell & Woolf 1997).

The repair process of the connective tissue around nerve is similar to that of ligament. Following a nerve injury, there is an increase in the collagen tissue within the perineurium and endoneurium, indicative of scar formation (Starkweather et al. 1978; Salonen et al. 1985). Additionally, it has been demonstrated in rat sciatic nerves that, 3 weeks after a nerve injury, there is a 28% reduction in nerve length (Clark et al. 1992). Common musculoskeletal injuries may also have an element of nerve damage to them. Ankle sprains commonly affect not only the ligamentous structures but also either the common peroneal nerve or sural nerve (Nitz et al. 1985; Johnston & Howell 1999). This could be either due to the direct inversion sprain causing a sudden increase in length of the nerve or secondary to healing and scar tissue formation of structures close to the nerve. Sunderland (1978) termed these conditions friction fibrosis.

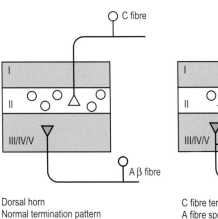

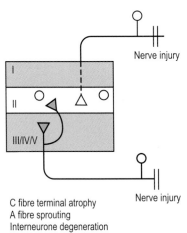

Figure 6.35 • Sprouting of A fibres into lamina II of the dorsal horn to replace atrophied C fibres (from Doubell et al. 1999, with permission).

In such conditions it may be that the nerve loses its ability to slide and glide through its interface (Butler 2000). Another example of restricted interface movement is the adhesion formation between lumbar nerve roots and the intervertebral foramina that can reduce the ability of the nerve to move (Goddard & Reid 1965). This can be caused by local pathological changes or may occur as a result of normal age-related changes (Goddard & Reid 1965).

Production of symptoms

Pain from a peripheral nerve can arise from its innervated connective tissue covering or from the axon itself. Where pain arises from the connective tissue it can be considered similar to pain arising from ligament or muscle, in the sense that nociceptors lying in the tissue can provoke symptoms. The pain coming from the connective tissue is therefore classified in the same way as joint and muscle pain, as mechanical or chemical pain, with chemical pain being further subdivided into inflammatory and ischaemic (Gifford 1998). Pain arising from the axon itself is termed neurogenic pain, and can be subdivided into peripheral or central neurogenic pain. Where pathology causes pain from the nerve, it can be referred to as neuropathic pain. The effects of nerve compression and CTS, discussed earlier, are examples of peripheral neurogenic or neuropathic pain. For further details on pain, the reader is advised to refer to Chapter 8.

Summary of nerve dysfunction

For a nerve to function optimally, there must be normal functioning of the relevant joints and muscles. Conversely, nerve dysfunction may in turn adversely affect joints and muscles. The physiological and mechanical mechanisms leading to nerve dysfunction have been explored. The next chapter discusses nerve treatment.

References

Adams, M.A., Burton, K., Dolan, P., et al., 2006. The biomechanics of back pain, second ed. Churchill Livingstone, Edinburgh.

Allmann, K.H., Horch, R., Uhl, M., et al., 1997. MR imaging of the carpal tunnel. Eur. J. Radiol. 25 (2), 141–145.

Bahns, E., Ernsberger, U., Janig, W., et al., 1986. Discharge properties of mechanosensitive afferents supplying the retroperitoneal space. Pflügers. Arch. 407, 519–525.

Bear, M.F., Connors, B., Paradiso, M., 2006. Neuroscience: exploring the Brain, third ed. Lippincott Williams and Wilkins, New York, pp. 254–255.

Bisby, M.A., 1982. Functions of retrograde axonal transport. Fed. Proc. 41 (7), 2307–2311.

Bland, J.D., 2007. Carpal tunnel syndrome. BMJ 18;335 (7615), 343–346.

Bogduk, N., 1997. Clinical anatomy of the lumbar spine and sacrum, third ed. Churchill Livingstone, New York.

Bove, G.M., Light, A.R., 1995. Unmyelinated nociceptors of rat paraspinal tissues. J. Neurophysiol. 73 (5), 1752–1762.

Breig, A., 1978. Adverse mechanical tension in the central nervous system. Almqvist & Wiksell, Stockholm.

Breig, A., Marions, O., 1963. Biomechanics of the lumbosacral nerve roots. Acta. Radiol. 1, 1141–1160.

Butler, D.S., 1991. Mobilisation of the nervous system. Churchill Livingstone, Melbourne.

Butler, D.S., 2000. The sensitive nervous system. Noigroup, Adelaide.

Buttermann, G.R., 2004. Treatment of lumbar disc herniation: epidural steroid injection compared with discectomy. A prospective, randomized study. J. Bone. Joint. Surg. Am. 86, 670–679.

Chaix, Y., Marque, P., Meunier, S., et al., 1997. Further evidence for non-monosynaptic group I excitation of motoneurones in the human lower limb. Exp. Brain Res. 115, 35–46.

Clark, W.L., Trumble, T.E., Swiontkowski, M.F., et al., 1992. Nerve tension and blood flow in a rat model of immediate and delayed repairs. J. Hand Surg. 17A, 677–687.

Colak, T., Bamaç, B., Gönener, A., et al., 2005. Comparison of nerve conduction velocities of lower extremities between runners and controls. J. Sci. Med. Sport 8 (4), 403–410.

Crow, J.L., Haas, B.M., 2001. The neural control of human movement. In: Trew, M., Everett, T. (Eds.), Human movement, an introductory text, fourth ed. Churchill Livingstone, Edinburgh, p. 69.

Dahlin, L.B., Lundborg, G., 1990. The neurone and its response to peripheral nerve compression. J. Hand Surg. 15B (1), 5–10.

Dahlin, L.B., McLean, W.G., 1986. Effects of graded experimental compression on slow and fast axonal transport in rabbit vagus nerve. J. Neurol. Sci. 72, 19–30.

Dahlin, L.B., Shyu, B.C., Danielsen, N., et al., 1989. Effects of nerve compression or ischaemia on conduction properties of myelinated and non-myelinated nerve fibres. An experimental study in the rabbit common peroneal nerve. Acta. Physiol. Scand. 136, 97–105.

Dellon, A.L., 1978. The moving two-point discrimination test: clinical evaluation of the quickly-adapting fiber/receptor system. J. Hand Surg. 3, 474–481.

Dellon, A.L., 1980. Clinical use of vibratory stimuli to evaluate peripheral nerve injury and compression neuropathy. Plast. Reconstr. Surg. 65 (4), 466–476.

Dellon, A.L., 1981. Evaluation of sensibility and re-education of sensation in the hand. Williams and Wilkins, Baltimore.

Dilley, A., Greening, J., Lynn, B., et al., 2001. The use of cross-correlation analysis between high-frequency ultrasound images to measure longitudinal median nerve movement. Ultrasound Med. Biol. 27 (9), 1211–1218.

Dilley, A., Lynn, B., Greening, J., et al., 2003. Quantitative in vivo studies of median nerve sliding in response to wrist, elbow, shoulder and neck movements. Clin. Biomech. 18 (10), 899–907.

Doubell, T.P., Woolf, C.J., 1997. Growth-associated protein 43 immunoreactivity in the superficial dorsal horn of the rat spinal cord is localized in atrophic C-fiber, and not in sprouted A-fiber, central terminals after peripheral nerve injury. J. Comp. Neurol. 386, 111–118.

Doubell, T.P., Mannion, R.J., Woolf, C.J., 1999. The dorsal horn: state-dependent sensory processing, plasticity and the generation of pain. In: Wall, P.D., Melzack, R. (Eds.), Textbook of pain, fourth ed. Churchill Livingstone, Edinburgh, pp. 165–181.

Dyck, P.J., Lais, A.C., Giannini, C., et al., 1990. Structural alterations of nerve during cuff compression. Proc. Natl. Acad. Sci. USA 87, 9828–9832.

Dyhre-Poulsen, P., Krogsgaard, M.R., 2000. Muscular reflexes elicited by electrical stimulation of the anterior cruciate ligament in humans. J. Appl. Physiol. 89, 2191–2195.

Elvey, R.L., 1986. Treatment of arm pain associated with abnormal brachial plexus tension. Aust. J. Physiother. 32, 224–229.

Epstein, B.S., 1966. An anatomic, myelographic and cinemyelographic study of the dentate ligaments. Am. J. Roentgenol. Radium Ther. Nucl. Med. 98 (3), 704–712.

Erel, E., Dilley, A., Greening, J., et al., 2003. Longitudinal sliding of the median nerve in patients with carpal tunnel syndrome. J. Hand Surg. [Br] 28 (5), 439–443.

Fallon, J.B., Bent, L.R., McNulty, P.A., et al., 2005. Evidence for strong synaptic coupling between single tactile afferents from the sole of the foot and motoneurons supplying leg muscles. J. Neurophysiol. 94, 3795–3804.

Fink, B.R., Cairns, A.M., 1982. A bioenergetic basis for peripheral nerve fiber dissociation. Pain 12 (4), 307–317.

Freeman, M.A.R., Wyke, B., 1967. Articular reflexes at the ankle joint: an electromyographic study of normal and abnormal influences of ankle joint mechanoreceptors upon reflex activity in the leg muscles. Br. J. Surg. 54 (12), 990–1001.

Fuchs, P.C., Nathan, P.A., Myers, L.D., 1991. Synovial histology in carpal tunnel syndrome. J. Hand Surg. 16A (4), 753–758.

Gandevia, S.C., Hall, L.A., McCloskey, D.I., et al., 1983. Proprioceptive sensation at the terminal joint of the middle finger. J. Physiol. (Lond) 335, 507–515.

Gelberman, R.H., Hergenroeder, P.T., Hargens, A.R., et al., 1981. The carpal tunnel syndrome. A study of carpal canal pressures. J. Bone Joint. Surg. Am. 63 (3), 380–383.

Gelberman, R.H., Szabo, R.M., Williamson, R.V., et al., 1983. Sensibility testing in peripheral-nerve compression syndromes, an experimental study in humans. J. Bone Joint. Surg. 65A (5), 632–638.

Gifford, L., 1998. Pain. In: Pitt-Brooke, J., Reid, H., Lockwood, J. et al. (Eds.), Rehabilitation of movement, theoretical basis of clinical practice. W B Saunders, London, pp. 196–232.

Goddard, M.D., Reid, J.D., 1965. Movements induced by straight leg raising in the lumbo-sacral roots, nerves and plexus, and in the intrapelvic section of the sciatic nerve. J. Neurol. Neurosurg. Psychiatry 28, 12–18.

Goldberg, J.M., Lindblom, U., 1979. Standardised method of determining vibratory perception thresholds for diagnosis and screening in neurological investigation. J. Neurol. Neurosurg. Psychiatry 42, 793–803.

Grafstein, B., Forman, D.S., 1980. Intracellular transport in neurons. Physiol. Rev. 60 (4), 1167–1283.

Greening, J., Smart, S., Leary, R., et al., 1999. Reduced movement of median nerve in carpal tunnel during wrist flexion in patients with non-specific arm pain. Lancet 354, 217–218.

Greening, J., Lynn, B., Leary, R., et al., 2001. The use of ultrasound imaging to demonstrate reduced movement of the median nerve during wrist flexion in patients with non-specific arm pain. J. Hand Surg. 26B (5), 401–406.

Grey, M.J., Ladouceur, M., Andersen, J.B., et al., 2001. Group II muscle afferents probably contribute to the medium latency soleus stretch reflex during walking in humans. J. Physiol. 534, 925–933.

Haftek, J., 1970. Stretch injury of peripheral nerve, acute effects of stretching on rabbit nerve. J. Bone Joint. Surg. 52B (2), 354–365.

Hough, A., Moore, A., Jones, M., 2000a. Doppler ultrasound measurement of median nerve motion. International Federation of Orthopaedic Manipulative Therapists 7th Scientific Conference Proceedings Abstract 62, p. 56.

Hough, A.D., Moore, A.P., Jones, M.P., 2000b. Peripheral nerve motion measurement with spectral Doppler sonography: a reliability study. J. Hand Surg. 25B (6), 585–589.

Hough, A.D., Moore, A.P., Jones, M.P., 2000c. Measuring longitudinal nerve motion using ultrasonography. Man. Ther. 5 (3), 173–180.

Hough, A.D., Moore, A.P., Jones, M.P., 2007. Reduced longitudinal excursion of the median nerve in carpal tunnel syndrome. Arch. Phys. Med. Rehabil. 88 (5), 569–576.

Howe, J.F., Loeser, J.D., Calvin, W.H., 1977. Mechanosensitivity of dorsal root ganglia and chronically injured axons: a physiological basis for the radicular pain of nerve root compression. Pain 3, 25–41.

Hromada, J., 1963. On the nerve supply of the connective tissue of some peripheral nervous system components. Acta. Anat. (Basel) 55, 343–351.

Indahl, A., Kaigle, A., Reikeras, O., et al., 1995. Electromyographic response of the porcine multifidus musculature after nerve stimulation. Spine 20 (24), 2652–2658.

Indahl, A., Kaigle, A.M., Reikeras, O., et al., 1997. Interaction between the porcine lumbar intervertebral disc, zygapophysial joints, and paraspinal muscles. Spine 22 (24), 2834–2840.

Inman, V.T., Saunders, J.B., 1942. The clinico-anatomical aspects of the lumbosacral region. Radiology 38, 669–678.

Inufusa, A., An, H.S., Lim, T.-H., et al., 1996. Anatomic changes of the spinal canal and intervertebral foramen associated with flexion–extension movement. Spine 21 (21), 2412–2420.

Jessell, T.M., Kelly, D.D., 1991. Pain and analgesia. In: Kandel, E.R., Schwartz, J.H., Jessell, T.M. (Eds.), Principles of neural science, third ed. Elsevier, New York, pp. 385–399.

Johansson, H., Sjolander, P., Sojka, P., 1986. Actions on gamma-motoneurones elicited by electrical stimulation of joint afferent fibres in the hind limb of the cat. J. Physiol. 375, 137–152.

Johnston, E.C., Howell, S.J., 1999. Tension neuropathy of the superficial peroneal nerve: associated conditions and results of release. Foot Ankle Int. 20 (9), 576–582.

Kandel, E.R., Schwarz, J.H., Jessel, T.M., 2000. Principles of Neural Science fourth ed. McGraw- Hill, New York.

Keir, P.J., Bach, J.M., Rempel, D.M., 1998. Fingertip loading and carpal tunnel pressure: differences between a pinching and a pressing task. J. Orthop. Res. 16 (1), 112–115.

Keir, P.J., Bach, J.M., Rempel, D., 1999. Effects of computer mouse design and task on carpal tunnel pressure. Ergonomics 42 (10), 1350–1360.

Kimura, J., 1983. Electrodiagnosis in diseases of nerve and muscle: principles and practice. F A Davies, Philadelphia.

Levin, S., Pearsell, G., Ruderman, R.J., 1978. Von Frey's method of measuring pressure sensibility in the hand: an engineering analysis of the Weinstein–Semmes pressure aesthesiometer. J. Hand Surg. 3, 211–216.

Louis, R., 1981. Vertebroradicular and vertebromedullar dynamics. Anatomica Clinica 3, 1–11.

Lundborg, G., 1970. Ischaemic nerve injury. Scand. J. Plast. Reconstr. Surg (Suppl 6).

Lundborg, G., 1975. Structure and function of the intraneural microvessels as related to trauma, edema formation, and nerve function. J. Bone Joint. Surg. 57A, 938–948.

Lundborg, G., 1988. Intraneural Microcirculation Orthopaedic Clinics of North America 19 (1), 1–12.

Lundborg, G., 2004. Nerve injury and repair, Regeneration, recontruction and cortical remodelling, second ed. Churchill Livingstone, Edinburgh.

Lundborg, G., Dahlin, L.B., 1992. The pathophysiology of nerve compression. Hand Clin. 8 (2), 215–227.

Lundborg, G., Dahlin, L.B., 1996. Anatomy, function, and pathophysiology of peripheral nerves and nerve compression. Hand Clin. 12 (2), 185–193.

Lundborg, G., Rydevik, B., 1973. Effects of stretching the tibial nerve of the rabbit. A preliminary study of the intraneural circulation and the barrier function of the perineurium. J. Bone Joint. Surg. 55B (2), 390–401.

Lundborg, G., Gelbermann, R.H., Minteer-Convery, M., et al., 1982. Median nerve compression in the carpal tunnel: functional response to experimentally induced controlled pressure. J. Hand Surg. 7 (3), 252–259.

Lundborg, G., Myers, R., Powell, H., 1983. Nerve compression injury and increased endoneurial fluid pressure: a 'miniature compartment syndrome'. J. Neurol. Neurosurg. Psychiatry 46, 1119–1124.

Lundborg, G., Rydevik, B., Manthorpe, M., et al., 1987. Peripheral nerve: the physiology of injury and repair. In: Woo, S.L.-Y., Buckwalter, J.A. (Eds.), Injury and repair of the musculoskeletal soft tissues. American Academy of Orthopaedic Surgeons, Park Ridge, Illinois, pp. 295–352.

Macefield, G., Gandevia, S.C., Burke, D., 1990. Perceptual responses to microstimulation of single afferents innervating joints, muscles and skin of the human hand. J. Physiol. (Lond) 429, 113–129.

MacNab, I., 1972. The mechanism of spondylogenic pain. In: Hirsch, C., Zotterman, Y. (Eds.), Cervical pain. Pergamon Press, Oxford, pp. 89–95.

Magee, D.J., 2002. Orthopaedic physical assessment, fourth ed. Saunders, Philadelphia.

Marchand-Pauvert, V., Nielsen, J.B., 2002. Modulation of non-monosynaptic excitation from ankle dorsiflexor afferents to quadriceps motoneurones during human gait. J. Physiol. 538, 647–657.

Marchand-Pauvert, V., Pierrot-Deseilligny, E., Rothwell, J.C., 1998. Role of spinal premotoneurones in mediating corticospinal input to forearm motoneurones in man. J. Physiol. 508, 301–312.

Marchand-Pauvert, V., Simonetta-Moreau, M., Pierrot-Deseilligny, E., 1999. Cortical control of spinal pathways mediating group II excitation to human thigh motoneurones. J. Physiol. 517, 301–313.

Marchand-Pauvert, V., Nicolas, G., Marque, P., et al., 2005. Increase in group II excitation from ankle muscles to thigh motoneurones during human standing. J. Physiol. 566, 257–271.

Marieb, E.N., 1995. Human anatomy and physiology, third ed. Benjamin/Cummings, San Francisco, California.

Martina, I.S.J., van Koningsveld, R., Schmitz, P.I.M., et al., 1998. Measuring vibration threshold with a graduated tuning fork in normal aging and in patients with polyneuropathy. J. Neurol. Neurosurg. Psychiatry 65, 743–747.

McCloskey, D.I., Macefield, G., Gandevia, S.C., et al., 1987. Sensing position and movements of the fingers. News Physiol. Sci. 2, 226–230.

McLellan, D.L., Swash, M., 1976. Longitudinal sliding of the median nerve during movements of the upper limb. J. Neurol. Neurosurg. Psychiatry 39 (6), 566–570.

Middleditch, A., Oliver, J., 2005. Functional anatomy of the spine, second ed. Butterworth Heinemann, Edinburgh.

Moberg, E., 1983. The role of cutaneous afferents in position sense, kinaesthesia, and motor function of the hand. Brain 106, 1–19.

Morishita, K., Murakami, G., Fujisawa, Y., et al., 2003. Anatomical study of blood supply to the spinal cord. Ann. Thorac. Surg. 76 (6), 1967–1971.

Nakamichi, K., Tachibana, S., 1995. Restricted motion of the median nerve in carpal tunnel syndrome. J. Hand Surg. 20B (4), 460–464.

Nitz, A.J., Dobner, J.J., Kersey, D., 1985. Nerve injury and grades II and III ankle sprains. Am. J. Sports Med. 13 (3), 177–182.

Noback, C.R., Ruggiero, D.A., Demarest, R.J., et al., 2005. The human nervous system: structure and function, sixth ed. Humana Press, Totowa, New Jersey.

Ochoa, J., Fowler, T.J., Gilliatt, R.W., 1972. Anatomical changes in peripheral nerves compressed by a pneumatic tourniquet. J. Anat. 113 (3), 433–455.

O'Connor, B.L., Palmoski, M.J., Brandt, K.D., 1985. Neurogenic acceleration of degenerative joint lesions. J. Bone Joint. Surg. 67A (4), 562–572.

Ogata, K., Naito, M., 1986. Blood flow of peripheral nerve effects of dissection, stretching and compression. J. Hand Surg. 11B (1), 10–14.

Okutsu, I., Ninomiya, S., Hamanaka, I., et al., 1989. Measurement of pressure in the carpal canal before and after endoscopic management of carpal tunnel syndrome. J. Bone Joint. Surg. Am. 71 (5), 679–683.

Oliver, J., Middleditch, A., 1991. Functional anatomy of the spine. Butterworth-Heinemann, Oxford.

Palastanga, N., Field, D., Soames, R., 2002. Anatomy and human movement: structure and function, fourth ed. Butterworth-Heinemann, Oxford.

Panjabi, M.M., White, A.A., 2001. Biomechanics in the musculoskeletal system. Churchill Livingstone, New York.

Petty, N.J., 2011. Neuromusculoskeletal examination and assessment: a handbook for therapists, fourth ed. Churchill Livingstone, Edinburgh.

Powell, H.C., Myers, R.R., 1986. Pathology of experimental nerve compression. Lab. Invest. 55 (1), 91–100.

Rempel, D.M., Diao, E., 2004. Entrapment neuropathies: pathophysiology and pathogenesis. J. Electromyogr. Kinesiol. 14 (1), 71–75.

Rempel, D., Dahlin, L., Lundborg, G., 1999. Pathophysiology of nerve compression syndromes: response of peripheral nerves to loading. J. Bone Joint. Surg. 81A (11), 1600–1610.

Ridehalgh, C., Greening, J., Petty, N.J., 2005. Effect of straight leg raise examination and treatment on vibration thresholds in the lower limb: a pilot study in asymptomatic subjects. Man. Ther. 10 (2), 136–143.

Rydevik, B., Lundborg, G., 1977. Permeability of intraneural microvessels and perineurium following acute, graded experimental nerve compression. Scand. J. Plast. Reconstr. Surg. 11, 179–187.

Rydevik, B., Lundborg, G., Bagge, U., 1981. Effects of graded compression on intraneural blood flow. An in vivo study on rabbit tibial nerve. J. Hand Surg. 6, 3–12.

Rydevik, B., Brown, M.D., Lundborg, G., 1984. Pathoanatomy and pathophysiology of nerve root compression. Spine 9 (1), 7–15.

Rydevik, B., Lundborg, G., Skalak, R., 1989. Biomechanics of peripheral nerves. In: Nordin, M., Frankel, V.H. (Eds.), Basic biomechanics of the musculoskeletal system, second ed. Lea & Febiger, Philadelphia, pp. 75–87.

Salonen, V., Lehto, M., Vaheri, A., et al., 1985. Endoneurial fibrosis following nerve transection. Acta. Neuropathol. (Berl) 67, 315–321.

Scadding, J.W., 2003. Complex regional pain syndrome. In: Melzack, R., Wall, P.D. (Eds.), Handbook of pain management: a clinical companion to Wall and Melzack's textbook of pain. Churchill Livingstone, Edinburgh, pp. 275–288.

Schaumburg, H.H., Spencer, P.S., Ochoa, J., 1983. The aging human peripheral nervous system. In: Katzman, R., Terry, R. (Eds.), The neurology of aging. F A Davies, Philadelphia, pp. 111–122.

Schwartz, J.H., 1991. Synthesis and trafficking of neuronal proteins. In: Kandel, E.R., Schwartz, J.H., Jessell, T.M. (Eds.), Principles of neural science, third ed. Elsevier, New York, pp. 49–65.

Seradge, H., Jia, Y.-C., Owens, W., 1995. In vivo measurement of carpal tunnel pressure in the functioning hand. J. Hand Surg. 20A, 855–859.

Simonetta-Moreau, M., Marque, P., Marchand-Pauvert, V., et al., 1999. The pattern of excitation of human lower limb motoneurones by probable group II muscle afferents. J. Physiol. 517, 287–300.

Smyth, M.J., Wright, V., 1958. Sciatica and the intervertebral disc, an experimental study. J. Bone Joint. Surg. 40A (6), 1401–1418.

Solomonow, M., Zhou, B.-H., Harris, M., et al., 1998. The ligamento-muscular stabilizing system of the spine. Spine 23 (23), 2552–2562.

Spindler, H.A., Dellon, A.L., 1982. Nerve conduction studies and sensibility testing in carpal tunnel syndrome. J. Hand Surg. 7 (3), 260–263.

Starkweather, R.J., Neviaser, R.J., Adams, J.P., et al., 1978. The effect of devascularization on the regeneration of lacerated peripheral nerves: an experimental study. J. Hand Surg. 3 (2), 163–167.

Stromberg, T., Dahlin, L.B., Brun, A., et al., 1997. Structural nerve changes at wrist level in workers exposed to vibration. Occup. Environ. Med. 54, 307–311.

Sunderland, S., 1978. Nerves and nerve injuries, second ed. Churchill Livingstone, Edinburgh, pp. 39, 680.

Sunderland, S., 1990. The anatomy and physiology of nerve injury. Muscle Nerve 13, 771–784.

Sunderland, S., Bradley, K.C., 1961. Stress–strain phenomena in human peripheral nerve trunks. Brain 84, 102–119.

Szabo, R.M., Chidgey, L.K., 1989. Stress carpal tunnel pressures in patients with carpal tunnel syndrome and normal patients. J. Hand Surg. Am. 14 (4), 624–627.

Szabo, R.M., Gelberman, R.H., Williamson, R.V., et al., 1983. Effects of increased systemic blood pressure on the tissue fluid pressure threshold of peripheral nerve. J. Orthop. Res. 1 (2), 172–178.

Tencer, A.F., Allen, B.L., Ferguson, R.L., 1985. A biomechanical study of thoracolumbar spine fractures with bone in the canal, part III, mechanical properties of the dura and its tethering ligaments. Spine 10 (8), 741–747.

Terenghi, G., 1995. Peripheral nerve injury and regeneration. Histol. Histopathol. 10, 709–718.

Todd, A.J., Koerber, R., 2006. Neuroanatomical substrates of spinal nociception. In: Wall and Melzack's textbook of pain, fifth ed. Churchill Livingstone, Edinburgh.

Topp, K.S., Boyd, B.S., 2006. Structure and biomechanics of peripheral nerves: nerve responses to physical stresses and implications for physical therapist practice. Phys. Ther. 86 (1), 92–109.

Turkof, E., Jurecka, W., Sikos, G., et al., 1993. Sensory recovery in myocutaneous, noninnervated free flaps: a morphologic, immunohistochemical, and electron microscopic study. Plast. Reconstr. Surg. 92, 238–247.

Vilensky, J.A., O'Connor, B.L., Brandt, K.D., et al., 1997. Serial kinematic analysis of the canine hindlimb joints after deafferentation and anterior cruciate ligament transection. Osteoarthritis Cartilage 5, 173–182.

von Piekartz, H., Bryden, L., 2001. Craniofacial dysfunction and pain: manual therapy, assessment and management. Butterworth-Heinemann, Oxford.

Wall, E.J., Massie, J.B., Kwan, M.K., et al., 1992. Experimental stretch neuropathy. Changes in nerve conduction under tension. J. Bone Joint. Surg. 74B (1), 126–129.

Williams, P.L., Warwick, R., 1980. Gray's anatomy, thirty-sixth ed. Churchill Livingstone, Edinburgh.

Williams, P.L., Bannister, L.H., Berry, M.M., et al., 1995. Gray's anatomy, thirty-eighth ed. Churchill Livingstone, New York.

Woolf, C.J., Shortland, P., Coggeshall, R.E., 1992. Peripheral nerve injury triggers central sprouting of myelinated afferents. Nature 355 (2), 75–77.

Wright, T.W., Glowczewskie, F., Wheeler, D., et al., 1996. Excursion and strain of the median nerve. J. Bone Joint. Surg. 78A (12), 1897–1903.

Zehr, E.P., Duysens, J., 2004. Regulation of arm and leg movement during human locomotion. Neuroscientist 10: 347–361.

Zehr, E.P., Komiyama, T., Stein, R.B., 1997. Cutaneous reflexes during human gait: electromyographic and kinematic responses to electrical stimulation. J. Neurophysiol. 77, 3310–3325.

Zehr, E.P., Stein, R.B., Komiyama, T., 1998. Function of sural nerve reflexes during human walking. J. Physiol. 507 (1), 305–314.

Zoech, G., Reihsner, R., Beer, R., et al., 1991. Stress and strain in peripheral nerves. Neuro-orthopaedics 10, 73–82.

7

Principles of nerve treatment

Colette Ridehalgh   Kieran Barnard

CHAPTER CONTENTS

There is no pure treatment for nerves, that is, treatment cannot be isolated to nerve alone: it will always, to a greater or lesser extent, affect joint and/or muscle tissues. Some sort of classification system for treatment is needed in order to have meaningful communication among and between clinicians, and this text follows the traditional classification of nerve, joint and muscle treatment. In this text a 'nerve treatment' is defined as a 'treatment to effect a change in nerve'; that is, the intention of the clinician is to produce a change in nerve and therefore it is described as a nerve treatment. Similarly, where a technique is used to effect a change in a joint, it will be referred to as a 'joint treatment', and where a technique is used to effect a change in muscle, it will be referred to as a 'muscle treatment'. Thus, techniques are classified according to which tissue the clinician is predominantly attempting to affect. This relationship of treatment of nerve, joint and muscle is depicted in Figure 7.1.

An example may help to illustrate the impurity of a nerve treatment technique. With the subject in supine, the clinician takes the hip into flexion, with the knee extended, and applies an oscillatory dorsiflexion movement to the ankle, with a view to mobilising the posterior tibial nerve/sciatic nerve. Further analysis of this movement reveals that this technique is not purely a nerve treatment: it also involves joints and muscles. There will be a sustained lengthening of the hip extensor and knee flexors. The oscillatory movement into dorsiflexion will cause talocrural dorsiflexion, which will cause movement at the inferior and superior tibiofibular joints. The movement will also cause oscillatory lengthening of the ankle plantarflexor muscles. It can readily be seen that this simple straight-leg raise (SLR) technique, which might be described as a neurodynamic (i.e. movement of nerve) treatment, also affects joint and muscle tissues. For this reason the technique could be used to effect a change in joint and/or muscle. The therapeutic effect of the SLR technique is likely to be a combined effect on nerve, joint and muscle.

The aim when treating nerve is to address the altered dysfunctional states highlighted in the previous chapter, namely to alter nerve conduction, promote optimum mobility and ultimately to reduce symptoms. Keeping in mind that there are a variety of ways to affect nerve tissue and that it is not possible to affect nerve without affecting joint and muscle structures also, Table 7.1 illustrates the diversity of techniques which may be employed to address altered nerve states. Given that there are clearly various ways of affecting nerve, when the clinician's aim is to target nerve tissue specifically,

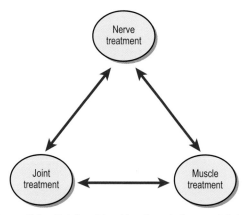

Figure 7.1 • Relationship of treatment of nerve, joint and muscle.

Table 7.1 Nerve dysfunction: aim of nerve treatment and treatment techniques

Nerve dysfunction	Aim of nerve treatment	Nerve treatment technique
Altered nerve conduction	Alter nerve conduction	Joint, muscle or nerve treatment techniques to affect the suspected interface tissue responsible for altered nerve conduction. Electrotherapy
Altered nerve motion	Restore normal motion	Longitudinal movements of the nerve using neurodynamic movements. Soft-tissue mobilisations
	Improve relationship with interface tissue	Joint mobilisations. Soft-tissue mobilisations
Production of symptoms	Reduce symptoms	Joint, muscle or nerve treatment techniques to affect nerve tissue. Soft-tissue mobilisations. Electrotherapy

there are broadly two ways to accomplish this: treating the global mobility of the nerve by encouraging it to move, slide and glide in relation to its surounding structures, and treating specific locations

(interfaces) along its course where nerve function may be compromised. It is the clinician's hope that these techniques will have both biomechanical and neurophysiological effects to help restore normal homeostasis, allowing the nerve to return to optimal function.

The following aspects of nerve treatment will be considered in this chapter:

- biomechanical effects of nerve treatment, including treatments aimed at increasing nerve excursion and nerve interface treatments
- neurophysiological effects of nerve treatment
- addressing the biopsychosocial aspects of symptoms
- modification, progression and regression of treatment.

Biomechanical effects of nerve treatment

Traditionally, neurodynamic tests have been advocated to explore tension within neuromeningeal tissue (Elvey 1986; Butler 1991). If neural tissue is not able to move and slide in relation to its surrounding structures, adverse tension may develop and the test may reproduce pain (Butler 1991; Shacklock 1995). Recent advances in pain science have, however, led to a more complex appreciation of neural dysfunction. Symptoms arising from the nervous system are now widely accepted to be a physiological as well as a mechanical phenomenon (Shacklock 1995; Hall & Elvey 1999; Butler 2000).

The SLR was the first recorded neurodynamic test. The test is widely attributed to the French physician Charles Lasègue (1816–1883), although the test was first described on paper in the 1881 medical thesis of Lasègue's student, J Forst. The original test was split into two parts. In the first part of the test, with the patient lying supine, the leg to be examined was elevated with the knee extended to the point of pain. In the second part of the test (which became known as Lasègue's test), the leg was elevated with the knee flexed and the knee was then gently extended to the point of pain (Rebain et al. 2002). A major problem with both parts of the test as described, however, is that it is not possible to establish whether the pain reproduced is emanating from neural tissue or from other local structures such as the hamstrings, or structures of the knee or hip complex. For this reason, the sensitising manoeuvres of ankle dorsiflexion, medial hip rotation and hip adduction can be added to the basic test to place increased mechanical force upon the nervous system, thereby biasing neural tissue more than non-neural tissue (Breig & Troup 1979; Butler 1991, 2000; Shacklock 1995; Boland & Adams 2000; Refshauge & Gass 2004). The reader is directed to the companion text (Petty 2011) for a more complete description of the neurodynamic tests.

A hierarchy of evidence indicating a positive test has been proposed to include the reproduction of symptoms, an asymmetry in range between the symptomatic and asymptomatic limb, and the change in symptoms with structural differentiation testing (Butler 2000). Neurodynamic examination procedures can be readily converted to treatment techniques by simply replicating the technique to target a given nerve and adding a treatment dose as described below. An important point to emphasise is that neural tissue may be easily provoked by treatment and there may be a latency effect whereby symptoms increase long after treatment has ceased. For this reason it is important to be closely guided by the patient's level of irritability.

Treatment aimed at restoring normal nerve mechanics

Treatment aimed at restoring normal nerve mechanics can be performed in much the same way as a passive stretch to a joint or a muscle, that is, the clinician applies a static or oscillatory force longitudinally through the nerve. As previously mentioned, nerves move, slide and glide in relation to their surrounding structures. When longitudinal force is placed through a given nerve therefore, the aim is not necessarily to stretch the nerve, as the nerve itself may not actually change in length, but rather to re-establish optimal mobility. As clinically it is not possible to know the amount of relative slide and strain occurring when longitudinal force is applied to a nerve, the term lengthening used throughout this section should be interpreted with caution. The dose of passive lengthening incorporates a number of factors, and is outlined in Table 7.2.

Position

This includes the general position of the patient, such as lying, sitting or standing, and the specific position of the body part – for example, the hip may be placed in medial rotation and then flexed. The nervous

---

Table 7.2 Treatment dose for passive mobilisation by the clinician and active movement by the patient

Factors	Passive mobilisation by the clinician	Active movement by the patient
Patient's position	e.g. supine	e.g. sitting, standing with heel of foot on a stool with knee extended
Direction of movement	e.g. hip flexion	e.g. active knee extension
Magnitude of force applied	Related to therapist's perception of resistance: grades I–V	Related to patient's perception of stretch
Amplitude of oscillation	Static or small or large	Static or small or large
Speed	Slow or fast	Slow or fast (if fast, may be referred to as ballistic)
Rhythm	Smooth or staccato	Smooth or staccato
Time	Of repetitions and number of repetitions	Of repetitions and number of repetitions
Symptom response	Short of symptom production Point of onset or increase in resting symptom Partial reproduction of symptom Full reproduction of symptom	Short of symptom production Point of onset or increase in resting symptom Partial reproduction of symptom Full reproduction of symptom

system is one whole organ from the head to the toes and to the hands, and so the clinician needs to consider carefully the positioning of the whole body. The choice of general and specific positioning will depend on a number of factors:

- the comfort and support of the patient
- the comfort of the clinician applying the technique
- accurate application of the technique
- the desired effect of the treatment
- whether weight-bearing or non-weight-bearing is desired
- to what extent the movement is to be functional
- to what extent symptoms are to be produced

Direction of movement

The predominant direction of movement can be broadly divided into longitudinal movement and transverse movement. An example of a predominantly longitudinal movement would be foot plantarflexion/dorsiflexion movement to effect a change in the common peroneal nerve, where the movement of plantarflexion will theoretically lengthen and dorsiflexion will theoretically shorten the nerve. An example of a transverse movement is at the carpal tunnel where during finger flexion, the nerve has to move transversely to avoid compression. It is worth emphasising that such a distinction between longitudinal and transverse movements may not be absolute: when a longitudinal force is applied to a nerve both longitudinal and transverse movement may occur.

Magnitude of force

The force applied by the clinician may be described using grades of movement (Magarey 1985, 1986; Maitland et al. 2005) in the same way as joint mobilisations. As a nerve is passively lengthened, resistance to movement will be felt by the clinician and this can be depicted on a movement diagram (Petty 2011). With physiological movements that lengthen nerve there is often minimal resistance early in the range of movement. For example, during the SLR, hip flexion will have little resistance in the early part of the range and the clinician may mark the onset of resistance (R$_1$) somewhere towards the end of the movement (Figure 7.2). Grades of movement are then defined according to the resistance curve. The grades of movement as defined in this text

are shown in Table 7.3; they are modified from Maitland et al. (2005) and Magarey (1985, 1986). The modification allows every possible position in range to be described (Magarey 1985, 1986), and each grade to be distinct from one another (Maitland et al. 2005). The choice of magnitude of force, like every other factor of treatment dose, depends on what the clinician is attempting to achieve. It has been

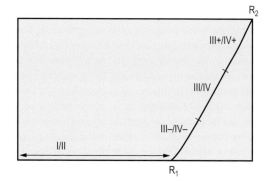

Figure 7.2 • A movement diagram depicting grades of movement for straight-leg raise (hip flexion, adduction and medial rotation, with knee extension). The onset of resistance (R$_1$) may be felt by the clinician somewhere towards the end of the movement, with R$_2$ depicting the end of range.

Table 7.3 Grades of movement

Grade	Definition
I	Small-amplitude movement short of resistance
II	Large-amplitude movement short of resistance
III−	Large-amplitude movement in the first third of resistance
IV−	Small-amplitude movement in the first third of resistance
III	Large-amplitude movement in the middle third of resistance
IV	Small-amplitude movement in the middle third of resistance
III+	Large-amplitude movement in the last third of resistance
IV+	Small-amplitude movement in the last third of resistance

continually emphasised in this text that it is not possible to move one structure, e.g. nerve, without in some way affecting another, e.g. joint or muscle. A thoughtful appreciation of resistance is therefore advised when examining neural tissue as it is unlikely that the resistance the clinician feels is from neural tissue alone. For example, a study of hamstring activity during the SLR in 29 asymptomatic subjects found that hip flexion to the onset of stretch in the posterior thigh significantly increased both medial and lateral hamstring electromyogram (EMG) activity ($P <0.01$; Barnard 2007). Furthermore, the individual addition of the sensitising movements of ankle dorsiflexion, hip medial rotation and hip adduction further increased hamstring activity ($P <0.01$). These findings may question the ability of the SLR to descriminate accurately between neural and non-neural structures (Barnard 2007). One tempting conclusion to draw from this is that muscle activity increases to protect neural tissue; however, to the authors' knowledge, such a reflex has not been demonstrated experimentally. By contrast, numerous other well-documented endogenous musculoskeletal and cutaneous reflex pathways might have the potential to increase hamstring activity during the SLR.

Amplitude of oscillation

The movement can be a sustained or oscillatory force. If the force is oscillated it is described as having a small or large amplitude, which is relative to the available range of any movement. The amplitude of oscillatory movement is described within the definition of grades of movement: grades I and IV are small-amplitude movements and grades II and III are large-amplitude movements. It is impossible for a truly sustained force to be applied to the tissues as there will always be some variation in the force, albeit very small. For this reason it is sometimes referred to in research articles as a quasistatic force; however, for the purposes of clinical practice the term static is used. Where a clinician applies a sustained force, the written clinical notes may use grades I, IV–, IV or IV+ with the word 'sustained' written prior to the grade; for example, treatment notes would read 'sustained grade IV–'. In this case the grade of movement is used only to denote where in resistance the force is applied. Alternatively, the clinician may write in words where in range s/he applied a sustained force. What is important, however, is not the choice of notation but the full description of the treatment dose.

It can be seen that, with an oscillatory force, grades of movement describe the magnitude of the force and the amplitude of oscillation. The choice of grade of movement is determined by the relationship of pain (or other symptom) and resistance through the range of movement. Where resistance limits the range of movement and there is minimal pain, a grade III+ or IV+ might be appropriate (Figure 7.3A). Where pain limits the range of movement and there is minimal resistance, a grade I or II may be appropriate (Figure 7.3B), so that no pain is produced. A grade III– or IV– may be chosen if the pain is not severe and not irritable and there is no caution related to the nature of the disorder. Where resistance limits the movement, and there is a significant amount of pain, or where pain limits the movement and there is a significant amount of resistance, the choice of grade will depend on the degree to which symptoms can be provoked (Figure 7.3C and D). For example, in Figure 7.3C, if a grade IV is chosen at about 50% of resistance, this would provoke an intensity of pain for the patient of about 3 out of 10 (where A is 0 and C is 10). If a grade IV is chosen for 7.3D, this would provoke about 4 out of 10, which may or may not be acceptable to the patient.

Speed and rhythm of movement

The speed of the movement can be described as slow or fast, and the rhythm as smooth or staccato (jerky); of course, these terms will apply only to oscillatory forces. Speed and rhythm go hand in hand: movements will tend to be slow and smooth, fast and smooth, or fast and staccato; it would be difficult to apply a slow staccato movement. The connective tissue in nerve is viscoelastic and is therefore sensitive to the speed of the applied force (Sunderland & Bradley 1961). A force applied quickly will produce less movement, provoking a greater stiffness; that is, the gradient of the resistance curve will be steep. On the other hand, a force applied more slowly will cause more movement as the stiffness is relatively less. If the intention of treatment is to maximise range of movement by lengthening connective tissue then a slow speed would seem preferable.

Time

In terms of treatment dose, time relates to the amount of time the nervous tissue is placed on a stretch, the number of times this is repeated and the frequency of the appointments.

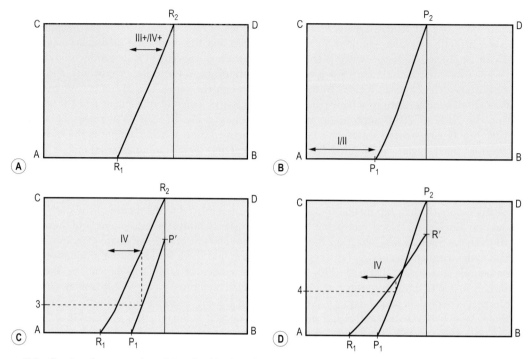

Figure 7.3 • Grades of movement are determined by the relationship of pain and resistance through the range of movement; this is depicted on a movement diagram. **A** Resistance limiting movement. **B** Pain limiting movement. **C** Resistance limiting movement with a significant amount of pain. **D** Pain limiting movement with a significant amount of resistance.

Symptom response

The clinician decides which symptom, and to what extent, is to be provoked during treatment. Choices include:

- no provocation
- provocation to the point of onset, or increase in resting symptoms
- partial reproduction
- total reproduction

The decision as to what extent symptoms are provoked during treatment depends on the severity and irritability of the symptom(s) and the nature of the condition. If the symptoms are severe, that is, the patient is unable to tolerate the symptom being produced, the clinician would choose not to provoke the symptoms. The clinician may also choose not to provoke symptoms if they are irritable, that is, once symptoms are provoked they take some time to ease. If, however, the symptoms are not severe and not irritable, then the clinician is able to reproduce the patient's symptoms during treatment, and the extent to which symptoms are reproduced will depend on the tolerance of the patient. The nature of the

condition may limit the extent to which symptoms are produced, such as a recent traumatic injury.

Treatment is progressed or regressed by altering appropriate aspects of the treatment dose: the patient's position, movement, direction of force, magnitude of force, amplitude of oscillation, speed, rhythm, time, temperature or symptom response. Progression and regression of each aspect of the treatment dose can be used (Table 7.4).

It is suggested that inexperienced clinicians alter only one aspect of treatment dose at an attendance so that they fully understand the value of the alteration; in this way they will quickly develop valuable clinical experience and clinical mileage, which will contribute to growth in their clinical learning skills. The immediate and more long-term effect of the alteration can then be evaluated by reassessment of the subjective and physical asterisks. Table 7.5 provides an example of how a treatment dose may be progressed and regressed. It can be seen in the last example that both speed and rhythm have been altered; these two factors are very closely linked and can be considered separately or together. Other aspects of treatment dose that are closely linked are the

Table 7.4 Progression and regression of treatment dose

Treatment dose	Progression	Regression
Position	Joint towards end of available range	Joint towards beginning of available range
Direction of force	More provocative	Less provocative
Magnitude of force	Increased	Decreased
Amplitude of oscillation	Decreased	Increased
Rhythm	Staccato	Smoother
Time	Longer	Shorter
Speed	Slower or faster	Slower
Symptom response	Allowing more symptoms to be provoked	Allowing fewer symptoms to be provoked

length of time for each repetition and the number of repetitions; these, together, provide a dose of time and so can be considered separately or together.

Active movement by the patient

The factors defining the treatment dose when patients apply their own treatment are exactly the same as the clinician applying a passive technique (Table 7.2). The only difference is that, in this instance, the patient is in total control of the movement and relies on his or her own perception of stretch and symptom production to determine the way the movement is carried out. The patient needs to be fully informed as to how to carry out the movement, that is, how forceful to be and to what extent to reproduce the symptoms. The clinician in this case takes on a more educational and advisory role.

An analysis of each neurodynamic test is provided below to offer a biomechanical basis for the use of these tests as treatment techniques.

The underlying effect of lengthening nerve

The effect of certain movements on nerve length and tension is largely a matter of logical deduction, based on the position of a nerve relative to the axis of the movement. If a nerve lies anterior to the axis of movement and the movement reduces the angle between the bones then it seems reasonable to suggest that the nerve will be slackened and tension will be reduced; if the movement increases the angle between the bones, then theoretically it makes sense that the nerve will be lengthened and the tension will be increased. However, there are variations in the pathway of nerves between individuals (Adkison et al. 1991), and the presence of pathology may further alter the response of tests and treatment (Butler 1991). In addition it is known that nerves are not held at length in normal resting positions and are

Table 7.5 Examples of how a neurodynamic treatment dose can be progressed and regressed

Regression	Dose	Progression	Explanation
In cervical extension did central PA C4 IV ×3 (1 minute) slowly and smoothly to partial reproduction of patient's neck pain	In cervical neutral did central PA C4 IV ×3 (1 minute) slowly and smoothly to partial reproduction of patient's neck pain	In cervical flexion did central PA C4 IV ×3 (1 minute) slowly and smoothly to partial reproduction of patient's neck pain	The starting position has been altered. It might be assumed that extension is a position of ease and flexion a more provocative position
In 90° knee flexion did medial glide tibiofemoral joint I ×3 (1 minute) slowly and smoothly short of P1	In 90° knee flexion did: medial glide tibiofemoral joint II slowly and smoothly ×3 (1 minute) short of P1	In 90° knee flexion did medial glide tibiofemoral joint III− ×3 (1 minute) slowly and smoothly short of P1	The grade of movement has been altered
Physiological plantarflexion III ×3 (1 minute) slowly and smoothly to full reproduction of ankle pain	Physiological plantarflexion III+ ×3 (1 minute) slowly and smoothly to full reproduction of ankle pain	Physiological plantarflexion III+ ×3 (1 minute) fast and staccato to full reproduction of ankle pain	Grade has been altered as a regression. Speed and rhythm have been altered as a progression

PA, posteroanterior.

wrinkled within the nerve bed. This suggests that, during movements which move them longitudinally, rather than tension being exerted on the nerve, the nerve may simply uncoil and then slide within the interface (Sunderland 1978; Kwan et al. 1992; Dilley et al. 2003). Nerves also exhibit a phenomenon known as convergence, whereby if a single joint is moved, the nerve on either side of the joint will move towards the joint (Topp & Boyd 2006). This means that there will be a section of the nerve close to the joint axis where no movement takes place. For these reasons, the clinician is wise to be cautious in assigning treatment to a particular nerve, or root level, and may often need to examine and treat patients in non-standard positions.

While it is known that lengthening a nerve beyond 15% (Clark et al. 1992) of its resting length results in nerve pathology, it is difficult to assess what percentage change in length is occurring during neurodynamic examination and treatment. It is conceivable that a change in nerve conduction would occur if lengthening of greater than 15% occurred during the technique. This does not seem to occur in asymptomatic individuals (Ridehalgh et al. 2005). Vibration threshold testing was performed on 30 asymptomatic subjects before, during and after a three-repetition, 30-second treatment of SLR with plantarflexion and inversion. Significant differences ($P < 0.05$) were not found between readings, suggesting that conduction of the large-diameter afferents (the first to show signs of minor nerve injury) was not altered; therefore, it seems unlikely that such detrimental changes in length occur during neurodynamic assessment and treatment.

There is not necessarily a direct relationship between length and tension; the degree to which lengthening increases tension, or shortening reduces tension, will depend on the ability of the nerve to move. If, for example, a nerve is fixed at one end, and is then pulled, there will be an increase in length with a gradual build-up in tension. If, on the other hand, a nerve is not fixed at either end, and a longitudinal pull is applied, the whole nerve may be free to move, relative to adjacent tissues, and until there is some resistance to this movement, tension within the nerve may not rise appreciably. This freedom of nerve to move relative to adjacent tissues is thought to be greater where a nerve is passing through tissues, and is least where nerve branches, where it pierces muscle or where it runs around a bone (Sunderland 1978).

The viscoelastic nature of nerve was observed in one small study using two cadavers (Reid 1987).

Repeated movements resulted in a reduction in nerve tension and the tension did not return to its original level, indicating the phenomenon of stress relaxation and hysteresis. It is not known whether this occurs with neurodynamic treatments.

The following text provides a useful anatomical and biomechanical basis of neurodynamic tests and treatment – but that is all it is: it does not necessarily explain the response of a test or treatment of a particular patient. The clinician applies this knowledge to patients and, using the concept of the permeable brick wall (Maitland et al. 2005), believes the response of the patient, regardless of whether or not it fits with anatomical or biomechanical knowledge of nerve movement. In this way, the clinician is free to explore movement fully and to treat any movement dysfunction that the patient may present with.

Passive neck flexion

Cervical flexion has been found to:

- reduce the length of the cervical region of the sympathetic trunk
- lengthen the spinal canal and neuroaxis in the cervical region (Reid 1960; Tencer et al. 1985)
- increase the tension in the neuroaxis in the cervical region (Reid 1960; Tencer et al. 1985)
- increase tension of the dural sac (Reid 1960; Tencer et al. 1985)
- move and tension the lumbosacral nerve roots (Breig & Marions 1963; Breig 1978).

Neurodynamic testing of the mandibular nerve involves upper cervical flexion and lateral flexion, with the addition of depression and contralateral deviation of the mandible for the lingual and mental nerves, and transverse movement of the mandible for the buccal and auriculotemporal nerves (von Piekartz & Bryden 2001). Neurodynamic testing of the facial nerve involves upper cervical flexion and lateral flexion, with ipsilateral rotation (von Piekartz & Bryden 2001). Further details are given elsewhere (von Piekartz & Bryden 2001).

Straight-leg raise

The movement of hip flexion with knee extension, with variable amounts of hip adduction and medial rotation, will lengthen and tense the sciatic nerve, the central nervous system neuroaxis as far as the brain, the upper-limb nervous system and the sympathetic trunk (Breig 1978; Butler 1991). During

SLR the L5–S1 nerve roots have been found to move distally between 0 and 5 mm, and the sciatic nerve at the exit from the pelvis between 3 and 10 mm (Goddard & Reid 1965; Smith et al. 1993). The nerve roots are lengthened about 2–4% from neutral to 60° SLR (Smith et al. 1993). Movement of the sciatic nerve has been found to occur immediately the foot is lifted up from the horizontal position, with little movement after 70° hip flexion (Goddard & Reid 1965). Moving the knee from flexion to extension is thought to cause the nervous system, distal to the knee, to move in a cephalad direction, and the nervous tissue proximal to the knee to move in a caudad direction (Figure 7.4). Behind the knee there is little movement, and this is considered to be a 'tension point'. Foot dorsiflexion, eversion and a combination of dorsiflexion and eversion have been found to increase the tension of the posterior tibial nerve (Daniels et al. 1998). Indeed, ankle dorsiflexion has been shown to increase sciatic strain during hip flexion in an asymptomatic population (Coppieters et al. 2006) and reduce the available range of hip flexion during the SLR in both asymptomatic and symptomatic populations (Gajdosik et al. 1985; Boland & Adams 2000).

The addition of hip adduction and medial rotation has been shown to increase tension in the sacral plexus in cadavers (Breig & Troup 1979; Coppieters et al. 2005), with the latter causing the sacral plexus to move 0–1 cm towards the greater sciatic foramen during the SLR (Breig & Troup 1979).

Passive knee bend

Side lie slump, hip extension with the knee flexed, lengthens the femoral nerve (L2/3/4 nerve roots) and will also apply tension to the neuroaxis and meninges (Dyck 1976; Davidson 1987). The hypothesised movement of the femoral nerve and neuroaxis during the slump passive knee bend is shown in Figure 7.5.

Slump

The full slumped position – sitting with the cervical spine and trunk in flexion, and with the hip in flexion, knee in extension and foot in dorsiflexion – is thought to lengthen and tense the central nervous

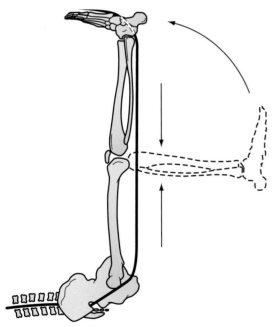

Figure 7.4 • Straight-leg raise. It is thought that the nervous system distal to the knee moves in a cephalad direction, and the nervous tissue proximal to the knee moves in a caudad direction. Behind the knee there is little movement, and this is considered to be a tension point. (After Butler 1991, with permission).

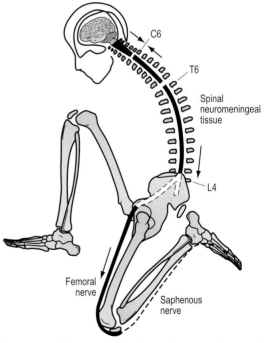

Figure 7.5 • Movement of the femoral nerve and neuroaxis during the slump passive knee bend (from Davidson 1987, with permission).

system and posterior tibial portion of the sciatic nerve. There is some evidence to suggest that the slump has a greater potential for lengthening and tensioning the nervous system than the proprioceptive neuromuscular facilitation or SLR movements (Massey 1986).

In asymptomatic subjects, the addition of foot dorsiflexion, hip medial rotation and cervical flexion were all found to reduce the available knee extension range of movement (Johnson & Chiarello 1997). Furthermore, cervical flexion has been shown to increase posterior-thigh pain during the slump examination and thigh pain reduces with cervical extension in an asymptomatic population (Lew & Briggs 1997). No measurement was made of nerve movement or tension in either study, so while these studies provide some support for these components in the slump, they do not validate their use.

Several studies have examined the clinical application of the slump test as a treatment modality for both spinal and peripheral pain. In one study of 30 patients with non-radicular low-back pain, Cleland et al. (2006) found that treatment with exercise, lumbar mobilisation and slump mobilisation significantly improved pain, disability and centralisation of symptoms when compared with exercise and lumbar mobilisation alone. Another study examining Australian Rules football players with signs of a hamstring tear found a large majority of players (76%) were found to have a positive slump test (Kornberg & Lew 1989). All the players were treated with traditional muscle treatment techniques, with one group also receiving slump treatment. The players who were treated with slump had a greater functional improvement than those treated only with traditional methods. In a later study, the slump test was found to cause an increase in sympathetic outflow to the lower limbs, causing vasodilation, and it was speculated that this may have been the underlying effect of the slump treatment of the Australian Rules footballer players (Kornberg & McCarthy 1992).

Similarly, a positive slump test was found in patients with an ankle inversion sprain (Pahor & Toppenberg 1996), and while the effect of treatment with slump was not carried out in the study, it seems reasonable to suggest that this would need to be addressed in the management of such patients.

The sympathetic slump test is carried out in long sitting with the trunk in left lateral flexion and rotation, and the cervical spine in left lateral flexion to affect the right side of the sympathetic trunk (Figure 7.6; Butler & Slater 1994). It has been shown

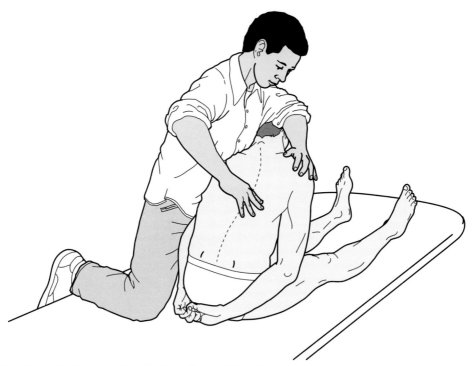

Figure 7.6 • Sympathetic slump (from Butler & Slater 1994, with permission).

in asymptomatic subjects that this position for 1 minute causes a large increase in skin conductance and a small decrease in temperature (compared with a placebo and control group), indicative of an increase in vasomotor activity and an increase in sympathetic activity (Slater et al. 1994). Furthermore, patients with symptoms suggestive of frozen shoulder, who were treated with a unilateral posteroanterior pressure to T6 for 1 minute in the sympathetic slump position, were found to have an increase in sympathetic nervous system (SNS) activity in the affected hand (Slater 1995). Interestingly, the treatment did not affect pain scores, pressure pain thresholds or neurodynamic testing.

Upper-limb neurodynamic tests

The following analysis of the effects of the upper-limb neurodynamic tests on nerve tension and nerve length uses a mixture of anatomical knowledge and research findings.

1. Cervical contralateral lateral flexion has been shown to increase the strain at the C5–T1 nerve roots (Reid 1987; Selvaratnam et al. 1988) and to alter the onset of pain in asymptomatic subjects (van der Heide et al. 2001). It has also been found to cause a small (0.3 mm) degree of nerve excursion (Dilley et al. 2003) and reduce the movement of the median nerve at the elbow by 5% (Hough et al. 2000).

2. Shoulder girdle depression has not been found to increase the tension in the brachial plexus (Reid 1987; Ginn 1988; Lewis et al. 1998), although when this is eliminated from the upper-limb tension test there is a large reduction in the developing tension in all the cords of the brachial plexus. Shoulder girdle depression with glenohumeral abduction increases the tension in the brachial plexus (Lord & Rosati 1971; Butler 1991).

3. Glenohumeral joint abduction causes an increase in the tension of the brachial plexus (Reid 1987; Ginn 1988) and causes about 15 mm of movement of the brachial plexus (Wilgis & Murphy 1986).

4. Horizontal extension at 90° glenohumeral abduction causes a slight reduction in tension in the brachial plexus (Ginn 1988).

5. Lateral rotation at 90° glenohumeral abduction causes a large reduction in the tension in all the cords of the brachial plexus (Reid 1987; Ginn 1988). The reduction in tension with lateral rotation is accompanied by an increase in tension in the biceps brachii muscle and, for this reason, is recommended as part of the test (Ginn 1988). Medial rotation has been found to reduce the tension in the ulnar nerve (Reid 1987).

6. Elbow extension has been found to increase tension significantly in the axilla (Kleinrensink et al. 1995; Lewis et al. 1998), at the elbow and at the wrist in comparison with 90° of elbow flexion (Kleinrensink et al. 1995). It is also thought that elbow extension increases the tension in the radial and median nerves, which lie anterior to the axis of rotation, while it decreases tension in the ulnar nerve (Reid 1987), as it lies posterior to the axis of rotation. The converse will occur: elbow flexion will increase tension in the ulnar nerve and decrease tension in the radial and median nerves (Reid 1987; Butler 1991).

7. Forearm supination and wrist extension each increase the tension on the median nerve at both the elbow and the wrist (Kleinrensink et al. 1995). From a neutral wrist position to 55° extension, the median nerve at the elbow has been found to move distally between 6 and 13 mm (Hough et al. 2000).

8. Wrist and finger extension will increase the length and tension of the median and ulnar nerves, and decrease tension in the radial nerve, and vice versa. Wrist extension has been found to increase the tension in the median nerve at both the elbow and wrist (Kleinrensink et al. 1995). The median nerve in the upper arm has been found to move distally about 7 mm on wrist and finger extension (McLellan & Swash 1976).

These studies support the component movements used in the upper-limb neurodynamic test for the median nerve (ULNT1). The use of horizontal extension does not appear to be useful to increase tension in the brachial plexus (Ginn 1988). Most research data in this area have been gathered from studies of the ULNT1.

Using buckle force transducers around the median nerve, just distal to the axilla of five cadavers, the typical order of movements of the ULNT1 was carried out while measuring the tension within the median nerve (Lewis et al. 1998). The position of neutral cervical spine, shoulder girdle depression, glenohumeral joint abduction and external rotation and forearm supination failed to cause an increase in median nerve tension (Lewis et al. 1998). When elbow extension was added, there was an increase in median nerve tension, and this was further increased with wrist extension and cervical contralateral lateral flexion.

Further support for the components of ULNT1 comes from an in vivo study of asymptomatic subjects (Coppieters et al. 2001). A starting position of 30° N longitudinal force to shoulder girdle depression, 90° glenohumeral abduction and external rotation was used. Additions of wrist extension, contralateral cervical lateral flexion and wrist extension with contralateral cervical lateral flexion each progressively reduced the available elbow extension and provoked more stretch or paraesthesia, mostly localised to the hand (Coppieters et al. 2001). No measurement was made of nerve movement or tension, so while the study provides some support for these components in the ULNT1 it does not validate their use.

In another cadaver study, changes in tension of the medial, lateral and posterior cords of the brachial plexus were explored during the ULNT1 in addition to tension changes in the median, radial and ulnar nerves just distal to the brachial plexus (Kleinrensink et al. 2000). Again buckle force transducers were used to measure tension. It was found that the ULNT1 created significant tension and selectively biased the median nerve as opposed to the radial and ulnar nerves. Furthermore, as might be expected with reference to the median nerve's origin (Palastanga et al. 1994), the ULNT1 generated more tension in the medial and lateral cord of the brachial plexus than the posterior cord. Interestingly, the authors concluded that the ULNT1 is a valid test for the median nerve, as it is both sensitive and specific: the test was sensitive because it was found to increase tension significantly in the target nerve; it was specific because it was not found to increase the tension significantly in the radial or ulnar nerves. The underlying assumption that it is an increase in neural tension which produces a positive test can, however, be challenged. With reference with the previously cited hierarchy of evidence indicating a positive test (Butler 2000), the underlying reason for performing the ULNT1 is not necessarily to create tension in the medial nerve but to reproduce the patient's symptoms. This may involve a physiological as well as a mechanical process. As a cadaver clearly cannot report symptoms, it would seem an assumption to postulate that increased neural tension would equate to a reproduction of symptoms. Kleinrensink et al. (2000) were, after all, not testing whether the

test was sensitive in detecting dysfunction but whether the test generated tension in neural tissue – they are not necessarily one and the same.

In asymptomatic subjects, the range of each component of arm movement during the ULNT1 of the left and right sides has been found to be the same (van der Heide et al. 2001). Treatment may be indicated, therefore, in patients with asymmetry (van der Heide et al. 2001). In addition, there appears to be a muscular response to the ULNT1 as a relationship has been demonstrated between increasing EMG activity of the upper fibres of trapezius and both increasing 'neural tension' (Balster & Jull 1997) and the onset of pain (van der Heide et al. 2001) during the test in asymptomatic populations. Furthermore, both symptomatic and asymptomatic limbs demonstrated a significant increase in shoulder girdle elevation force during the ULNT1 (Coppieters et al. 2003). Taking all these studies into account, it may be that treatment of the nervous system may also need to address this muscle component.

It is worth noting that the differing methodologies used between studies makes comparisons very difficult. Most studies have used cadavers, which clearly alters the biomechanical propeties of the nerves, and, as previously mentioned, no symptom response is possible during the test procedures. Interestingly, a more recent study utilising ultrasound imaging technology to examine nerve strain in vivo would suggest that the total excursion and strain of the nerve during certain manoeuvres may be much less than previously found in cadaver studies (Dilley et al. 2003). The reason for this is not clear, but could be related to the altered biomechanical properties of nerves in cadavers, or the indirect way in which strain has been calculated by Dilley et al. (2003).

Sliding techniques

Nerve sliding techniques are thought to produce the greatest possible nerve excursion whilst producing minimal strain in the target nerve (Butler 2000; Coppieters et al. 2004; Shacklock 2005; Coppieters & Alshami 2007; Coppieters & Butler 2008). The aim of these techniques is essentially the same as the more traditional 'tensioning' techniques, i.e. to glide the nerve bed relative to the surrounding structures to induce positive biomechanical and neurophysiological effects to help restore normal homeostasis and allow the nerve to return to optimal function. As less strain is thought to occur than during tensioning techniques, these techniques may be particularly useful when treating a severe and/or irritable condition. A sliding technique is performed by lengthening the nerve bed at one end of the nerve whilst simultaneously shortening the nerve bed at the other end of the nerve. In so doing, the clinician can imagine the nerve sliding proximally and distally. For example, when attempting a sliding technique to affect the median nerve, with the patient in the ULNT1 position, the cervical spine may be side-flexed contralaterally whilst the wrist is simultaneously flexed. The cervical spine may then be side-flexed ipsilaterally whilst the wrist is simultaneously extended.

Despite their advocation, it is only recently that the biomechanical and clinical efficacy of sliding techniques has been scrutinised. Two recent in vitro biomechanical studies appear to provide evidence that sliding techniques do indeed produce large nerve excursion without significant increases in nerve strain (Coppieters & Alshami 2007; Coppieters & Butler 2008). In the most recent of these studies, longitudinal excursion and strain of the medial and ulnar nerves during tensioning and sliding movements were examined in two embalmed cadavers (Coppieters & Butler 2008). The median nerve was tensioned by extending the elbow and wrist, whilst the sliding manoeuvre consisted of elbow extension with wrist flexion and vice versa. The ulnar nerve was tensioned by extending the wrist, flexing the elbow and abducting the shoulder, whilst the sliding manoeuvre consisted of elbow extension with shoulder abduction and vice versa. Although there was no statistical confirmation of the trends identified, the sliding techniques produced more excursion than the tensioning techniques whilst producing less strain. For example, the median nerve sliding technique produced 12.6 mm of excursion and a 0.8% increase in strain at the wrist, compared with the tensioning technique, which produced 6.1 mm of excursion and a 6.8% increase in strain at the wrist. Along with the small sample size and lack of statistical confirmation, a major limitation of this study was that it was performed on cadavers and it is not clear if these findings would accurately reflect nerve excursion and strain in vivo. Although more research is needed, this study provides a welcome addition to the small body of work which appears to advocate sliding techniques to maximise nerve excursion whilst minimising nerve strain. Whether to 'tension' or 'slide' nerve tissue depends largely on the forces the clinician wishes to impart and on the severity and irritability of the

condition. Ultimately it is the close monitoring and reassessment of treatment which will determine the effectiveness of the technique.

Nerve interface treatments

Nerve interface treatments refer to the treatment of specific locations (interfaces) along the course of a nerve where nerve function may be compromised as it winds its way around bone, or through muscle or fascia. Examples of possible nerve interfaces where function may be compromised include the median nerve passing beneath the flexor retinaculum of the wrist into the carpal tunnel, the sciatic nerve piercing the piriformis muscle, the common peroneal nerve passing around the superior tibiofibular joint and the tibial nerve passing through the tarsal tunnel into the foot. If a nerve becomes entrapped and loses its ability to move, slide and glide within the interface, the aim of treatment may often be to move the interface relative to the nerve. For example, a patient may have signs of L5 nerve root compression, comprising pain in the lumbar spine with posterolateral calf pain, reduced sensation to fine touch over the posterolateral calf, together with weakness of the big toe extensors. The SLR test position of hip flexion, knee extension and foot dorsiflexion may be limited to 45° hip flexion, reproducing the patient's pain, with the pain increased on cervical flexion, giving a positive SLR. In addition, there may be positive findings on passive accessory movements of the lumbar spine; for example, the patient's back and calf pain may be reproduced with a unilateral posteroanterior pressure on L5 with a caudad inclination. It could be speculated in this scenario that the pain may be emanating from the nerve root as it exits the intervertebral foramen at the L5/S1 level and so the accessory movement is being used as a neurodynamic interface treatment. In this example, it could be argued that treating the interface to offload the neural structures may be a priority to improve the mechanics of the nerve root. A longitudinal neurodynamic treatment could then be used to address the restricted SLR and re-establish optimum neural mobility if required. Following each intervention, the objective markers of altered sensation and strength and restricted SLR would need to be reassessed to establish the effectiveness of the technique.

Another example of an interface treatment may be treatment of a patient whose symptoms suggest a mild carpal tunnel syndrome. Treatment may be aimed at increasing the space within the carpal tunnel to reduce the compression on the median nerve. For example, joint accessory movements may be applied to the carpal bones (Tal-Akabi & Rushton 2000). Interestingly, 1 minute of wrist and finger flexion and extension at a rate of 30 cycles per minute has been found to reduce carpal tunnel pressure for up to 15 minutes (Seradge et al. 1995). If this effect occurred in a patient group it could reduce symptoms.

It has been suggested that, when an interface pathology is suspected, longitudinal mobilising techniques are contraindicated and any treatment should not provoke pain (Hall & Elvey 2004). Whilst it is advisable to proceed with caution, it is the authors' opinion that it is often extremely difficult to establish with certainty that the patient's symptoms are emanating from a compromised interface. As with any soft-tissue dysfunction, correctly establishing the patient's level of severity and irritability should be the predetermining factor in establishing whether the clinician wishes to reproduce the patient's symptoms partially or fully (Maitland et al. 2005).

Soft-tissue mobilisation

Hunter (1998) has coined the phrase 'specific soft-tissue mobilisation' (SSTM). It is essentially the application of manual force to soft tissue, which traditionally has been employed for muscle and ligament; however, it could also be applied to nerve. SSTM may be applied in the plane of the nerve (Figure 7.7) and at right angles to the site of dysfunction (Hunter 1998). For example, SSTM may be applied over the piriformis muscle to effect a change in the sciatic nerve, or to the supinator muscle to effect a change in the posterior interosseous nerve. Various parameters may be altered to adapt the technique according to the force the clinician wishes

to impart, taking into account factors such as the pathology, stage of healing and the degree of severity and irritability. One such parameter is relative nerve length: force could be applied with the nerve in a relaxed position, or with the nerve in a more lengthened position. for example, the common peroneal nerve could be treated with the hip in neutral or at end-of-range hip flexion (with knee extension), with the addition of hip adduction and ankle plantarflexion. The technique could also be applied with an isometric, concentric or eccentric muscle contraction.

The decisions to be made by the clinician, in terms of treatment dose, include the patient's position, movement, direction, magnitude of force applied, amplitude of oscillation, speed and rhythm of movement, time and symptom response. Table 7.6 provides a summary of the treatment options, and is identical to the treatment dose for joint and muscle.

The underlying effect of soft-tissue mobilisation is not yet known. Soft-tissue mobilisation is considered to be appropriate following soft-tissue injury,

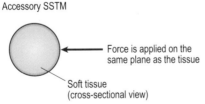

Accessory SSTM

Force is applied on the same plane as the tissue

Soft tissue
(cross-sectional view)

Figure 7.7 • Direction of force and position of force for accessory specific soft-tissue mobilisation (SSTM) to a nerve (from Hunter 1998, with permission).

Table 7.6 Treatment dose for specific soft-tissue mobilisation

Factors	Variables
Patient's position	e.g. prone, side lie, sitting
Movement	Physiological movement Accessory movement or a mixture of accessory and physiological
Direction of force applied	e.g. medial transverse, lateral transverse, anteroposterior, posteroanterior, caudad, cephalad
Magnitude of force applied	Related to therapist's perception of resistance: grades I–V
Amplitude of oscillation	None: sustained (quasistatic) Small: grades I and IV Large: grades II and III
Speed	Slow or fast
Rhythm	Smooth or staccato
Time	Of repetition and number of repetitions
Symptom response	Short of symptom production Point of onset or increase in resting symptom Partial reproduction of symptom Full reproduction of symptom

especially during the regeneration and remodelling phase of healing (Hunter 1998). During the regeneration and remodelling phases, soft-tissue mobilisation is thought to enhance collagen synthesis and cross-linkage development, promote the orientation of collagen fibres along functional lines of stress, and promote 'normal' viscoelastic behaviour (Hunter 1998). It is also proposed that SSTM is beneficial for degenerative lesions by stimulating an inflammatory response that initiates healing (Hunter 1998).

Neurophysiological effects of nerve treatment

As with all treatment techniques, the effects of treatment will incorporate not only biomechanical effects, but also therapeutic neurophysiological effects. The aim of both nerve movement and nerve interface treatments is to restore normal homeostasis. As well as restoring normal nerve movement, it has been hypothesised that nerve treatment may also positively affect endoneurial fluid pressure and intrafascicular capillary flow, reduce neural oedema, and normalise axoplasmic flow and A and C fibre afferent activity (Butler 2000; Shacklock 2005; Nee & Butler 2006). There is, however, also a growing research base to suggest the mobilising soft tissue can have a significant hypoalgesic effect, and this is now explored.

Descending inhibition of pain

The immediate hypoalgesic effect of manual therapy has been well documented (Vicenzino et al. 1994; Wright 1995; McGuiness et al. 1997; Vincenzino et al. 1998; Sterling et al. 2001; Schmid et al. 2008). It had been widely theorised that this phenomenon can be explained by the 'gate control theory' (Melzack & Wall 1965), which proposes that large-diameter myelinated afferent neurons inhibit nociceptive afferent activity at spinal cord level. Subsequent research has also highlighted the presence of a multifaceted endogenous pain control system utilising a number of neuronal systems. The periaqueductal grey (PAG) area has been found to be particularly important in the control of nociception. Neurones from the PAG project to the dorsal horn, having a descending control of nociception (Figure 7.8). Neurones also project upwards to the medial thalamus and orbital frontal cortex, suggesting that the PAG may also have an ascending control of

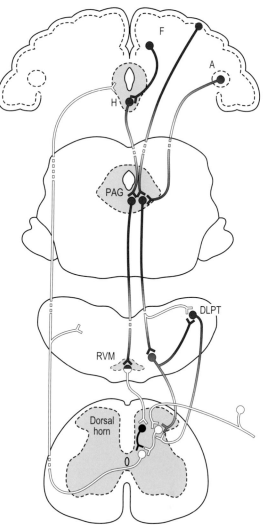

Figure 7.8 • Pain-modulating pathway. Periaqueductal grey (PAG) receives input from the frontal lobe (F), the amygdala (A) and the hypothalamus (H). Afferents from PAG travel to the rostral ventromedial medulla (RVM) and the dorsolateral pontomesencephalic tegmentum (DLPT) and on to the dorsal horn. The RVM has bidirectional control of nociceptive transmission. There are inhibitory (filled) and excitatory (unfilled) interneurones. (From Fields & Basbaum 1999, with permission).

nociception (Fields & Basbaum 1999). The PAG has two distinct regions: the dorsolateral PAG (dPAG) and the ventrolateral PAG (vPAG).

dPAG

The dPAG runs to the dorsolateral pons and ventrolateral medulla, which is involved in autonomic control (Fields & Basbaum 1999). In the rat, stimulation of the dPAG causes analgesia, increased blood pressure, increased heart rate, vasodilation of the hind-limb muscles and increased rate and depth of respiration, and coordinated hind limb, jaw and tail movements, suggesting increased activity of the SNS and alpha motor neurones (Lovick 1991). The neurotransmitter from dPAG is noradrenaline (norepinephrine) and the analgesic effect appears to mediate morphine analgesia of mechanical nociceptor stimuli (Kuraishi et al. 1983). At the spinal cord dPAG causes inhibition of substance P from peripheral noxious mechanical stimulation (Kuraishi 1990).

vPAG

The vPAG mainly runs to the nucleus raphe magnus. In the rat, stimulation of vPAG causes analgesia with decreased blood pressure, decreased heart rate, vasodilation of the hind-limb muscles and reduced hind-limb, jaw and tail movements, suggesting inhibition of the SNS and inhibition of alpha motor neurones (Lovick 1991). The neurotransmitter used in vPAG is serotonin and the analgesic effect appears to mediate morphine analgesia of thermal nociceptive stimuli (Kuraishi et al. 1983). At the dorsal horn vPAG inhibits the release of somatostatin produced by peripheral noxious thermal stimulation (Kuraishi 1990). These mechanisms have been linked to the behaviour of an animal under threat, which initially acts with a defensive flight-or-fight response followed by recuperation (Fanselow 1991; Lovick 1991); this is summarised in Figure 7.9.

Noxious stimuli can cause activation of the descending control system (Yaksh & Elde 1981; Fields & Basbaum 1999), which may reduce nociceptive transmission. Noxious stimulation has been found to cause release of enkephalins at the supraspinal and spinal levels (Yaksh & Elde 1981). It has also been found that stimulation of the spinothalamic tract, transmitting nociceptive information from one foot, can be inhibited by noxious input from the contralateral foot, hand, face or trunk (Gerhart et al. 1981). It has been suggested that this may explain the relief of pain with acupuncture and pain behaviours such as biting your lip and banging your head against a wall (Melzack 1975). Production of pain during neurodynamic treatment may also activate the descending control system.

The proposed mechanism by which nerve mobilisations relieve pain is outlined in Figure 7.10 (Wright

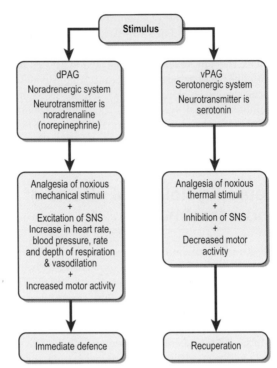

Figure 7.9 • Descending inhibition of mechanical nociception from the dorsolateral periaqueductal grey (dPAG: noradrenergic system) and thermal nociception from the ventrolateral periaqueductal grey (vPAG: serotonergic system). SNS, sympathetic nervous system.

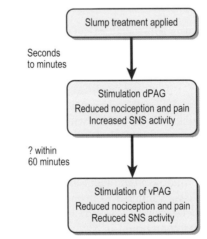

Figure 7.10 • Proposed mechanism whereby a neurodynamic treatment, such as a slump, reduces pain (Wright 1995). dPAG, dorsolateral periaqueductal grey; vPAG, ventrolateral periaqueductal grey; SNS, sympathetic nervous system.

1995). It is suggested that nerve mobilisations almost immediately stimulate the dPAG to cause hypo-algesia, and a few minutes later vPAG is stimulated (Takeshige et al. 1992). There are a number of research studies that support the proposal by Wright (1995); these studies have investigated the immediate effects of joint mobilisation on noxious mechanical and thermal thresholds and SNS activity. In a number of the studies noxious mechanical thresholds have been measured using a digital pressure algometer, and nox-ious thermal thresholds have used a contact thermode system (Wright 1995). Increased SNS activity has been measured indirectly by measuring a decrease in skin temperature and an increase in skin conductance (due to a decrease in skin resistance). Skin temperature has been measured using an AT42 skin temperature monitor (Autogenic Advanced Technology, Chicago) and skin conductance has been measured using an AT64 skin conductance monitor (Autogenic Advanced Technology, Chicago).

A number of studies have found that joint mobi-lisations have an immediate hypoalgesic effect on mechanical nociceptor activity and/or increased SNS activity. In two separate randomised, double-blind, placebo-controlled trials, the application of passive mobilisation in the form of a centrally applied grade III posteroanterior to C5 and a grade III lateral glide technique to C5/6 applied to asymptomatic volunteers were shown to produce significant ($P \leq$ 0.05) sympathoexcitatory effects; respiratory rate, heart rate and systolic and diastolic blood pressure were all shown to rise (McGuiness et al. 1997; Vicenzino et al. 1998). An earlier study by Vicenzino et al. (1994) found that adding a neural mobilisation component (ULNT1 and 2b) whilst performing a grade III lateral glide technique to C5 also resulted in a increase in skin conductance, suggesting a sym-pathoexcitatory response. A further randomised, double-blind, placebo-controlled trial has been carried out by Stirling et al. (2001). This time 30 subjects with mid to low cervical spine pain were included in the study. It was found that a grade III unilateral posteroanterior glide to C5/6 produced a significant increase in skin conductance ($P \leq$ 0.0002) coupled with significant hypoalgesia; pres-sure pain thresholds on the side of treatment were shown to increase ($P = 0.0001$) and resting visual analogue pain scale scores were shown to decrease ($P = 0.049$). Although the majority of the research examining decending control systems has looked pri-marily at joint treatment, it may be that nerve treat-ment techniques have a similar effect.

Addressing the biopsychosocial aspects of symptoms

Injury, or the perception of injury, produces anxiety and fear (Craig 1999). Who has ever injured them-selves, however minimally, and not experienced an emotional reaction? The psychological aspects of pain sometimes focus on 'emotional individuals' or on chronic pain patients. However, all of us will have a cognitive and emotional response to injury, because injury interrupts our lives. There is never a right time for an injury: it will always be, to a greater or lesser degree, a nuisance to us. That 'nuisance' will drive our emotional reactions. It seems reasonable to sug-gest, therefore, that all patients with neuromusculos-keletal dysfunction will have thoughts and feelings about their problem, and it would be an oversight on the part of the clinician not to enquire about this. This enquiry involves the clinician understanding the patient's thoughts and feelings. This is no easy task, and to do it well requires a high level of skill in active listening. Active listening involves putting our own thoughts, beliefs and feelings to one side and choosing instead to hear what the patient has to say. It involves trying to understand patients and their world, through their eyes, and trying to avoid the all-too-easy error of reinterpreting through our eyes. It requires the clinician to listen with compassion and patience, and without judgement. It involves the clinician using words carefully and meaningfully, and using open-ended questions, to search for information, until understanding is reached. It involves sensitive verbal and non-verbal communication, thus encouraging safe and open communication. This is a tall order, but the benefits of truly being able to come alongside the patient will far outweigh the effort of developing these skills.

The use of 'yellow flags' was devised specifically for acute low-back pain to identify beliefs, emotions and behaviours that may contribute to long-term disability (Watson & Kendall 2000). Screening ques-tionnaires (Main & Waddell 1999) have been devised; these, like all questionnaires, have major limitations. Questions provide a superficial, and sometimes false, understanding of the problem – as anyone who has filled in any questionnaire knows only too well. For example, when a question asks: 'How much have you been bothered by feeling depressed in the last week?' and the recipient answers on a 0–10 scale from 'not at all' to 'extremely', little information is gleaned from this; there may be a wide variety of factors underlying the given score. For this reason, if a questionnaire is used, a discussion with the patient will also be necessary to understand the problems faced by the patient (Watson & Kendall 2000). The questionnaire can be useful to provide the clinician with aspects to discuss with the patient; however, there is a danger that it becomes a mechanistic form-filling exercise. It is worth remembering that the clinical management of patients is fundamentally based on human relationships, which are not normally enriched by form-filling!

Following the enquiry of the patient as to his or her thoughts and feelings, two further steps are recommended: education and exposure (Vlaeyen & Crombez 1999). Education involves the clinician carefully facilitating the patient's understanding of the problem. How this is carried out with patients will vary according to a number of factors, such as patients' prior knowledge, thoughts and beliefs and how they feel about the problem. All the listening skills discussed above will be imperative in this process. The ability of the clinician to be honest is important. The clinician needs to explain the problem to the patient in a careful way. There is a world of difference between 'The pain in your back is from the disc' and 'I think the pain in your back could be coming from the disc'. The former explanation suggests that you know that the pain is coming from the disc, and yet there is overwhelming evidence that you cannot make such claims; it has been estimated that a definite diagnosis of the pathology can be made in only about 15% of cases (Waddell 1999). Furthermore, there is a long-term problem with being so confident as the patient may, in the future, have a recurrence of the same pain and may see another clinician who may say 'The pain in your back is from your sacroiliac joint'. The patient is aware that this is a repeat episode and now, quite rightly, begins to have doubts about the ability of these two clinicians. This will be a familiar story to experienced clinicians who will have come across patients who have received perhaps three, four or even more confident 'diagnoses' of the same problem and who come to you depressed, cynical and disillusioned with the medical profession.

The final aspect is exposure, which involves careful and graded exposure to the movements or postures that provoke pain (Vlaeyen & Crombez 1999). While this is designed for chronic pain patients who learn to avoid movements and posture through fear (Waddell & Main 1999; Moseley 2003), it may also be an important part of the treatment of acute tissue damage. Using movements and postures in a careful, controlled and graded way may help to avoid long-term movement dysfunctions.

Modification, progression and regression of treatment

The continuous monitoring of the patient's subjective and physical asterisks guides the entire treatment and management programme of the patient. The clinician judges the degree of change with treatment and relates this to the expected rate of change from the prognosis, and then decides whether or not a treatment needs to be altered in some way. The nature of this alteration can be to modify the technique in some way, to progress the treatment or regress the treatment. Regardless of which alteration is made, the clinician makes every effort to determine what effect this alteration has on the patient's subjective and physical asterisks. In order to do this, the clinician alters one aspect of treatment at a time and reassesses immediately to determine the value of the alteration.

The clinician may modify the treatment given to a patient by altering an existing treatment, adding a new treatment or stopping a treatment. At all times the treatment should have the functional goals of the patient in mind. Altering an existing treatment involves altering some aspect of the treatment dose, discussed earlier. The immediate and more long-term effect of the alteration is then evaluated by reassessment of the subjective and physical asterisks; this process is outlined in Figure 7.11. The clinician then decides whether, overall, the patient is better, the same or worse, relating this to the prognosis. For instance, if a quick improvement was expected, but only some improvement occurred, the clinician may progress treatment. If the patient is worse after treatment, the dose may be regressed in some way, and if the treatment made no difference at all, then a more substantial modification may be made. Before discarding a treatment it is worth making sure that it has been fully utilised, as it may be that a much stronger or much weaker treatment dose may be effective.

Summary

This chapter has outlined the principles of nerve treatment. The reader is directed to Chapter 8 for further background information on pain, and Chapter 9 for broad principles underpinning patient management.

Figure 7.11 • Modification, progression and regression of treatment.

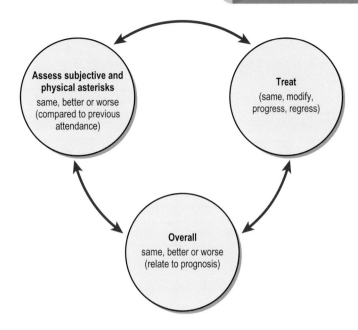

References

Adkison, D.P., Bosse, M.J., Gaccione, D.R., et al., 1991. Anatomical variations in the course of the superficial peroneal nerve. J. Bone Joint Surg. 73A (1), 112–114.

Balster, S.M., Jull, G., 1997. Upper trapezius muscle activity during the brachial plexus tension test in asymptomatic subjects. Man. Ther. 2, 144–149.

Barnard, K., 2007. The effect of the straight leg raise and sensitising manoeuvres on hamstring muscle activity. Unpublished MSc Thesis.

Boland, R., Adams, R., 2000. Effects of adding ankle dorsiflexion to passive straight leg raising in patients with low back pain. Aust. J. Physiother. 46 (3), 191–200.

Breig, A., 1978. Adverse mechanical tension in the central nervous system. Almqvist & Wiksell, Stockholm.

Breig, A., Marions, O., 1963. Biomechanics of the lumbosacral nerve roots. Acta Radiologica 1, 1141–1160.

Breig, A., Troup, J.D.G., 1979. Biomechanical considerations in the straight-leg-raising test, cadaveric and clinical studies of the effects of medial hip rotation. Spine 4 (3), 242–250.

Butler, D.S., 1991. Mobilisation of the nervous system. Churchill Livingstone, Melbourne.

Butler, D., 2000. The sensitive nervous system. Noigroup, Adelaide.

Butler, D.S., Slater, H., 1994. Neural injury in the thoracic spine: a conceptual basis for manual therapy. In: Grant, R. (Ed.), Physical therapy of the cervical and thoracic spine, second ed. Churchill Livingstone, New York, pp. 313–338.

Clark, W.L., Trumble, T.E., Swiontkowski, M.F., et al., 1992. Nerve tension and blood flow in a rat model of immediate and delayed repairs. J. Hand Surg. 17A, 677–687.

Cleland, J.A., Childs, J.D., Palmer, J.A., et al., 2006. Slump stretching in the management of non-radicular low back pain: a pilot clinical trial. Man. Ther. 11 (4), 279–286.

Coppieters, M.W., Alshami, A.M., 2007. Longitudinal excursion and strain in the median nerve during novel nerve gliding exercises for carpal tunnel syndrome. J. Orthop. Res. 25 (7), 972–980.

Coppieters, M.W., Butler, D.S., 2008. Do 'sliders' slide and 'tensioners' tension? An analysis of neurodynamic techniques and considerations

regarding their application. Man. Ther. 13 (3), 213–221.

Coppieters, M.W., Stappaerts, K.H., Everaert, D.G., et al., 2001. Addition of test components during neurodynamic testing: effect on range of motion and sensory responses. J. Orthop. Sports Phys. Ther. 31 (5), 226–237.

Coppieters, M.W., Stappaerts, K.H., Wouters, L.L., et al., 2003. Aberrant protective force generation during neural provocation testing and the effect of treatment in patients with neurogenic cervicobrachial pain. J. Manipulative Physiol. Ther. 26, 99–106.

Coppieters, M.W., Bartholomeeusen, K.E., Stappaerts, K.H., 2004. Incorporating nerve-gliding techniques in the conservative treatment of cubital tunnel syndrome. J. Manipulative Physiol. Ther. 27 (9), 560–568.

Coppieters, M.W., Kurz, K., Mortensen, T.E., et al., 2005. The impact of neurodynamic testing on the perception of experimentally induced muscle pain. Man. Ther. 10 (1), 52–60.

Coppieters, M.W., Alshami, A.M., Babri, A.S., et al., 2006. Strain and excursion of the sciatic, tibial, and plantar nerves during a modified straight leg raising test. J Orthop Res. 24 (9), 1883–1889.

Craig, K.D., 1999. Emotions and psychobiology. In: Wall, P.D., Melzack, R. (Eds.), Textbook of pain. fourth ed. Churchill Livingstone, Edinburgh, pp. 331–343.

Daniels, T.R., Lau, J.T.-C, Hearn, T.C., 1998. The effects of foot position and load on tibial nerve tension. Foot Ankle Int. 19 (2), 73–78.

Davidson, S., 1987. Prone knee bend: an investigation into the effect of cervical flexion and extension. In: Dalziell, B.A., Snowsill, J.C. (Eds.), Proceedings of the Manipulative Therapists'. Association of Australia, 5th Biennial Conference, pp. 236–246.

Dilley, A., Lynn, B., Greening, J., et al., 2003. Quantitative in vivo studies of median nerve sliding in response to wrist, elbow, shoulder and neck movements. Clin. Biomech. 18 (10), 899–907.

Dyck, P., 1976. The femoral nerve traction test with lumbar disc protrusions. Surg. Neurol. 6, 163–166.

Elvey, R.L., 1986. Treatment of arm pain associated with abnormal brachial plexus tension. Aust. J. Physiother. 32, 224–229.

Fanselow, M.S., 1991. The midbrain periaqueductal gray as a coordinator of action in response to fear and anxiety. In: Depaulis, A., Bandler, R. (Eds.), The midbrain periaqueductal gray matter. Plenum Press, New York, pp. 151–173.

Fields, H.L., Basbaum, A.I., 1999. Central nervous system mechanisms of pain modulation. In: Wall, P.D., Melzack, R. (Eds.), Textbook of pain. fourth ed. Churchill Livingstone, Edinburgh, pp. 309–329.

Gajdosik, R.L., LeVeau, B.F., Bohannon, R.W., 1985. Effects of ankle dorsiflexion on active and passive unilateral straight leg raising. Phys. Ther. 65 (10), 1478–1482.

Gerhart, K.D., Yezierski, R.P., Giesler, G.J., et al., 1981. Inhibitory receptive fields of primate spinothalamic tract cells. J. Neurophysiol. 46 (6), 1309–1325.

Ginn, K., 1988. An investigation of tension development in upper limb soft tissues during the upper limb tension test. In: Proceedings of the

International Federation of Orthopaedic Manipulative Therapists' Conference. Cambridge, England, pp. 25–26.

Goddard, M.D., Reid, J.D., 1965. Movements induced by straight leg raising in the lumbo-sacral roots, nerves and plexus, and in the intrapelvic section of the sciatic nerve. J. Neurol. Neurosurg. Psychiatry 28, 12–18.

Hall, T.M., Elvey, R.L., 1999. Nerve trunk pain: physical diagnosis and treatment. Man. Ther. 4 (2), 63–73.

Hall, T.M., Elvey, R.L., 2004. Management of mechanosensitivity of the nervous system in spinal pain syndromes. In: Boyling, G., Jull, G. (Eds.), Grieves Modern Manual Therapy. third ed. Churchill Livingstone, Edinburgh, pp. 413–431.

Hough, A., Moore, A., Jones, M., 2000. Doppler ultrasound measurement of median nerve motion. International Federation of Orthopaedic Manipulative Therapists 7th Scientific Conference Proceedings, Abstract 62, p. 56.

Hunter, G., 1998. Specific soft tissue mobilization in the management of soft tissue dysfunction. Man. Ther. 3 (1), 2–11.

Johnson, E.K., Chiarello, C.M., 1997. The slump test: the effects of head and lower extremity position on knee extension. J. Orthop. Sports Phys. Ther. 26 (6), 310–317.

Kleinrensink, G.J., Stoeckart, R., Vleeming, A., et al., 1995. Mechanical tension in the median nerve. The effects of joint positions. Clin. Biomech. 10 (5), 240–244.

Kleinrensink, G.J., Stoeckart, R., Mulder, P.G., et al., 2000. Upper limb tension tests as tools in the diagnosis of nerve and plexus lesions. Anatomical and biomechanical aspects. Clin. Biomech. 15 (1), 9–14.

Kornberg, C., Lew, P., 1989. The effect of stretching neural structures on grade one hamstring injuries. J. Orthop. Sports Phys. Ther. 6, 481–487.

Kornberg, C., McCarthy, T., 1992. The effect of neural stretching technique on sympathetic outflow to the lower limbs. J. Orthop. Sports Phys. Ther. 16 (6), 269–274.

Kuraishi, Y., 1990. Neuropeptide-mediated transmission of nociceptive information and its regulation. Novel

mechanisms of analgesics. Yakugaku Zasshi 110 (10), 711–726.

Kuraishi, Y., Harada, Y., Aratani, S., et al., 1983. Separate involvement of the spinal noradrenergic and serotonergic systems in morphine analgesia: the differences in mechanical and thermal algesic tests. Brain Res. 273, 245–252.

Kwan, M.K., Wall, E.J., Massie, J., et al., 1992. Strain, stress and stretch of peripheral nerve. Rabbit experiments in vitro and in vivo. Acta Orthop. Scand. 63 (3), 267–272.

Lew, P.C., Briggs, C.A., 1997. Relationship between the cervical component of the slump test and change in hamstring muscle tension. Man. Ther. 2 (2), 98–105.

Lewis, J., Ramot, R., Green, A., 1998. Changes in mechanical tension in the median nerve: possible implications for the upper limb tension test. Physiotherapy 84 (6), 254–261.

Lord, J.W., Rosati, L.M., 1971. Thoracic outlet syndromes. In: CIBA Clinical Symposia, vol. 23. issue 2. Ciba Pharmaceutical, New Jersey, pp. 20–23.

Lovick, T., 1991. Interactions between descending pathways from the dorsal and ventrolateral periaqueductal gray matter in the rat. In: Depaulis, A., Bandler, R. (Eds.), The midbrain periaqueductal gray matter. Plenum Press, New York, pp. 101–120.

Magarey, M.E., 1985. Selection of passive treatment techniques. In: Proceedings of 4th Biennial Conference of the Manipulative Therapists'. Association of Australia, Brisbane, pp. 298–320.

Magarey, M.E., 1986. Examination and assessment in spinal joint dysfunction. In: Grieve, G.P. (Ed.), Modern manual therapy of the vertebral column. Churchill Livingstone, Edinburgh, pp. 481–497.

Main, C.J., Waddell, G., 1999. Psychological distress. In: Waddell, G. (Ed.), The back pain revolution. Churchill Livingstone, Edinburgh, pp. 173–186.

Maitland, G.D., Hengeveld, E., Banks, K., et al., 2005. Maitland's vertebral manipulation, seventh ed. Butterworth-Heinemann, Oxford.

Massey, A.E., 1986. Movement of pain-sensitive structures in the neural canal. In: Grieve, G.P. (Ed.), Modern manual therapy of the vertebral column. Churchill Livingstone, Edinburgh, pp. 182–193.

McGuiness, J., Vicenzino, B., Wright, A., 1997. Influence of a cervical mobilisation technique on respiratory and cardiovascular function. Man. Ther. 2 (4), 216–220.

McLellan, D.L., Swash, M., 1976. Longitudinal sliding of the median nerve during movements of the upper limb. J. Neurol. Neurosurg. Psychiatry 39, 566–570.

Melzack, R., 1975. Prolonged relief of pain by brief, intense transcutaneous somatic stimulation. Pain 1, 357–373.

Melzack, R., Wall, P.D., 1965. Pain mechanisms: a new theory. Science 150, 971–979.

Moseley, L., 2003. A pain neuromatrix approach to patients with chronic pain. Man. Ther. 8 (3), 130–140.

Nee, B.J., Butler, D., 2006. Management of peripheral neuropathic pain: Integrating neurobiology, neurodynamics, and clinical evidence. Physical Therapy in Sport 7 (1), 36–49.

Pahor, S., Toppenberg, R., 1996. An investigation of neural tissue involvement in ankle inversion sprains. Man. Ther. 1 (4), 192–197.

Palastanga, N., Field, D., Soames, R., 1994. Anatomy and Human Movement, second ed. Butterworth Heinmann, Oxford.

Petty, N.J., 2011. Neuromusculoskeletal examination and assessment, a handbook for therapists, fourth ed. Elsevier, Edinburgh.

Rebain, R., Baxter, G.D., McDonough, S., 2002. A systematic review of the passive straight leg raising test as a diagnostic aid for low back pain. Spine 27 (17), E388–E395.

Refshauge, K., Gass, E., 2004. Musculoskeletal Physiotherapy: Its Clinical Science and Evidence-Based Practice, fourth ed. Butterworth-Heinemann, Oxford.

Reid, J.D., 1960. Effects of flexion–extension movements of the head and spine upon the spinal cord and nerve roots. J. Neurol. Neurosurg. Psychiatry 23, 214–221.

Reid, S.A., 1987. The measurement of tension changes in the brachial plexus. In: Proceedings of the fifth Biennial Conference of the Manipulative Therapists'. Association of Australia, Melbourne, pp. 79–90.

Ridehalgh, C., Greening, J.B., Petty, N.J., 2005. The effect of straight leg raise examination and treatment on vibration threshold in the lower limb. Man. Ther. 10 (2), 136–143.

Schmid, A., Brunner, F., Wright, A., et al., 2008. Paradigm shift in manual therapy? Evidence for a central nervous system component in the response to passive cervical joint mobilisation. Ma. Ther. 13 (5), 387–396.

Selvaratnam, P.J., Glasgow, E.F., Matyas, T., 1988. The strain at the nerve roots of the brachial plexus. J. Anat. 161, 260.

Seradge, H., Jia, Y.-C., Owens, W., 1995. In vivo measurement of carpal tunnel pressure in the functioning hand. J. Hand Surg. 20A, 855–859.

Shacklock, M.O., 1995. Neurodynamics. Physiotherapy 81 (1), 9–16.

Shacklock, M.O., 2005. Clinical neurodynamics: A new system of musculoskeletal treatment. Elsevier/Butterworth Heinemann, Edinburgh.

Slater, H., 1995. An investigation of the physiological effects of the sympathetic slump on peripheral sympathetic nervous system function in patients with frozen shoulder. In: Shacklock, M.O. (Ed.), Moving in on pain. Butterworth-Heinemann, Australia.

Slater, H., Vicenzino, B., Wright, A., 1994. 'Sympathetic slump': the effects of a novel manual therapy technique on peripheral sympathetic nervous system function. Journal of Manual and Manipulative Therapy 2 (4), 156–162.

Smith, S.A., Massie, J.B., Chesnut, R., et al., 1993. Straight leg raising, anatomical effects on the spinal nerve root without and with fusion. Spine 18 (8), 992–999.

Stirling, M., Jull, G., Wright, A., 2001. Cervical mobilisation: concurrent effects on pain, sympathetic nervous system activity and motor activity. Man. Ther. 6 (2), 72–81.

Sunderland, S., 1978. Nerves and nerve injuries, second ed. Churchill Livingstone, Edinburgh.

Sunderland, S., Bradley, K.C., 1961. Stress–strain phenomena in human peripheral nerve trunks. Brain 84, 102–119.

Takeshige, C., Sato, T., Mera, T., et al., 1992. Descending pain inhibitory system involved in acupuncture analgesia. Brain Res. Bull. 29, 617–634.

Tal-Akabi, A., Rushton, A., 2000. An investigation to compare the effectiveness of carpal bone mobilisation and neurodynamic mobilisation as methods of treatment for carpal tunnel syndrome. Man. Ther. 5 (4), 214–222.

Tencer, A.F., Allen, B.L., Ferguson, R.L., 1985. A biomechanical study of thoracolumbar spine fractures with bone in the canal, part III, mechanical properties of the dura and its tethering ligaments. Spine 10 (8), 741–747.

Topp, K.S., Boyd, B.S., 2006. Structure and biomechanics of peripheral nerves: nerve responses to physical stresses and implications for physical therapist practice. Phys. Ther. 86 (1), 92–109.

van der Heide, B., Allison, G.T., Zusman, M., 2001. Pain and muscular responses to a neural tissue provocation test in the upper limb. Man. Ther. 6 (3), 154–162.

Vicenzino, B., Collins, D., Wright, A., 1994. Sudomotor changes induced by neural mobilisation techniques in asymptomatic subjects. Journal of Manual and Manipulative Therapy 2 (2), 66–74.

Vicenzino, B., Cartwright, T., Collins, D., et al., 1998. Cardiovascular and respiratory changes produced by lateral glide mobilization of the cervical spine. Man. Ther. 3 (2), 67–71.

Vlaeyen, J.W.S., Crombez, G., 1999. Fear of movement/(re)injury, avoidance and pain disability in chronic low back pain patients. Man. Ther. 4 (4), 187–195.

von Piekartz, H., Bryden, L., 2001. Craniofacial dysfunction and pain: manual therapy, assessment and management. Butterworth-Heinemann, Oxford.

Waddell, G., 1999. Diagnostic triage. In: Waddell, G. (Ed.), The back pain revolution. Churchill Livingstone, Edinburgh, p. 9.

Waddell, G., Main, C.J., 1999. Beliefs about back pain. In: Waddell, G. (Ed.), The back pain revolution. Churchill Livingstone, Edinburgh, pp. 187–202.

Watson, P., Kendall, N., 2000. Assessing psychological yellow flags. In:

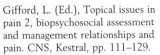
Gifford, L. (Ed.), Topical issues in pain 2, biopsychosocial assessment and management relationships and pain. CNS, Kestral, pp. 111–129.

Wilgis, E.F.S., Murphy, R., 1986. The significance of longitudinal excursion in peripheral nerves. Hand Clin. 2 (4), 761–766.

Wright, A., 1995. Hypoalgesia post-manipulative therapy: a review of a potential neurophysiological mechanism. Man. Ther. 1 (1), 11–16.

Yaksh, T.L., Elde, R.P., 1981. Factors governing release of methionine enkephalin-like immunoreactivity from mesencephalon and spinal cord of the cat in vivo. J. Neurophysiol. 46 (5), 1056–1075.

Principles of managing pain

8

Chris Murphy

CHAPTER CONTENTS

Introduction

This chapter aims to introduce the reader to the science and clinical management of pain. Relevant neurophysiology is first introduced in a simplified format before being applied to explain the pain gate theory. The physiological cascade of events that transpire following an injury are discussed and integrated with the relevant social and psychological factors which influence the clinical presentation. The information is applied throughout so the reader can understand how patients with similar injuries might present completely differently. The consequences of persistent pain are discussed and the physiological mechanisms underpinning these highlighted so treatment interventions can be clinically reasoned. Finally, the various sections are drawn together to highlight treatment principles you might use to assist in your clinical management of patients in pain.

A note on how to read this chapter

Much like a thriller novel, you want to know who did it and how? However, if you simply read the last page you will have missed out on the story and, as a result, you might not understand how the final conclusion was reached. With this in mind I would ask that you read this chapter from start to finish. This does not need to be completed in one sitting but do not leave it too long until you finish it. Once you have done that please consider how you will remember it; this might be by making up your own stories or analogies. When you have done that read it again and reinforce your own creations so the information sticks in your mind.

A brief history of pain

The modern era of pain

Until the 1960s, the scientific and medical viewpoint on pain was that it functioned as a warning system. Its presence indicated damage or disease in the body tissues, i.e. if something hurt, there was something wrong and vice versa.

However, clinical observations reported in the literature challenged this theory. Well-known examples included:

- patients who presented with fatal malignant tumours that did not hurt (Melzack & Wall 1988)
- patients who presented at accident and emergency with little or no pain in the presence of obvious injury (Melzack & Wall 1988)
- soldiers injured in the frontline of war frequently did not complain of enough pain to warrant painkillers (analgesics) (Beecher 1956).

When an injured person presented complaining of little or no pain it was observed that (Melzack & Wall 1988):

- distraction was not a factor
- the individual was aware of the injury
- the reduction or absence of pain was limited to the injured area
- the individual felt pain eventually, maybe minutes or hours later.

As these findings could not be adequately explained by existing theories, a revision of underpinning scientific knowledge was required. As a result, Ronald Melzack, a Canadian psychologist, and Patrick Wall, a British physician, proposed the pain gate theory (Melzack & Wall 1965; Melzack 1999). In the 1960s Melzack & Wall proposed that pain was not hard-wired but was highly modifiable via the central nervous system, especially at the dorsal horn and the brain.

To understand the pain gate theory, we need to consider the basic neurophysiology that underpins the sensation of pain.

The neurophysiology of pain

We do not have pain nerves

Before considering this it is important to dismiss the misconception of the pain nerve. It is common to encounter references to pain nerves. If you look in books you will find them (Caudill 2008), you will probably hear clinicians discussing them and they are to be found on the internet (The Web of the Back 2009). It is important to recognise quickly that these are incorrect: pain nerves do not exist and to refer to them does little to help you or your patients understand pain. If we do not have pain nerves, it begs the question, what nerves do we have and what messages do they carry?

Sensory nerves carry sensory information

Different types of nerves convey sensory information from the body tissues to the central nervous system (Kandell et al. 2000). They detect sensations such as touch, pressure, temperature changes and different chemicals, especially those released during inflammation or ischaemia. The different sensory nerves are commonly classified according to the speed at which electrical impulses, or action potentials, travel along them. This is known as their conduction speed. The common nerves to remember are A beta (Aβ), A delta (Aδ) and C nerves. Their conduction speed is dependent on various factors such as their width (diameter) and whether they are insulated with myelin (myelinated). The wider and more insulated they are, the faster they are. Of these, Aβ have the fastest conduction speed, then Aδ, and finally C are the slowest as they are thin and have no myelin insulation.

Action potentials in sensory nerves are generated in response to stimuli

Sensory nerves run from the body tissues to the dorsal horn in the spinal cord. These are often called sensory afferent nerves (Kandell et al. 2000). Different sensations, e.g. mechanical, thermal and chemical, may activate their respective specialised receptors which are situated on the outer surface of the end of the nerve in the tissues. Activation of these receptors changes the electrical charge within the end of the nerve by allowing charged ions to flow across the nerve membrane. When this electrical charge is raised above a certain threshold (activation threshold), an action potential is generated inside the nerve. This process of creating an electrical signal from a physical stimulus is known as transduction. The common receptors are:

- mechanical: these respond to pressure and stretch
- thermal: these respond to changes in temperature
- chemical: these respond to chemicals, especially those released during inflammation or ischaemia.

The channels (ion channels) in these different receptors are opened in response to their specific stimuli. It is worth noting that some receptors can be multimodal; this simply means that ion channels can open in response to a range of stimuli, e.g. mechanical and thermal and chemical (Figure 8.1).

Another way to picture the stimulus and its specific receptor is like a key approaching the lock on a closed door. If the right key (stimulus) fits the right door lock (receptor) it unlocks it and the door can momentarily open (ion channel opens) (Figure 8.2). As this occurs positively charged ions flow through (Julius & Basbaum 2001; Woolf & Ma 2007). This results in an increase in the electrical charge across the membrane on the end of the nerve. If this rises above the activation threshold, an action potential may be generated, which then travels along the nerve. Different types of sensory nerves have

different receptors (locks), which respond to different stimuli (keys).

Receptors on the membranes of sensory nerves are continually being made and replaced. They are produced by the cell body of the nerve and are slowly transported along the nerve to their chosen location (Kandell et al. 2000). They are then slotted into place, or inserted, in the membrane of the nerve and are then ready to respond to their respective stimulus. When a nerve is described as expressing certain receptors, this refers to the production and insertion of these receptors on its membrane. For example, a nerve expressing receptors for mechanical stimuli can convert mechanical stimuli into action potentials. As receptors are being removed and replaced every few days, this allows for a highly adaptable dynamic system (Kandell et al. 2000).

Sensory nerves carry innocuous and nociceptive messages

Sensations that do not cause damage to the body, e.g. light touch, vibration and gentle stretch, are detected by receptors on the large-diameter, fast-conducting, Aβ nerves. These stimuli are known as innocuous stimuli. As innocuous stimuli can be very subtle, the receptors on Aβ nerves have a low stimulation threshold. The light touch of a feather on your skin would be enough to activate them.

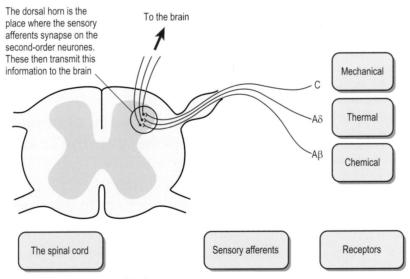

Figure 8.1 • Sensory afferent nerves and their receptors.

Door is locked   **Door is unlocked**

Figure 8.2 • The lock-and-key analogy.

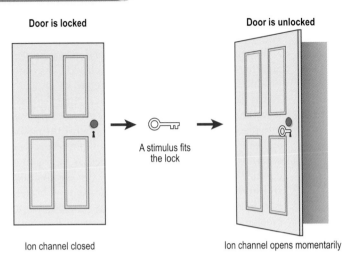

A stimulus fits
the lock

Ion channel closed   Ion channel opens momentarily

Sensations that could cause or have caused damage to the body are detected by receptors on the smaller-diameter, slower-conducting Aδ and C nerves. These sensations might be heavy pressure, extremes of temperature or the chemicals released during inflammation or ischaemia. These stimuli are known as noxious stimuli. As noxious stimuli are usually of greater intensity, Aδ and C nerves have a high stimulation threshold. As it might take a burn or a strong poke to activate them, consider them as being harder to excite. That is, normally it takes a greater stimulus for them to be activated than a receptor with a lower stimulation threshold such as those on the Aβ nerves (Melzack & Wall 1988; Julius & Basbaum 2001).

Receptors that respond to noxious stimuli (or nociception) are known as nociceptors and these are expressed by Aδ and C nerves. These nerves then transmit this noxious information or, the term more commonly used, nociceptive information. This information indicates to the dorsal horn that something is happening that could cause, or has caused, damage to the tissues. An example of this information might be a point of rapidly increasing skin temperature, which may cause a burn, or the chemicals released during inflammation. As Aδ and C nerves respond to nociception and transmit nociceptive information they are known as nociceptive nerves (Julius & Basbaum 2001; Woolf & Ma 2007).

The above information is summarised in Box 8.1.

> ### Box 8.1
>
> #### A summary of the different sensory nerves
>
> The different types of sensory afferent nerves carry their messages at different speeds. The specialised receptors on the end of them, when activated by their specific stimuli, allow ions to flow into the nerve at that point. The result, if enough ions flow to cause an action potential to be generated is action potentials travel along the nerve to the dorsal horn in the spinal cord. The receptors on Aβ nerves are easy to stimulate (low-threshold) and these carry messages relating to non-threatening or innocuous stimuli. The receptors on Aδ and C nerves take a greater stimulus to excite them (high threshold) and they carry messages about stimuli that can threaten the tissues, e.g. hot and cold, heavy pressure and chemicals, especially those released during inflammation. These various stimuli are known as nociception. The nerves which carry this nociceptive information are referred to as nociceptive nerves.

The pathway of nerves from the periphery to the brain

The path of the action potential from the periphery to the brain

The destination for information travelling in these sensory nerves is the dorsal horn in the spinal cord and then on to the brain. To reach the brain, the message, in the form of action potentials, needs to pass from nerve to nerve. Against what was proposed back in the 17th century (Melzack & Wall 1988), there is no single nerve that takes messages from the periphery to the brain. Instead there are a number of nerves, with each passing its messages on to the next at the point where they join or connect. The point at which one nerve connects to another is known as a synapse.

The action potentials in the sensory afferent nerves travel from one end in the tissues to the other end, the presynaptic membrane, which is in the dorsal horn. The arrival of these action potentials may cause chemicals (neurotransmitters), such as glutamate, to be released from the presynaptic membrane into the synaptic space between it and the next nerve (Figure 8.3).

They travel across the gap between the two nerves and connect to their receptor on the end of the next nerve (postsynaptic membrane). As with our stimuli and receptors, imagine these neurotransmitters as keys trying to find their respective receptors or locks. If the key fits the lock and it binds to its receptor, the door (ion channel) briefly opens and positively charged particles flow through into the end of the next nerve (the second-order neurone). If enough doors are opened on the postsynaptic membrane to raise its charge above its activation threshold, an action potential is generated. The second-order neurone then conducts this action potential to the next nerve. This continues from nerve to nerve until it reaches the brain. For a review of the

neurophysiological events underpinning the generation of action potentials please refer to Martini (2006).

It may be helpful to consider the message passing along the sensory nerve as the first runner in a relay. The point where the first runner reaches the end of his length and passes the baton to the next runner is the synapse. If the postsynaptic membrane activation threshold is reached and an action potential is generated in the second-order neurone, the baton would be considered as having been successfully passed on. The runner on the second leg, in the form of the action potential in the second-order neurone, then sets off on a sprint from the postsynaptic membrane along the second-order neurone.

Pain is all in our head

We have considered the generation of action potentials in response to different stimuli. These messages travel in the sensory nerves to the brain and it is within the brain that the sensation of pain is generated. 'No brain, no pain' (Jensen et al. 2008 p. 195).

For the brain to produce what we call sensations or 'feelings', it considers information from a number of sources. Using hunger as an example, the brain will gather various pieces of information, e.g. feedback from the liver, the blood, the stomach and the eyes (e.g. the clock telling us it is lunchtime), and, as a result of all these, it may decide we should eat

Figure 8.3 • The synapse between the sensory afferent and the second-order neurone.

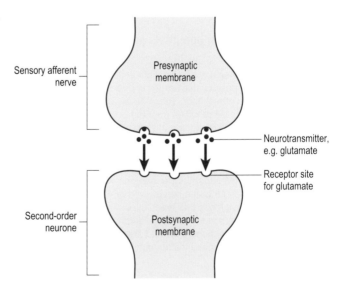

and so we may experience the sensation of hunger. However, sensory information is not the whole picture: context, emotion and knowledge will strongly influence this decision process. The brain may have come to the conclusion that we need to eat but it may not be helpful to feel hungry if you are perhaps in the middle of an important presentation. Hence, the feeling of hunger may be delayed until afterwards when you may then experience it and act accordingly. The brain makes us experience hunger in an effort to look after us from a nutritional point of view. You might consider the experience of hunger as a warning signal that we need to eat because the brain perceives we need food. It does this using the sensory information available to it along with multiple other factors before deciding what we will feel.

Pain, like hunger, is a sensation produced by the brain. The incoming messages from the nociceptive nerves are processed in conjunction with other factors, including knowledge, beliefs, emotional state and past experience. The result of this complex interaction may be the sensation of pain. Pain might be thought of as a warning signal that we need to take action because the brain perceives the body is being threatened (Woolf & Ma 2007). The absence of pain in the injured soldiers observed by Beecher (1956) is a powerful demonstration that pain, like other sensations, can be temporarily delayed and the relationship between pain and damage is not fixed.

A summary of the above information can be found in Box 8.2.

Box 8.2

A summary of action potentials and nociception

A delta (Aδ) and C sensory afferent nerves conduct nociceptive messages from the tissues to their synapses situated within the dorsal horn. These cause neurotransmitters to be released from the presynaptic membrane. If a sufficient amount of neurotransmitters find their respective receptors on the postsynaptic membrane of the next nerve (second-order neurone) the activation threshold is reached. An action potential is then generated in the second-order neurone which travels along the length of the nerve.

When nociceptive messages reach the brain they are processed in conjunction with multiple factors, including knowledge, beliefs, emotional state and past experience. The combination of all these factors may result in the sensation of pain.

The pain gate theory

In the 1960s Melzack & Wall (1965) proposed the pain gate theory. Part of their theory stated that the messages travelling in the Aδ and C sensory afferent nerves could be inhibited at the dorsal horn. To understand what is meant by inhibited, let us recap and expand on our existing descriptions of nerves.

We have considered the generation of action potentials in response to stimuli. These travel to the presynaptic membrane and cause neurotransmitters to be released into the synapse. If the state of 'readiness' of the presynaptic membrane to release neurotransmitters was reduced, the arriving action potentials would cause less or maybe no neurotransmitters to be released. There may then not be enough to trigger an action potential in the second-order neurone. If this were to happen, the information arriving from the periphery via the Aδ and C nerves would be blocked or inhibited from being passed on. The correct term for this is that the nerves have been presynaptically inhibited.

If we use our analogy of runners in a relay race, imagine the message approaching the presynaptic membrane as the first runner nearing the end of his sprint. With inhibition of the presynaptic membrane, as he reaches the change-over point (the synapse), he is unsuccessful in passing the baton to the next runner and as a result the next runner cannot begin to sprint.

Melzack & Wall (1965) proposed that the messages coming into the spinal cord from the Aδ and C nerves were presynaptically inhibited. They stated that the source of the inhibition was via activity in the Aβ nerves which conduct innocuous stimuli, e.g. touch. In simple terms, they scientifically explained what children discover for themselves every day – if you rub something better, it does not hurt as much.

A neural mechanism to explain pain relief achieved by manual therapy

From a therapeutic point of view, this offered an explanation as to why therapies that touched or rubbed the body, e.g. massage and manual therapy techniques, could reduce pain. The non-threatening or innocuous Aβ input to the spinal cord presynaptically inhibited the threatening or nociceptive information travelling in the Aδ and C nerves. By reducing the nociceptive input reaching the brain, pain relief may be experienced. Using this principle, an electrical therapy was developed called transcutaneous electrical nerve stimulation or TENS. TENS is a small battery-powered unit producing high-frequency electrical pulses which, when applied over an area, stimulate the local Aβ nerves. The pain-relieving effects of this cheap and simple method are still widely utilised today in many areas of pain management, including childbirth (Dowswell et al. 2009) and chronic pain (Nnoaham & Kumbang 2008).

The limitations of the pain gate theory

Despite advancing scientific thought and therapeutic interventions, the pain gate theory could not explain all clinical presentations. Examples of these are patients in whom light touch has the opposite effect and is excruciatingly painful or those for whom TENS does not work (Nnoaham & Kumbang 2008). To understand these, we need to appreciate the physiological events that transpire when we hurt ourselves and especially those that occur when pain persists.

The physiological events following an injury

To consider the physiological consequences following an injury we will use the example of a sprained ankle. The events occurring in the tissues, the dorsal horn and the brain in response to the initial injury will be discussed. In addition to this, the changes that occur with ongoing nociception and pain will be briefly included. The following text is drawn from various references (Melzack & Wall 1988; Rice 1998; Kandell et al. 2000; Ji et al. 2003; van Griensven 2005).

Physiological events in the tissues following an injury

Initially, at the point of injury, the tissues are stretched and may be damaged by the ankle sprain. The mechanical stretch may stimulate the receptors on the Aδ and C nerves, causing action potentials to be sent to the dorsal horn, indicating that something that threatens the body has happened in the tissues.

As a result of any tissue injury, chemicals will be released by the damaged cells. These chemicals initiate inflammation, the first step in the normal healing process. There are a multitude of inflammatory chemicals and collectively they are referred to as 'the inflammatory soup' (Rice 1998). The key chemicals you may read about are histamine, bradykinin, prostaglandins and serotonin (Watson 2009). Aside from activating the chemical receptors, some of the chemicals in the inflammatory soup also sensitise the receptors on the end of the surrounding sensory nerves. When sensitised, the receptors are more easily stimulated (lowered activation threshold) and they produce a greater number of action potentials than normal for the same stimulus. The net result is that more nociceptive messages are generated in the Aδ and C nerves.

A commonly observed key clinical finding resulting from this sensitisation is that a stimulus that is normally painful is now more painful. This can be understood by the brain, via the dorsal horn, receiving more nociceptive messages for a given stimulus due to the nociceptors being more easily stimulated and generating more action potentials. This phenomenon is known as hyperalgesia. When this occurs in the tissues as a result of the local sensitisation, it is called primary hyperalgesia.

The inflammatory soup and the repeated stimulation of the nociceptors cause chemicals such as substance P and calcitonin gene-related peptide (CGRP) to be released from the ends of the nociceptive nerves into the surrounding tissues. These chemicals further stimulate the inflammatory process.

In addition to the nociceptors that respond immediately, there are nociceptors which in normal life do not respond to any stimuli. These might be thought of as dormant and they are called silent nociceptors (Schmidt et al. 1995). When these silent nociceptors are exposed to the inflammatory soup they wake up and, being multimodal, respond to all the same stimuli as the other nociceptors, e.g. mechanical, thermal AND chemical. This increase in the number of available receptors offers a further explanation for the physiological mechanisms underpinning primary hyperalgesia (Schmidt et al. 1995).

The net result of these various physiological events is a rising level of nociceptive messages being conducted along the Aδ and C nerves from the injured tissues to the dorsal horn.

Summary of physiological events in the tissues following injury

Following tissue injury, nociceptors in the vicinity are triggered to fire by the traumatic mechanical deformation of the tissues and inflammatory soup of

Box 8.3

An alternative analogy to explain physiological events in the tissues

Imagine, following an injury, the various receptors in the body tissues are children. Naturally, children cry out when an injury occurs; in this case, their cries are via action potentials which travel from the periphery to the dorsal horn. This needs to be thought of as Dad.

The first that Dad (the dorsal horn) knows of the injury is that some of the children are crying. At this stage he is not sure why, only that something problematic has happened in the tissues. As time passes this crying may get louder and it may disturb other sleeping children who wake up and start crying as well.

chemicals. The repeated firing and the inflammatory soup sensitise the nociceptors, which leads to a greater number of action potentials and the release of substance P and CGRP from the Aδ and C nerves. The net result of these changes is primary hyperalgesia.

An alternative analogy summarising these may be found in Box 8.3.

Physiological events in the dorsal horn following an injury

The nociceptive messages produced following an injury travel along the Aδ and C nerves to the dorsal horn. The dorsal horn acts as a relay station passing the nociceptive messages from the periphery on to the brain.

At the dorsal horn, incoming nociceptive messages may be inhibited, as described earlier with reference to the pain gate theory. Presynaptic inhibition of the afferent Aδ and C nociceptive activity may be produced by activity in the Aβ nerves. Research has shown that this inhibition can be produced, or mediated, by an inhibitory interneurone. This is a separate nerve that connects the Aβ nerve and the Aδ and C nerves. Stimulation of the inhibitory interneurone by activity in the Aβ nerve causes inhibition to occur in the Aδ and C nerves.

If the nociceptive barrage to the dorsal horn from the periphery continues, much like the tissues, it may become sensitised and this can occur within a few minutes following an injury (Woolf & Ma 2007). There are a number of different mechanisms proposed to bring about this central sensitisation (Sandkuhler 2007): the key ones to consider are long-term potentiation (which includes wind-up) and physical changes in the dorsal horn.

Long-term potentiation

Long-term potentiation is a broad term used in neuroscience. In relation to the dorsal horn, it needs to be thought of as the synapses between the sensory afferent nerves and the second-order neurones becoming better at passing on the messages they receive (Sandkuhler 2007). For our running analogy, the baton is passed on more easily.

One method by which this occurs is that of wind-up. This is the process of sensitisation which is mediated by the activation of a receptor called the N-methyl-D-arginine (NMDA) receptor. Currently wind-up has been observed only in animal studies (van Griensven 2005). Whilst clinically, it does seem to be true, the research evidence to confirm this in humans is lacking.

Action potentials arriving in Aδ and C nerves cause the release of the neurotransmitter glutamate into the synapse. Glutamate normally fits the lock on a receptor known as an α-amino-3-hydroxyl-5-methyl-4-isoxazole-propionate (AMPA) receptor and it potentially could fit another receptor, the NMDA receptor. However, the NMDA receptor is normally obstructed or plugged by a magnesium ion. Following the ankle injury, as a result of the ongoing nociceptive messages arriving from the periphery, this plug is removed (Costigan & Woolf 2000). Both the AMPA and the NMDA receptors are then possible receptor sites for glutamate. Glutamate binding to the NMDA receptor causes a greater flow of ions across the postsynaptic membrane. This results in an action potential being more easily generated in the second-order neurone. With continuing stimulation, as in the periphery, chemicals are released by the sensitised second-order neurone into the synapse, which causes the sensory afferent nerve to release even more glutamate (Costigan & Woolf 2000). This further enhances sensitisation and leads to a greater output of nociceptive messages travelling to the brain.

The net result of these changes is that a single nociceptive message in the sensory afferent nerve now produces even more messages in the second-order neurones (Costigan & Woolf 2000).

Physical changes in the dorsal horn with central sensitisation

With ongoing nociception, it has been observed that physical changes occur in the dorsal horn (Costigan & Woolf 2000). These include:

- death of the inhibitory interneurones
- sprouting of the Aβ nerves into areas where normally only Aδ and C nerves synapse.

The former results in reduced inhibition and the latter may result in touch and pressure being mistakenly interpreted as nociceptive information, which might itself cause pain. When an innocuous stimulus, such as touch, is perceived as being painful, this is termed allodynia.

Consequences of central sensitisation

It can now begin to be seen how nociceptive messages from the periphery may be modified. Depending on the extent of these changes, they begin to explain why different patients with similar injuries might report different symptoms.

For simplicity, when considering the nerves that sensory afferents synapse with, the term second-order neurone has been used. To understand clinical presentations we need to consider second-order neurones as being either nociceptive-specific (NS) or wide-dynamic-range (WDR) neurones. WDR neurones are also referred to as WDR cells.

- NS neurones pass on the nociceptive messages from the C nerves.
- WDR neurones receive messages from Aβ, Aδ, C and the inhibitory interneurones.

The WDR neurone receives inputs from a number of different nerves; some of these may be inhibitory and some may stimulate it. Depending on the balance of inputs the WDR neurone receives, it may or may not pass on a nociceptive message. If it receives relatively more stimulation, nociceptive messages are passed on. If it receives more inhibition, nociceptive messages are not passed on.

If sensitised by the processes discussed, second-order neurones might amplify incoming nociceptive input, which could result in hyperalgesia. Hyperalgesia as a result of central sensitisation is referred to as secondary hyperalgesia. Remember, primary hyperalgesia is hyperalgesia which occurs due to sensitisation of the end of the sensory afferents by the inflammatory soup. Hyperalgesia experienced in areas distant from any initial injury may indicate central sensitisation of the dorsal horn.

If the WDR neurone is sensitised, the Aβ input to it may be a pathway by which an innocuous stimulus could produce nociceptive messages and pain. As mentioned above, when an innocuous stimulus, such as touch, is perceived as being painful, this is termed allodynia. The easiest way to observe this in the body is when you have burnt yourself. After a little while, touching the area around the burn, sometimes centimetres away, may be tender or painful. A lesson here

for clinical practice is that something may be painful to touch but it does not necessarily mean there is damage there.

Summary of physiological events in the dorsal horn following injury

Stretching and damage to the local tissues with an ankle sprain results in nociceptive input being received in the dorsal horn, via the sensory afferent nerves. The second-order NS neurones receive C nerve input and the WDR neurones receive inputs from Aβ, Aδ, C and the inhibitory interneurones. Prolonged stimulation induces long-term potentiation, which includes wind-up and physical changes within the dorsal horn. This results in a greater output in the second-order neurone for a given input. In the injured tissues a painful stimulus may now elicit more pain for the same input (hyperalgesia). This occurs due to primary and secondary hyperalgesia. Allodynia, or pain with an innocuous stimulus, may also be observed due to sensitisation of the WDR neurone.

With continued nociception, physical changes in the dorsal horn collectively result in the dorsal horn developing the capacity to report far greater levels of nociception for a given input. This is due to sensitisation and a reduction in inhibition.

An alternative analogy summarising this may be found in Box 8.4.

Box 8.4

An alternative analogy to explain physiological events in the dorsal horn

The children (the receptors in the tissues) are crying out to Dad (the dorsal horn) and faithfully he passes the message on to the brain (Mum) that something has happened (via action potentials). With children the usual advice is to rub it better; this may help a bit and if so, it might prevent Mum having to be continually bothered. However, if that isn't entirely effective and the children keep crying then Dad might start to listen more attentively to the children. He might become sensitive to their cries and as the situation winds him up he raises his voice in telling Mum what's happening. This heightened state of affairs will eventually have an impact on the other children nearby and just a cough, not even crying, from them might send Dad off into a frenzy, shouting to Mum that something is happening with them.

Physiological events in the brain following an injury

Whilst separated out here for illustrative purposes, the reality is that, if an injury is sustained, nociceptive information quickly arrives at the brain. Within this narrative, we will not consider the huge variety of locations to which the nociceptive information is distributed in the brain. For a review the reader is guided to Treede et al. (1999). As briefly raised earlier, incoming nociception is processed in conjunction with a variety of factors, including context, memory, emotions, thoughts, mood and beliefs (Tracey & Mantyh 2007). The dimensions that contribute to the pain experience are considerable; some of these are shown in Figure 8.4. These combine together and influence the reaction to an injury and the pain experienced.

To understand how these factors combine within the brain, Melzack (2002) proposed a conceptual model called 'the neuromatrix', now more commonly referred to as the pain matrix (Tracey & Mantyh 2007). In this, the various components combine to produce a certain pattern of electrical activity in the brain which constitutes the pain experience for that patient at that time. This is known as a neurosignature and this may be very different for different people who share the same injury. The longer an individual is in pain, the more reinforced the pain neurosignature becomes and the more easily it runs. This might become a problem when the pain neurosignature is triggered very easily or it will not switch off. Remember, the neurosignature will be made up from multiple brain areas, including the other senses.

One might now start to imagine how the mere sight of someone else bending over or lifting something might be enough to trigger the pain neurosignature in a patient with persistent pain.

The mechanisms underpinning the wide variety of reactions to pain

Our discussion has alluded to the clinical observation that the variety of possible responses to pain is considerable and differs from person to person. We will now consider how the brain can quickly create this great range of reactions to pain. These will be briefly discussed under the following headings:

- descending pain inhibition
- the sympathetic nervous system (SNS)
- the endocrine system
- the musculoskeletal system
- descending pain facilitation
- supraspinal changes.

Descending pain inhibition

This refers to inhibition of nociceptive messages at the dorsal horn via descending nerves from the brain.

Melzack & Wall (1965) also proposed that nociceptive activity at the level of the dorsal horn can be further modified by nerves that run from the brain to the dorsal horn. The mechanism for this is via them stimulating the local release within the dorsal horn of powerful natural analgesics (painkillers) called opioids. These may temporarily completely block or inhibit the nociceptive messages arriving in the sensory afferents (Tracey & Mantyh 2007).

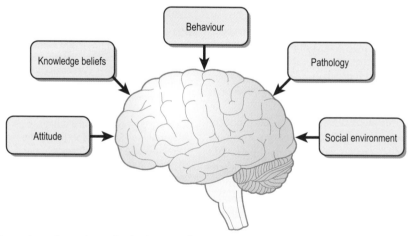

Figure 8.4 • The various dimensions of pain that contribute to the pain experience.

The observation of people experiencing a temporary absence of pain despite significant injury could hypothetically be explained via this mechanism.

The sympathetic nervous system

The SNS, part of the autonomic nervous system, innervates a range of structures, including the blood vessels, viscera, heart and muscles. Activity in the SNS is increased in the presence of pain. The result of this activity is the release of the hormone nor-adrenaline (norepinephrine) from the ends of the sympathetic nerves. The effect of noradrenaline is to prepare the body for action. This is achieved by raising blood pressure and heart rate and increasing the blood supply and energy available for use in the muscles. In addition, it triggers the release of the hormone adrenaline (epinephrine), leading to further widespread sympathetic effects. These changes in response to stressful situations are commonly summarised as the flight or fight reaction (Gifford & Thacker 2002).

The presence of persistent pain prolongs this stress reaction, which may cause associated cardio-vascular and digestive problems. For a fuller description of the SNS with respect to pain, please see Gifford & Thacker (2002).

The endocrine system

In response to stress via connections through the SNS, the hormone cortisol may be released into the blood from the hypothalamus (Gifford & Thacker 2002). This hormone both facilitates the release of energy for use in the muscles and inhibits the inflammatory process. This may be a useful short-term measure in focusing resources for action, e.g. running off a busy road. However, as inflammation is the first stage of the healing process, its inhibition may lead to delayed or poor healing of injured tissues.

The musculoskeletal system

Pain has the power to change how we move (Vlaeyen & Linton 2000). A sprained ankle may make us limp to protect the limb. This may be beneficial in the short term to prevent further nociception and reduce the load on healing tissue in the early stages of repair. A continued avoidance of movements that were pre-viously painful may lead to a fear that pain will be experienced on reattempting them. This fear of movement is commonly referred to as kinesophobia (Kori et al. 1990). As a result, limitations in the frequency of movement may cause a reduction in physical fitness (Vlaeyen & Linton 2000). It could be hypothesised that weakness and stiffness may then develop and result in further musculoskeletal problems, nociception and possibly more pain.

Descending pain facilitation

While the brain can turn down or block incoming nociception, it can also turn it up or enhance it (Wiech et al. 2008). Whilst far less understood than descending pain control, it may play a role in facilitating and maintaining central sensitisation (Vera-Portocarreroa et al. 2006).

Supraspinal changes

You may remember from your training that the body is represented in the brain on sensory maps, which help define how the brain 'sees' the body. These are often represented visually by the funny-looking man with skinny small legs, large lips, huge hands and an out-of-proportion head, known as homunculus man. What is now understood is that these maps are dynamic and changeable, especially in the presence of ongoing pain (Flor 2003; Apkarian et al. 2004). If these change as a result of pain, the brain may no longer 'see' the painful part of the body in the same way. As the brain uses these maps to help plan and execute movements, it has been theorised that move-ment patterns may change and these may contribute toward perpetuating the problem (Moseley 2007a). Interestingly, there is early evidence that, when asked to draw their lumbar spine, those with low-back pain cannot find the part that hurts in their mind and as a result their drawings are incomplete (Moseley 2008).

Summary of physiological events in the brain following injury

Nociceptive information generated from our sprained ankle is directed to multiple locations in the brain and is integrated with numerous other fac-tors. The amount of pain experienced and the response to the pain may vary enormously from patient to patient. The various reactions may be mediated by a number of different physiological mechanisms, including:

- Nociceptive input from the periphery may be inhibited by the secretion of opioids.
- Noradrenaline, adrenaline and cortisol may be secreted.

Box 8.5

An alternative analogy to explain physiological events in the brain

Dad has passed messages to Mum that the children are crying. Mum weighs up the situation based on all the information she has available to her, including experience, emotion and beliefs. If her conclusion is that that it is trivial and doesn't need a big response she might reassure Dad, and tell to him to not worry her about the crying, it will pass and isn't that important. She might also make sure the children have little reason to complain by doing all the things that encourage them to calm down and stop crying. The result is that any ongoing whimpers gradually reduce and disappear. There is no need to get hearts racing and all stressed for very long.

Alternatively, what if Mum overreacted slightly and she did worry excessively? She might then start getting hot and bothered, heart racing and blood pressure rising. By encouraging different movements thinking these might help recovery e.g limping, the children might calm down temporarily but with time they start to moan again. If she felt it necessary, despite Dad already being sensitised to the situation, she might further encourage him to respond to any murmur from the children. The net result now is that she is on alert, as is Dad, and the children are crying louder than ever.

- Movement patterns may be altered to protect the painful body part.
- The sensory maps of the body may be altered with persistent pain.
- The brain may facilitate the transmission of the nociceptive information at the dorsal horn.

An alternative analogy summarising these may be found in Box 8.5.

Harnessing the power of the mind with pain can be powerful

We have so far alluded to a number of physiological processes occurring from the point of injury through to the brain with little discussion of the influence of conscious thought or action. As you might imagine, these are powerful avenues by which clinicians can work with patients to facilitate recovery. Reassurance and clear explanations of what pain really means may reduce fear (Moseley 2004). This may limit activity in the SNS and prevent the secretion of cortisol, preventing possible interruptions to the healing process. Maintenance of normal movement may further encourage healing via application of therapeutic

stresses which guide the healing process (Watson 2009). These movements may reduce or alleviate fear of movement and any associated reductions in fitness caused by limiting physical activity (Vlaeyen & Linton 2000). The above changes, if successful in maintaining movement and alleviating pain, may hypothetically prevent changes in the sensory maps and facilitate recovery.

By understanding the possible physiological consequences of pain, the clinician might adapt his or her treatment plan to optimise recovery and prevent problems before they develop. Skills such as relaxation might be employed as a result of clinical reasoning, e.g. teaching relaxation to reduce SNS activity (Payne 2005). These may be especially useful when symptoms have persisted and further problems of central sensitisation now coexist. Knowledge of these physiological mechanisms may bring insight as to those that dominate the clinical presentation and could be best targeted with treatment.

Pain mechanisms

The method by which nociceptive messages are generated and modified has been discussed with strong reference to nociceptive input as a result of a tissue injury.

Pain resulting from such an injury is commonly termed nociceptive pain. In addition, nociception may originate from an injury to a nerve itself and pain experienced as a result of that is termed peripheral neurogenic pain. Finally, nociception may be enhanced by changes in the dorsal horn, which we have discussed under central sensitisation.

It will be helpful in your clinical reasoning to understand how each of these different mechanisms may present. This knowledge may then be used to target the most effective treatment programme. In addition, we need to consider the terms referred pain and acute and chronic pain to contextualise them within our discussion.

Nociceptive pain

Nociceptive pain can be thought of as the everyday pain we all experience, i.e. bruises, burns, strains and sprains. It results from nociceptive messages generated following an injury or pathology in the body tissues. Following this the body would be expected to go through a normal healing process to repair the damage. As healing occurs, nociception from the healing tissue should reduce and disappear within the expected healing time (Watson 2009).

Symptoms

Symptoms that may indicate the presence of nociceptive-mediated pain are as follows (van Griensven 2005):

- Specific movements, sometimes when held, aggravate the pain whilst others ease the pain.
- There are clearly defined borders to the pain.
- There is an on/off pattern of pain with specific postures or activities.
- Findings from physical examination tests are consistent.
- The pain reduces in line with the expected healing time.
- It responds well to manual and electrical treatments directed at reducing nociception.
- It responds well to simple painkillers (analgesics).
- With inflammation there may be redness/swelling and increased temperature.
- Pain due to ischaemia from prolonged postures will improve with postural correction.

Clinical consideration

For the clinician dealing with acute injuries, the assessment findings listed may be commonplace. As time passes from the point of injury, the additional local and central changes previously discussed may cloud the clinical presentation. Sensitisation in the dorsal horn may result in allodynia which may produce false positives on physical tests, i.e. a test may produce pain where there is no injury or pathology. Manual treatment may be applied, in the expectation that it will decrease pain via the pain gate theory, but symptoms may be increased due to central sensitisation. This may confuse the clinician and dishearten the patient.

It is important to approach any patient presenting with an injury with an open mind. It is important to consider not only the nociception from the tissues but also to be aware of possible central sensitisation. This is to be suspected if symptoms do not fit your expectations based on the history or the results from physical tests are confusing.

Conversely, the role of ongoing nociception in longer-standing problems must not be ignored. As nociception can maintain central sensitisation, one should not discount possible sources of nociception

such as scar tissue, shortened muscles or stiff joints (Costigan & Woolf 2000). Whilst the clinical picture may well be complicated by central changes, carefully applied local treatments may improve tissue strength, length and quality. These may be useful in the management of these patients through a reduction in nociception, which may contribute towards a reduction in central sensitisation.

Peripheral neurogenic pain

This is pain generated as a result of damage to peripheral nerves. The term neuropathic pain is often used interchangeably with neurogenic pain, the difference being that neurogenic pain may be transitory in nature, i.e. it does not last as long (IASP 2009).

Damage to a nerve can be thought of as ranging from quickly compressing it, e.g. banging your funny bone, to forcefully stretching or cutting it. The extent of the damage will, to a certain extent, dictate the symptoms experienced. For a comprehensive review please see van Griensven (2005).

Damage anywhere along the length of the nerve can cause action potentials to be generated at the point of injury, which can then travel both up and down the nerve. Some may travel along the nerve towards the dorsal horn as they normally would. The others may go 'the wrong way' down the nerve toward the periphery. Action potentials terminating in the periphery cause the release of substance P and CGRP from the end of the nerve (White & Helme 1985). These chemicals have strong effects and from our previous discussion we know they encourage the inflammatory response. This inflammatory response can be maintained by these chemicals even in the absence of any local tissue damage. This is known as neurogenic inflammation (Black 2002).

Another response of a nerve following damage is the manufacture of more receptors, which are then inserted along the nerve within the locality of the damage. A consequence of these additional receptors is that action potentials can be generated spontaneously (ectopic action potentials) (Woolf & Ma 2007). The dorsal horn and brain interpret these messages as nociceptive activity originating from where the nerve terminates in the periphery. Symptoms may then be felt and reported there, despite the absence of tissue pathology. Some of these new receptors may be sensitive to adrenaline (adrenergic), which is released via SNS activity during stressful situations and which may then cause nociception and pain.

Symptoms

The symptoms of pain mediated by a peripheral neurogenic source may include (van Griensven 2005):

- a history of trauma to a nerve; this may include surgery
- a continuation of the pain beyond the normal timescale of healing
- sudden bursts of pain for no obvious reason
- pain that does not fit a normal on/off pattern with aggravating and easing movements
- difficulty in describing the pain
- numbness or altered sensation, e.g. pins and needles
- increased pain when stressed
- a lack of response to simple analgesics, e.g. paracetamol.

Clinical considerations

Peripheral neurogenic pain may have an underlying musculoskeletal cause, e.g. compression by scar tissue or a tight muscle. In these situations addressing these structures may bring resolution to the symptoms (see Chapter 7 for further information).

A challenging aspect of managing peripheral neurogenic pain is the fact that it does not respond well to simple analgesics. Interestingly, other medications such as antidepressants and anticonvulsants can be extremely useful in controlling peripheral neurogenic pain when prescribed in doses lower than would be used for their original condition (Ross 2004).

Central sensitisation

This refers to a state in which the neurones in the dorsal horn become sensitised to input from the periphery. Clinically this leads to a reduction in pain thresholds, hyperalgesia and allodynia in areas adjacent to the original injury (Ji et al. 2003).

These changes, like those observed with peripheral neurogenic pain, can manifest in a wide variety of symptoms. As a result, they may not always make sense to both patient and clinician.

Common features which can help identify central sensitisation are (van Griensven 2005):

- the continuation of pain beyond the normal timescale of healing
- pain that does not fit a normal on/off pattern with aggravating and easing movements

- exaggerated pain response to a given stimulus or pain in response to a normally non-painful stimulus
- a difficultly in describing the pain
- a lack of response to simple analgesics, e.g. paracetamol
- a history of failed, or lack of improvement with, conventional treatments
- pain expanding into areas adjacent to the original site of injury/pain.

It must be noted that a number of these symptoms overlap with peripheral neurogenic pain. As a result, it may not be possible to differentiate between the two in a patient presenting with a mixed pattern of symptoms.

Clinical considerations

Determining the contribution of central sensitisation to patients' symptoms is not a simple objective task. One needs to consider the timescale in which symptoms have been present: the longer past the expected healing time, the more central sensitisation should be suspected in maintaining symptoms. The highly irritable patient is an example in which a given input produces a significant reaction. Central sensitisation may well be suspected here. A knowledge of associated musculoskeletal and visceral structures innervated by the same and adjacent spinal level may assist in determining the presence of central sensitisation. Alterations in their function and the presence of allodynia or hyperalgesia in them may lead you to suspect central sensitisation.

If central sensitisation is suspected, a confident but cautious approach to examination and treatment is recommended to prevent exacerbating a patient's symptoms.

Referred pain

Referred pain is pain reported in an area separate from where suggested 'causal' pathology is located. Pain commonly labelled as referred may be hypothetically explained as resulting from peripheral neurogenic pain affecting the nerve innervating the structures reported as painful, e.g. sciatica. Other clinical examples cannot be explained by such mechanisms, e.g. the arm pain experienced during a heart attack. Numerous mechanisms have been proposed to explain this phenomenon. The coming together (convergence) of inputs from somatic structures (muscles, ligaments) and visceral structures in the dorsal horn is the most common. This is simplistic, explained by the brain becoming confused as to where the nociceptive input has come from. Unfortunately, none of the various theories proposed to date explain all the clinical findings associated with referred pain (van Griensven 2005).

The lesson for practice is always to perform a thorough clinical examination and maintain a knowledge of the various structures innervated by each spinal level.

Acute and chronic pain

Patients in pain are often labelled as being either acute or chronic, with recent-onset pain being labelled as acute and pain present for longer than 3 months being chronic (Waddell 2004). These terms may cause confusion with respect to the treatments you might expect to use as these will depend on the clinical presentation, which may vary enormously. See Box 8.6 for two patient presentations, one acute and one chronic.

Box 8.6

Clinical presentations of an acute and a chronic pain patient

As you read about the patients below, consider the physiological mechanisms at the tissues, dorsal horn and brain that may explain the presentation. Once you have done that consider your treatment options based on your thoughts regarding the underlying neurophysiology.

Patient 1

An acute pain patient presents to you with a sprained ankle which happened 2 days earlier. The patient is non-weight-bearing on crutches with a cold foot which is exquisitely painful to touch. The patient has minimal active movement in the foot and reports a high level of pain on any movement. Palpation of the whole foot causes pain with only light touch. X-rays taken 2 days ago indicate no fracture and the history suggests minimal to moderate trauma.

Patient 2

A chronic pain patient presents to you with a sprained ankle which happened 2 years earlier. The patient is fully weight-bearing with a normal-coloured foot and no temperature differences. The patient has full range of movement except for some stiffness at the end of dorsiflexion. There is thickening and tenderness on palpation of the lateral ligaments. X-rays taken at the time of injury reported no fracture. The history of original trauma was minimal to moderate and the patient reported it had settled very quickly but had been continually bothered by a small amount of pain experienced when going down stairs.

Guidelines for the treatment of pain

The following uses the knowledge discussed to draw out principles that may help to guide the effective management of a patient in pain. The other chapters in this book will expand on these and consider possible treatment options.

The tissues and the peripheral nerves

After an injury the inflammatory process is followed by the regeneration phase, which sees growth of new blood vessels and the laying down of new collagen. The result of this process is the restoration of mechanical strength and function to the area (Watson 2009). Treatments aimed at improving the quality and function of healing tissue and peripheral nerves may be applied. These may come from either the patient or the clinician (e.g. massage, mobilisations, exercise). From a pain perspective, a key underlying neurophysiological aim of these treatments is to reduce nociceptive input to the dorsal horn.

An awareness of the central influences on healing, such as cortisol and altered activity due to fear avoidance, must not be overlooked. With these in mind, treatments aimed at the dorsal horn and the brain should be used in conjunction with tissue-based therapies. See below for details.

The dorsal horn

The goal of treatments directed at the dorsal horn may be classified under one of the following:

- reducing peripheral nociception arriving at the dorsal horn, which can serve to maintain central sensitisation
- enhancing inhibition at the sensitised spinal segment.

The first is discussed above. Enhancing inhibition at a sensitised segment may be addressed using the pain gate theory. Local manual treatments might be utilised to encourage inhibition, e.g. TENS, massage. However, if the local area is too tender to touch or touch causes pain, a different approach is needed. The answer might lie in using your knowledge of other structures that synapse at a similar spinal level. The stimulation of these other structures, especially skin and muscle, may, via massage or stretching, be used to provide input to the spinal level and enhance inhibition. As you consider the various other chapters consider the effect the treatments discussed will have and how they might be utilised to achieve this treatment goal.

The brain

The role of the brain in combining nociception with various psychological factors has been emphasised. Whilst not featured strongly in this text, the influence of social factors in the experience of pain should be remembered (Waddell 2004). Clinicians need to be mindful of these factors, whatever the length of time someone has been in pain. Therapeutic intervention directed at the brain should aim to:

- prevent or improve associated disability
- reduce descending facilitation
- maximise descending inhibition
- prevent central sensitisation and supraspinal changes.

In addition to the methods already discussed, we can broadly summarise further treatment options which target the brain under the following headings:

- addressing faulty thoughts and beliefs
- teaching and encouraging recovery behaviours
- supplying good-quality understandable information that benefits the patient

The concept of yellow flags will be briefly discussed within the first section.

Addressing faulty thoughts and beliefs

Negative thoughts such as imagining things to be far worse than reality are referred to as catastrophising and these have the power to limit recovery (Nicholas 2009). An example of catastrophising might be a patient who experiences back pain when lifting a small box. She might then quickly conclude that if she cannot lift a box she will be unable to pick up her children and eventually might end up in a wheelchair. These thought progressions, although not always logical, can and do happen very quickly and patients may be unaware of this process.

These thoughts can sometimes be facilitated by poor or inaccurate knowledge or anxiety. With this in mind, take a moment to think how you could explore and challenge these within your scope of practice. See Box 8.7 for ideas on some questions you might find it useful to ask.

Box 8.7

Questions to explore poor or inaccurate knowledge

- What have other professionals and friends or family told you is wrong?
- What do you think is going to happen over time?
- What can you do to help yourself?
- What do your family and friends think is happening?

Engaging, challenging and coaching resistant patients is a topic often dealt with only briefly during undergraduate training. As an active skill, it needs to be practised and whilst it can be done alone you may benefit from regular reflection with colleagues on both the successes and problems you are experiencing.

The addressing of faulty thoughts and beliefs needs to be extended to other family members. An awareness of family members and significant others who play a role in your patient's life can be important (Leonard et al. 2006). Any therapeutic value from your interaction with the patient may quickly be challenged and undermined if the patient returns to a family environment in which therapeutic messages are not reinforced. Worse still, poor thoughts and behaviours may be encouraged, further limiting recovery and maintaining disability. The importance of engaging and educating relatives, partners and close friends cannot be understated (Leonard et al. 2006). If not possible directly, it might be wise to raise this through your discussions with the patient.

Embrace yellow flags and explore patients' thoughts and beliefs

Any clinician in practice today will hear mention of a number of different-coloured flags, e.g. red, yellow, black and blue flags. These are frequently discussed within the context of low-back pain (Kendall et al. 1997). Please refer to Main & Spanswick (1999) for a fuller discussion.

For our discussion we will only consider yellow flags. These are psychological risk factors shown to be predictors for the development of chronic low-back pain, i.e. back pain which lasts longer than 3 months (Waddell 2004). They have been embraced in various therapeutic settings since their introduction over 10 years ago (Kendall et al. 1997; Sowden et al. 2006). Screening for them has been recommended in various low-back pain guidelines (Royal College of General Practitioners 1999; NICE 2009).

Broadly, they include:

- attitudes and beliefs about pain
- a lack of behaviour that encourages recovery
- the reaction to failed treatments
- fear associated with activity and work.

It would be useful for you to familiarise yourself with the relevant topics for yellow flags so you might briefly explore these areas in your clinical encounters. Whilst developed within the scope of low-back pain management, there are important lessons to draw which we can apply in patients presenting with pain in other areas. See Box 8.8 for a summary of the most important yellow flags that predict poor outcome in those with low-back pain. Questions are then included which will help you elicit this information in a clinical scenario. Although not validated for research purposes, these can easily be adapted for any patient in pain and they may provide insight into those thoughts and beliefs that may be barriers to recovery.

Using these factors will help you gain more insight in identifying those patients in whom you suspect pain may persist. If you do suspect a patient's thoughts or behaviour might limit his or her recovery, ask your colleagues what they would do. It is likely you will get a range of answers. Who is right? Well, in different situations they all might be. The core

value to take forward is to use simple questions that engage patients and elicit their perspective on their condition. These then serve as a base on which to clarify and correct faulty beliefs.

Be careful when taking a subjective examination. Do not miss out on engaging with the patient you are talking to. Most of us want to feel listened to, understood, reassured, empowered, cared for and hopeful. These are my words; please change them to those you wish to develop in your practice with patients. Aside from the questions in Boxes 8.7 and 8.8 it can be insightful to ask a patient:

- Why do you think you are experiencing what you are?
- How do you see the future in relation to your pain?
- Do you expect to recover from this?

All of these questions may provide valuable information which might have been missed previously in a symptom-based subjective assessment.

Teaching and encouraging recovery behaviours

The goal here is to encourage your patient to engage in behaviours that promote recovery and limit disability.

From a nutritional perspective, we are told eating fruit and vegetables is recommended. With exercise, we are told regular exercise is good for us. What happens when it hurts? Commonly, a reaction with those in pain is to avoid activities that hurt (Vlaeyen & Linton 2000). In the short term this may be useful but, as time progresses, it brings with it problems of disuse. Through reduced movement individuals may become weaker, stiffer and less fit. In addition, repeated experiences of being unable to do something in a painfree manner may increase fear of pain and lead to them avoiding that activity (fear avoidance) (Vlaeyen & Linton 2000). Quickly, one can see how people might become stuck in a rut without good practical advice.

A principle utilised for years in pain management programmes has been that of starting off with a manageable amount of an activity or exercise and slowly building it up. This is referred to as pacing, graded exposure or graded exercise. Pacing can apply to both functional tasks, e.g. sitting, and strengthening and stretching exercises. The principles and methods of pacing are helpful in managing not only those with chronic pain but all patients in pain (Nicholas et al. 2000).

Patients may stir up symptoms if an exercise regime is completed too vigorously. By starting them

---

Box 8.8

Predictors of poor outcome and identifying questions

The following factors have been found to be important in identifying those patients with low-back pain who are less likely to recover from a recent episode of low-back pain (Sowden et al. 2006).

- The presence of back pain is harmful or potentially severely disabling
- Tendency to low mood and withdrawal from social interaction
- An expectation that passive treatments rather than active participation will help
- Low self-efficacy (the belief that you can do something or succeed in something)

Simple questions to help identify these factors are:

- What do you understand to be the cause of your back pain?
- What are you expecting will help you?
- How is your family and your employer responding to your back pain?
- What are you doing to cope with your back pain?
- Do you think you will return to work and, if so, when?

Box 8.9

Setting a baseline and pacing up activities

Ask your patient to time how long s/he can perform a functional activity or note how many repetitions of an exercise s/he can perform before feeling any pain or discomfort. Ask the patient to repeat this process the next day. Total these two figures and take an average of them, then reduce this average figure by 20%. The final figure serves as an estimate of the patient's activity level baseline which, it is hoped, the patient can complete without discomfort. When the patient reaches this baseline, s/he stops the activity or exercise and does something else. Activity therefore becomes time- or repetition-based as opposed to symptom-based. The aim is to increase this steadily by set increments, e.g. increasing the sitting baseline by 1 minute every 3 days or increasing an exercise by a repetition every 2 days.

slowly and respecting symptoms, repetitions may be paced up and the associated benefits will reinforce the message that exercise is helpful. Patient self-help books often contain detailed examples of this method and are worth reading (Nicholas et al. 2000). See Box 8.9 for a simple description that you might utilise in clinical practice.

For those with low-back pain, historically taking to your bed was a strategy for managing back pain. However, research has shown that this is not the case and staying active is a better strategy (Waddell et al. 1997). Interestingly, catastrophising and fear of injury separated out those who stayed in bed and those who stayed active. After a year the people who took to their beds for longer were still more disabled (Verbunt et al. 2008). Imagine yourself to be a patient with back pain and you are advised not to go to bed. What do you do instead? Advising someone not to do something may be fine; however, make sure you equip patients with what they can or should be doing instead. Giving tips regarding posture and simple adaptations may help by making functional tasks less painful or easier, e.g. pacing. Behind the scenes, the goal is to encourage activity, limit nociception and prevent further central sensitisation.

This aspect of treatment is more than just teaching skills – it requires a personal interaction with your patient. Reinforcing or encouraging good behaviours is important. Your words of encouragement might register not only in the conscious but in the subconscious as well. Praise patients who have followed guidelines, do not criticise when they have made a

mistake but guide them on making a better choice next time. Think of yourself as a coach building them up and guiding them on a path to recovery. What tone of voice should you use? Which words of encouragement? You might consider asking patients what they would appreciate. Remember, any clinical encounter is a two-way process; the goal is to work alongside the patient with each of you doing your bit. Both you and they need to know that for the best result (Goldingay 2006a, b).

Supplying good-quality understandable information that benefits the patient

Recent guidelines on managing low-back pain emphasises that good communication with patients is essential and evidence-based written information tailored to their need should be supplied (NICE 2009).

Patients are often given anatomical and pathological explanations for their pain via advice, back schools and consumer publications. We need to be discerning that the benefits derived from information supplied are as intended. Unpublished research has shown that anatomical descriptions, as given in many back schools, may actually increase fear of movement (Moseley, 2008 personal communication). This is thought to be as a result of patients perceiving that pain equals damage, which could encourage negative thoughts or catastrophisation. Explanations of pain physiology to patients demonstrated improvements in beliefs about pain and gains in physical measures (Moseley 2004). These were thought to be as a result of a reduction in fear about moving. You might now be able to hypothesise the physiological pathways by which this effect is mediated from the previous information.

Publications that present pain in an accessible format for patients are plentiful but, be warned, check them before recommending them. A pathological focus may be dominant (Burn et al. 2007), which from our discussions may not be ideal, depending on the message patients need to hear. That is not to say that you must not give an anatomical explanation. I would recommend you check with patients what any information supplied actually means to them and what lessons they may have learnt. Do not assume that patients have taken the intended meaning from what they have read or what you have said (Daykin 2006).

To illustrate this further, imagine someone had ongoing pain and was told the following:

- The scan of the patient's spine showed it was degenerating and some of the bones were collapsing. How do you think the patient would feel?
- If the patient did some exercises and it made the pain worse, the patient was told to stop those exercises immediately. What might that communicate?
- Following no improvement with treatment a patient was told there was nothing more that could be done. What future might the patient imagine?

Now imagine alternative explanations:

- The patient was told the scan showed normal changes in the spine associated with the patient's age. What now?
- The patient was sore after exercising and was told this may have been some training pain or the patient had attempted a few more than s/he could currently tolerate. As a result s/he simply needed to reduce the number to a comfortable level before steadily increasing again. Is that a positive message?
- Others who have been in the same situation made slow but steady progress and could often achieve the goals they set for themselves. Even running a marathon, if that was their goal!

Remember, you can be a strong influence in decreasing a patient's anxiety and fears. Conversely, poor wording and explanations could unintentionally increase anxiety (Klaber Moffett et al. 2006). Your explanations should reflect the principles detailed in Box 8.10.

Box 8.10

Principles to employ when talking to patients

Within your explanations use the following principles:
- Choose words that are simple
- Forget your technical terms
- Give analogies that people can relate to which normalise and play down the threat of symptoms
- Try not to use emotive words such as collapsed, crushed, snapped or permanent
- Compare investigation findings, e.g. X-rays, with those found in normal individuals with no pain or symptoms
- Emphasise how robust and strong bones, discs, muscles and other body tissues are
- Use stories of people in similar situations who have improved

Your explanations may be the difference in making them understand they are not alone and there is hope, rather than the opposite, more disheartening scenario. One can now immediately see a direct therapeutic role for reassurance of the patient and you could hypothesise how this might be changing the patient's symptoms. As in life, telling the patient not to worry will likely achieve little. A logical, empathetic approach with appropriate reasoning throughout may be the turning point for a patient. This can be easily imagined where the underlying driver for the patient's lack of improvement is the associated complications mediated by the brain via its various output mechanisms.

The power of metaphor

Communicating sometimes complex facts may seem daunting to the novice clinician. A powerful tool, often used in coaching and available to all, which can help enormously is that of metaphor. Metaphor is anything that uses analogies to create new meaning – an obvious example is our Mum, Dad and child examples in the boxes earlier in this chapter. An analogy is where something is recreated in a different way which might be more accessible and hence holds greater meaning. See Moseley (2007b) for a wealth of ideas.

Another example might be using the neurosignature to teach patients about the various factors that combine to produce the experience of pain. For those who like music, you might talk about a pain tune that plays too much or too readily (Butler & Moseley 2003). For the gastronomic, a dynamic pain dish that overpowers; for the visual, a living pain picture or collage that dominates. To give a working model of treatment, for these examples, one might respectively talk of varying the instruments, adjusting the herbs or spices or replacing one scene for another. These might be ways by which complex information may be made accessible to patients. Normalising things may make them seem a lot less threatening (Moseley 2004). This may require creativity on your part in conjunction with time and practice. It cannot be learnt from a book.

Summary: principles of treatment

The various stages of the healing process aim to restore mechanical and functional integrity to an injured area. Physical and electrical modalities may be clinically reasoned and applied to optimise this process. The principles of the pain gate theory and treating areas that share the same spinal innervations as a painful area may facilitate inhibition at the dorsal horn and reduce nociceptive input to the brain. Recognition and addressing of risk factors for chronicity and the provision of clear advice in setting and progressing baselines of activity can maintain and encourage physical recovery and a return to work.

The clinician needs to develop a wide remit of skill in communication to build both empathy and trust in patients and to help them understand knowledge which can prevent disability and improve existing symptoms.

What haven't we covered?

Despite covering a number of topics, pain is a huge topic and there are a number of issues and conditions that have not been touched on. Some of these are complex regional pain syndrome, the placebo effect, pain management clinics and peripheral neuropathy. However, from the knowledge covered here the reader should easily be able to embrace further knowledge.

Closing thoughts

Pain is a challenge, both to those experiencing it and to those treating it. For both clinicians and patients, information that is accurate and understandable can help alleviate their fear surrounding this topic.

Remember, pain is a multidimensional problem and physiotherapy is not the only profession actively involved in addressing it. You may wish to explore the other resources you have access to and, as always, keep your ears and eyes open for new developments.

The path between pathology, physiology and ultimately presentation is full of variations which may easily mislead. However, sound underpinning knowledge will hopefully bring greater understanding and the freedom to question. It is hoped that, using the information in this chapter, a more fruitful clinical journey may be enjoyed by both the clinician and patient. Go and enjoy the challenge of pain: your patients will thank you for it.

References

Apkarian, A.V., Sosa, Y., Levy, R.M., et al., 2004. Chronic back pain is associated with decreased prefrontal and thalamic grey matter density. J. Neurosci. 24 (46), 10410–10415.

Beecher, H.K., 1956. Relationship of significance of wound to pain experienced. J. Am. Med. Assoc. 162, 1609–1612.

Black, P.H., 2002. Stress and the inflammatory response: a review of neurogenic inflammation. Brain Behav. Immun. 16 (6), 622–653.

Burn, L., Sinel, M., Deardorff, W.W., 2007. Treating your back and neck pain for dummies. John Wiley, Chichester.

Butler, D., Moseley, G.L., 2003. Explain pain. NOI Group, Adelaide.

Caudill, M.A., 2008. Managing pain before it manages you. Guilford Press, New York.

Costigan, M., Woolf, C.J., 2000. Pain: molecular mechanisms. J. Pain 1 (3), S35–S44.

Daykin, A., 2006. Communication within therapeutic encounters: message received and understood? In: Gifford, L. (Ed.), Topical issues in pain. CNS Press, Falmouth, pp. 89–104.

Dowswell, T., Bedwell, C., Lavender, T., et al., 2009. Transcutaneous electrical nerve stimulation (TENS) for pain relief in labour. Available online at: http://www.cochrane.org/reviews/en/ab007214.html (accessed 1 September 2009).

Flor, H., 2003. Cortical reorganisation and chronic pain: implications for rehabilitation. J. Rehabil. Med. 35 (5), S66–S72.

Gifford, L., Thacker, M., 2002. A clinical overview of the autonomic nervous system, the supply to the gut and mind–body pathways. In: Gifford, L. (Ed.), Topical issues in pain 3. CNS Press, Falmouth, pp. 21–52.

Goldingay, S., 2006a. Communication and assessment: the skills of information gathering. In: Gifford, L. (Ed.), Topical issues in pain 5. CNS Press, Falmouth, pp. 69–88.

Goldingay, S., 2006b. Communication and assessment: what are the issues for physiotherapists? In: Gifford, L. (Ed.), Topical Issues in Pain 5, 1st edn, CNS Press, Falmouth, pp. 55–68.

IASP, 2009. Available online at: http://www.iasp-pain.org/AM/Template. cfm?Section=Pain_Definitions &Template=/CM/HTMLDisplay. cfm&ContentID=1728 (accessed 8 September 2009).

Jensen, M.P., Hakimian, S., Sherlin, L. H., et al., 2008. New insights into neuromodulatory approaches for the treatment of pain. J. Pain 9 (3), 193–199.

Ji, U., Kohno, T., Moore, K.A., et al., 2003. Central sensitization and LTP: do pain and memory share similar mechanisms? Trends Neurosci. 26 (12), 696–705.

Julius, D., Basbaum, A.I., 2001. Molecular mechanisms of nociception. Nature 413 (6852), 203–210.

Kandell, E.R., Schwartz, J.H., Jessell, T. M., 2000. Principles of neural science, fourth edn. McGraw-Hill Medical, New York.

Kendall, N.A.S., Linton, S.J., Main, C.J., 1997. Guide to assessing psychosocial yellow flags in acute low back pain: risk factors for long-term disability and work loss. Accident Rehabilitation and Compensation Insurance Corporation of New Zealand and the National Health

Committee, Wellington, New Zealand.

Klaber Moffett, J., Green, A., Jackson, D., 2006. Words that help, words that harm. In: Gifford, L. (Ed.), Topical issues in pain 5. CNS Press, Falmouth, pp. 105–126.

Kori, S.H., Miller, R.P., Todd, D.D., 1990. Kinisophobia: a new view of chronic pain behaviours. Pain Manag. 35–43.

Leonard, M.T., Cano, A., Jahanson, A.B., 2006. Chronic pain in a couples context: a review and integration of theoretical models and empirical evidence. J. Pain 7 (6), 377–390.

Main, C.J., Spanswick, C.C., 1999. Pain management: an interdisciplinary approach. Churchill Livingstone, Edinburgh.

Martini, F.H., 2006. Fundamentals of anatomy and physiology, seventh ed. Pearson Benjamin Cummings, San Francisco.

Melzack, R., 1999. From the gate to the neuromatrix. Pain 6, S121–S126.

Melzack, R., 2002. Gate control theory: on the evolution of pain concepts? In: Gifford, L. (Ed.), Topical issues in pain 3. CNS Press, Falmouth, pp. 3–20.

Melzack, R., Wall, P.D., 1965. Pain mechanisms: a new theory. Science 150 (3699), 971–978.

Melzack, R., Wall, P.D., 1988. The challenge of pain, second ed. Penguin, London.

Moseley, G.L., 2004. Evidence for a direct relationship between cognitive and physical change during an education intervention in people with chronic low back pain. Eur. J. Pain 8, 39–45.

Moseley, G.L., 2007a. Reconceptualising pain according to modern pain science. Phys. Ther. Rev. 12, 169–178.

Moseley, G.L., 2007b. Painful yarns. Dancing Giraffe Press, Oxford.

Moseley, G.L., 2008. I can't find it! Distorted body image and tactile dysfunction in patients with chronic back pain. Pain 140, 239–243.

NICE, 2009. Available online at: http://www.nice.org.uk/CG88fullguideline (accessed 8 September 2009).

Nicholas, M.K., 2009. Reductions in catastrophising before fear of movement. Pain 145, 6–7.

Nicholas, M., Molloy, A., Tonkin, L., et al., 2000. Manage your pain. ABC Books, Sydney.

Noaham, K.E., Kumbang, J., 2008. Transcutaneous electrical nerve stimulation (TENS) for chronic pain. Cochrane Database Syst. Rev. (2), CD003222. DOI: 10.1002/14651858.CD003222.pub2.

Payne, R., 2005. Relaxation techniques, third ed. Churchill Livingstone, Edinburgh.

Rice, A.S.C., 1998. Recent developments in the pathophysiology of acute pain. Acute Pain 1 (2), 27–36.

Ross, E.L., 2004. Hot topics: pain management. Hanley and Belfus, Philadelphia.

Royal College of General Practitioners, 1999. Clinical guidelines for the management of acute low back pain. Royal College of General Practitioners, London.

Sandkuhler, J., 2007. Understanding LTP in pain pathways. Available online at: http://www.molecularpain.com/content/pdf/1744-8069-3-9.pdf.

Schmidt, R., Schmelz, M., Forster, C., et al., 1995. Novel classes of responsive and unresponsive C nociceptors in human skin. J. Neurosci. 15, 333–341.

Sowden, M., Hatch, A., Gray, S., et al., 2006. Can four key psychosocial risk factors for chronic pain and disability (yellow flags) be modified by a pain management programme: a pilot study. Physiotherapy 92, 43–49.

The Web of the Back, 2009. Available online at http://www.espalda.org/english/divulgativa/dolor/causas/comoaparece/nervios.asp.

Tracey, I., Mantyh, P.W., 2007. The cerebral signature for pain perception and its modulation. Neuron 55, 377–391.

Treede, R., Kenshalo, D., Jones, A., 1999. The cortical representation of pain. Pain 79 (2), 105–111.

van Griensven, H., 2005. Pain in practice. Butterworth Heinemann, Oxford.

Vera-Portocarreroa, L.P., Zhanga, E.T., Ossipova, M.H., et al., 2006. Descending facilitation from the rostral ventromedial medulla maintains nerve injury-induced central sensitization. Neuroscience 140 (4), 1311–1320.

Verbunt, J.A., Sieben, J., Vlaeyen, J.W.S., et al., 2008. A new episode of low back pain: who relies on bed rest? Eur. J. Pain 12, 508–516.

Vlaeyen, J.W.S., Linton, S.J., 2000. Fear-avoidance and its consequences in chronic musculoskeletal pain: a state of the art. Pain 85, 317–332.

Waddell, G., 2004. The back pain revolution. Churchill Livingstone, Edinburgh.

Waddell, G., Feder, G., Lewis, M., 1997. Systematic reviews of bed rest and advice to stay active for acute low back pain. Br. J. Gen. Pract. 47, 647–652.

Watson, T., 2009. Tissue repair. Available online at: http://www.electrotherapy.org/downloads/Modalities/tissue%20repair.pdf.

White, D., Helme, R.D., 1985. Release of substance P from peripheral nerve terminals following electrical stimulation of the sciatic nerve. Brain. Res. 336, 27–31.

Wiech, K., Ploner, M., Tracey, I., 2008. Neurocognitive aspects of pain perception. Trends. Cogn. Sci. 12 (8), 306–313.

Woolf, C.J., Ma, Q., 2007. Nociceptors – noxious stimulus detectors. Neuron 55 (2), 353–364.

Principles of patient management

9

Ann Moore

CHAPTER CONTENTS

Introduction

There can be no greater privilege bestowed on a clinician than the unqualified trust of individual patients who are seeking to maintain or improve their health status. As clinicians, we are potentially in this position throughout our working lives. It is the responsibility of every clinician to ensure that this trust is well founded by maintaining excellence in all aspects of the clinician's role.

This book has set out to help clinicians along the sometimes complex road of clinical decision-making by offering the reader a comprehensive background to joint, muscle and nerve function and dysfunction. It also reviews and contextualises the principles of the treatment strategies that may be employed by a clinician when aiding patients recovering from either single or multiple tissue dysfunction.

This chapter is devoted to exploring the principles of patient management in its broadest sense. It commences with an overview of terminology used in the 'treatment context', explores the patient–clinician relationship, the responsibilities within the relationship and the issues surrounding this relationship. The chapter then expands to include a discussion of the treatment event itself, and it concludes with an

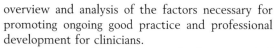

overview and analysis of the factors necessary for promoting ongoing good practice and professional development for clinicians.

It is not possible within a single chapter to deal comprehensively with all the issues raised. Rather, this chapter is concerned with raising the profile of concepts, idealisms and philosophies not usually harmonised in pure neuromusculoskeletal therapy courses or textbooks. It is hoped that this chapter will help to enrich the clinician's practice by presenting an eclectic approach to overall patient management.

By the end of this chapter readers may be struck by the complexity of the role encompassed by the clinician, and some may view the process of maturation into an expert clinician as a difficult journey. An old Taoist saying may be helpful here: 'A thousand-mile journey starts with one small step' (cited by Hoff 1982).

The stimulus constantly provided by patients, their carers and relatives, and the integration of the varied concepts addressed in this chapter, may help to sustain readers in their journey and ease the apprehension in these first early steps. It is important that each clinician enjoys the privilege of working with patients and also reaps every benefit that these working relationships have to offer both the patient and clinician.

Patient management defined

In this text the term 'patient management' has been used throughout. It is important here to clarify what is meant by this term. Synonyms for management include: administration, care, command, conduct, control, direction, guidance, handling, manipulation and supervision (Collins Thesaurus 1995). It is acknowledged that the term 'patient management', and the majority of synonyms associated with it, implies a very passive role for the patient and a paternalistic approach to the patient by the clinician. This is not the philosophy held by the author, and the term 'patient management' is used only in recognition of the common usage of these terms in general clinical practice. The context of debate surrounding 'patient management' is explored further in this chapter. The author's preferred approach is for patient-focused care with a strong emphasis on the therapeutic relationship.

Synonyms for 'therapeutic' are ameliorative, beneficial, corrective, good, healing, remedial and restorative, and synonyms for relationship include

association, bond, communication, conjunction, exchange, kinship, liaison, link and rapport (Collins Thesaurus 1995). These words would seem to imply more active participation from both parties engaged in the therapeutic relationship and celebrate the positive benefits which may occur from that working relationship.

The central importance of patients to the health service and health care providers has gained political momentum in the UK since the publication in 1997 of the government's white paper *The NHS: Modern and Dependable* (Secretary of State for Health 1997) and, later, *The NHS Plan* (Department of Health 2000), which affirmed that patients are the most important people in the health service. This document also acknowledged that, for patients, their importance in the health arena may not always be apparent and that patients often feel 'talked at rather than listened to' (Department of Health 2000 p. 88). The recommendations set out in *The NHS Plan*, and of relevance to this chapter, were for:

- more information for patients
- greater patient choice
- health services to become more patient-centred.

Later in the same year the National Health Service (NHS) document (NHS Executive 2000) *Meeting the Challenge – a Strategy for the Allied Health Professions* further emphasised the need for patient-focused care. From 1 April 1999, in the UK all NHS bodies had a new statutory duty of clinical governance placed upon them. Clinical governance places a duty on all health professionals to ensure that the level of service they deliver to patients is satisfactory, consistent and responsive. Essentially, clinical governance is about health service providers ensuring and guaranteeing quality of health care through a system of processes which include (Secretary of State for Health 1998):

- clear lines of responsibility and accountability being in place for the overall quality of clinical care
- a comprehensive programme of quality improvement activities being in place, including support for the use of evidence and the application of evidence-based practice in everyday health care activities
- continuing professional development being available for all health workers
- programmes being in place which are aimed at meeting the development needs of individual

health professionals and the service needs of the organisation, which are regularly monitored

- effective monitoring of clinical care with high-quality systems for clinical record keeping and the collection of relevant information
- processes being in place for assuring the quality of clinical care
- clear policies aimed at managing risk in health care
- procedures for all professional groups for identifying and remedying poor performance.

In essence, all health professionals have an individual and statutory responsibility to engage with clinical governance. For individuals this means taking a lead in the delivery of quality care, demonstrating that quality of care is being provided and sharing initiatives and ideas for best practice with others. It also means that individual practitioners have a duty to undertake continuing professional development (NHS Executive 1999) and that patients and health care organisations will increasingly expect practitioners to base their practice on the best-quality evidence available.

Clinical governance sits alongside a number of other NHS policies, for example:

- National Service Frameworks
- NHS performance and assessment frameworks
- health improvement programmes.

Clinical governance policy also sits alongside two statutory bodies that are outside the NHS but closely associated with it. They are the National Institute for Health and Clinical Excellence (NICE), which provides national evidence-based clinical guidelines and information on good practice, and the Commission for Health Improvements (CHI). CHI has been set up to provide national leadership in the principles of clinical governance and to undertake a programme of reviews within each NHS trust to ensure that clinical governance arrangements are in place and are working (Swage 2000).

All health professionals have a statutory duty to acquaint themselves with the quality systems/clinical governance arrangements existing within their own area of practice. For up-to-date information on clinical governance procedures readers are advised to visit the NHS Executive or the Department of Health websites or, alternatively, to use their local hospital trust's website or clinical governance office.

More recently *The Next Stage Review – Our NHS, Our Future* (Department of Health 2008a) set out a new vision for the future of the NHS in the UK

which strives to improve the quality of patient care, the provision of a more personalised health service and with clinicians themselves leading change, whilst making the best use of local resources.

A further report, *Framing the Contribution of Allied Health Professionals – Delivering High-Quality Care* (Department of Health 2008b) promotes self-referral to improve ease of access to allied health professional services, the use of minimum data sets to monitor referral waiting times together with the future introduction of a quality metric system whereby health professionals will increasingly utilise a standard set of outcome measures to determine the effectiveness and efficiency of their service provision.

Finally, *High-quality Care for All* (Department of Health 2008c) emphasises the importance of partnership working, patient empowerment, the use of quality metrics, raising standards of care, safeguarding quality and developing innovation in health care through strong leadership.

From the prolific documentation published in recent years by the Department of Health it is clear it is vital that all health professionals and especially those such as first contact practitioners, as is the case for musculoskeletal therapists, engage with the new agenda of priorities in order to play a part in securing a strong position for the physiotherapy profession in health care provision.

Important messages are, firstly, that future health commissioning will be based on local health needs, and therefore it is important for all services to assess what needs are, or are likely to be, in relation to the services currently offered. Secondly, a case will need to be made in each locality as to how physiotherapy meets current health priorities. It is vital that all practitioners continue to comply with clinical governance procedures and accept the accountability of their own actions and the outcomes of the service that they provide. This is particularly the case for those therapists in high-level posts within the NHS, particularly consultants who have gained more autonomy in practice over the years, but of course with autonomy in practice comes greater accountability.

Standards of proficiency – the Health Professions Council

In most countries there are minimum standards of proficiency that must be met in order for an individual practitioner to enter and be maintained on the health professions/physiotherapy register. In the UK the standards of proficiency have been developed in order to protect members of the public and to ensure high standards of care. These standards place the patient at the centre of practice and include statements relating to:

- professional autonomy and accountability
- professional relationships, including working and communicating with patients and their carers
- identification and assessment of health and social care needs
- formulation and delivery of plans and strategies for meeting health and social care needs
- critical evaluation of the impact of, or response to, the registrant's actions.

The standards also indicate that registrants must have knowledge, understanding and skills of profession-specific practice and be able to modify these for specific individuals and understand the need to establish and maintain a safe practice environment (Health Professions Council 2003a).

The Chartered Society of Physiotherapy and other national professional bodies relating to physiotherapy who publish their own rules of professional conduct also include a strong emphasis on patient-focused care (Chartered Society of Physiotherapy 2002).

The need for the patient to be the central focus of any clinical interaction is therefore underpinned by a body of government legislation, regulatory body standards and professional standards and guidelines. All clinicians need to be acquainted with, and to engage fully with, these frameworks, which are laid down in order to ensure safe and competent clinical practice.

Models of care

Historically, physiotherapy practice was well rooted in the medical/biological model of care, and paternalism was a strong characteristic of clinical behaviour within the therapeutic relationship. Paternalism has been defined as 'a refusal to accept or acquiesce in another person's wishes, choices or actions for that person's benefit' (Singleton & McLaren 1995). Historically, paternalism has been associated with individual patients being the passive recipients of health care. Clearly, with the growth of consumerism, the dramatic rise in the availability of health-related information and the political frameworks in which health services function, the paternalistic/biomedical

model of care has given way to an autonomy model which emphasises the rights of individuals in decision-making (Singleton & McLaren 1995). This situation, in which trust and respect for an individual's autonomy exist, would appear to be a vital foundation of the therapeutic relationship; hence, joint decision-making (between the patient and clinician) with regard to treatment strategies and short- and long-term goal-setting are becoming the norm in physiotherapy and in other health care practices. The benefits of the shift to more joint decision-making are increasingly being demonstrated. For example, Neistadt (1995) showed that collaboration on treatment goal-setting can reduce the length of hospital stays and achieve better outcomes in attaining goals.

In practice there is probably a spectrum of paternalistic and autonomous activities which take place in each clinical intervention involving both clinicians and patients. Occasionally it may be necessary for the clinician to assume a paternalistic role, focusing on the patient's condition with the patient's interests at heart and with very little importance placed on the patient's concerns, issues and beliefs. In modern health care practices this may be seen most frequently when clinicians are dealing with emergency situations in which time is of the essence in order to save life.

Barr & Threlkeld (2000) believe that the more contemporary view of health care is to see patients and clinicians as partners in designing interventions to achieve the best outcome while contextualising the problem within the patient's life situation. Clinicians dealing with patients with neuromusculoskeletal dysfunction are in an excellent position to develop such partnerships with patients because of the nature of the work that they do, i.e. having a strong focus on helping patients return to their pre-injury, or pre-pathological, states and because largely their patients do not need emergency interventions.

Patient-centred care and clinician-centred care lie at two ends of a continuum. There may be times – for example, if a patient is very ill or in considerable pain – when clinician-centred care is the only option in the initial stages, leading to more patient-centred care later in the treatment programme when the patient takes full responsibility for managing his or her own condition. The balance between patient- and clinician-centredness between these two ends of the continuum is complex and varies from patient to patient and clinician to clinician and is perhaps best demonstrated diagrammatically in Figure 9.1, which illustrates the patient care continuum.

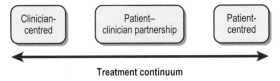

Figure 9.1 • The patient care continuum.

Stewart & Roter (1989) described several different types of doctor–patient relationship (Figure 9.2). These authors observed that paternalism has been, in the past, the most common model adopted by doctors but that, in the late 1980s, greater patient control was taking place and thus more mutuality occurred when both doctors and patients brought knowledge, experience and expectations to the relationship. Similar developments have occurred in other health care practices – not least in neuromusculoskeletal therapy. The clinician, in Stewart & Roter's model, also brings clinical skills and clinical knowledge, and the clinical interaction can be seen as a joint venture with both parties exchanging information and ideas. In some circumstances the relationship may be reversed, producing what Stewart & Roter (1989) described as a consumerist relationship in which the patient takes a more active role and the doctor a fairly passive role, for example when patients request a second opinion. A fourth type of relationship occurs when the patient continues to be in a passive role while the doctor also attempts to reduce some control of the consultation. Stewart & Roter (1989) indicate that different types of relationship may be appropriate at different stages of illness/treatment, as previously described. In the context of patient-focused care, in the early stages, the interaction may be more clinician-centred, moving later into a patient–clinician partnership mode. The interaction then becomes more exclusively patient-centred as the patient learns to take

control of the condition. At this point both the clinician and the patient prepare for the patient's discharge and future self-management (if necessary), either to maintain symptoms and signs at an acceptable level or to keep the condition from recurring. The patient-centred model emphasises the physical, personal and social aspects of the patient's condition (Jette 1994).

Ewles & Simnett (2003) proposed a number of ways in which clinicians can help their patients to take more control over their health and develop more autonomy. First, they can encourage individuals to make decisions and resist the urge to take over. Second, they can encourage individuals to think things out for themselves (this may take much longer than simply telling them!). Third, they can respect any unusual ideas that individuals may have about their health. In addition, Ewles & Simnett (2003) advocated acceptance of individuals rather than judging them.

According to Ewles & Simnett (2003), when we accept an individual it means the following:

- recognising that the individual's knowledge and beliefs have emerged from his or her own life experiences, whereas the clinician's have been modified and extended by professional education and experience
- understanding one's own knowledge, beliefs, values and standards
- understanding the patient's knowledge, beliefs, values and standards from the patient's point of view
- recognising that you (the clinician), your patients and others you work with may differ in knowledge, beliefs, values and standards
- recognising that these differences do not imply that you, as the clinician, are a person of greater worth than your patients/clients.

Figure 9.2 • Clinician–patient therapeutic relationships (adapted from Stewart & Roter 1989).

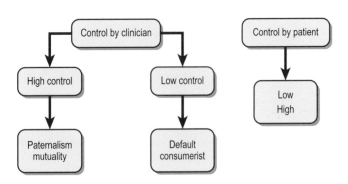

A partnership between a clinician and a patient can only exist if there is an atmosphere of mutual trust and openness, and this can be brought about by encouraging patients to ask questions and discuss issues openly. It is also important to ask patients for their views and opinions about treatment and related matters, and for the clinician then to accept and respect these views. Often it is helpful to let patients know that you, as a clinician, have learnt something from them, however small that may be. Finally, Ewles & Simnett (2003) believe that encouraging and fostering patients to share knowledge and experience with each other, if possible, is very helpful and appropriate in helping them to become more informed participants in the therapeutic partnership.

The importance of understanding and interacting with patients and their belief systems in order to highlight the relationship between psychosocial aspects of care and the biomedical aspects of care was emphasised by Jones et al. (2002), who discussed two contemporary models of health and disability: a model for organising clinical knowledge and a model for aiding reasoning strategies within the clinician. Additionally, the reader is referred to Waddell's biopsychosocial model of back pain (Figure 9.3), which can be applied to many neuromusculoskeletal dysfunctional states. This model shows clearly the relationship between pain, the patient's attitudes and beliefs, psychological distress and the illness behaviours which may emanate from

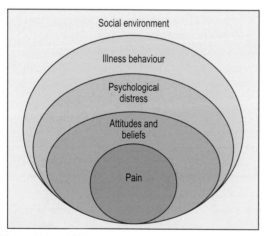

Figure 9.3 • A biopsychosocial model of the clinical presentation and assessment of low-back pain and disability at one point in time (reproduced from Waddell et al. 1984, with permission from the BMJ Publishing Group).

chronic pain states and the interaction and possible influences of the social environment. The importance of this model is that it highlights the need for clinicians to explore as many of the identified dimensions as possible with their patients during the course of their interactions with them.

The patient's needs and expectations of treatment and management

Patients consulting clinicians will do so bringing with them expectations of the clinician, the therapy they will receive, the outcome of treatment, the position of the clinician within the multidisciplinary team, the hospital, their own role within their treatment and rehabilitation and expectations about other issues.

For clinicians, it is important to understand that patients will have varied expectations which may differ from the clinician's own expectations in relation to the proposed treatment and its outcome.

When establishing a therapeutic relationship between the clinician and the patient, patients must feel comfortable in sharing their expectations and beliefs about their condition and the therapy they may receive. Clinicians should use both non-verbal and verbal communication when trying to identify what their patients' expectations are at an early stage in the patient–clinician consultation and the needs that they hope will be fulfilled during treatment (Jensen & Lorish 1994).

The patient's needs

Patients may have specific needs which they hope will be fulfilled by their treatment and by the clinician. The concept of need is brought to the fore mainly in the health promotion literature. Ewles & Simnett (2003), citing Bradshaw (1972), presented three types of need which are appropriate to discuss here:

1. normative need
2. felt need
3. expressed need.

Normative need

Normative need is usually defined for patients by experts (in this case, the clinician), based on their own value judgements. Opinions regarding normative need, however, will vary from expert to expert.

For example, safe lifting and handling information – which is thought by experts to be a need for one occupational group – may not be transferable from one working environment to another and the opinions of the experts may differ from those of the patients who may use this information.

Felt need

Felt needs are the needs in which people identify what they want. For example, a patient with low-back pain may feel the need for some information on lifting and handling procedures. Felt needs, however, are limited to people's knowledge about what could be available to them. For example, patients may not know about all the types of therapy that are available to them as they have not been exposed to information about the full range of treatments that currently exist (Ewles & Simnett 2003).

Expressed need

Expressed need is what people say they need, i.e. a felt need which has been turned into an expressed request or demand. For example, a patient may demand exercises to help with low-back pain (Ewles & Simnett 2003).

It is important to note here that not all of the patient's felt needs will be turned into expressed needs as the patient may lack motivation or assertiveness to do this. In some situations, in which the clinician adopts a paternalistic approach to care, patients may not be given the opportunity to express their needs fully.

It is also important to note that patients may have based their expressed needs on a limited amount of information, or on misinformation, and the expressed needs may conflict with the clinician's perceived normative needs! For example, a patient may have decided that she needs a certain form of therapy suggested by a friend who appears to have a similar problem, but the clinician may feel that the kind of therapy demanded is inappropriate. It is therefore essential that, in the spirit of partnership, these expressed needs are discussed in full to enable each party to understand fully the view of the other and come to a consensus decision about the most appropriate way forward.

Evidence is growing that patients who are well informed about their treatment, and the reasons for it, and who are involved in decisions about their care do better than those who do not share in the decision-making process (Brody et al. 1989). However, there is also evidence that clinicians may not be taking full advantage of the potential for patient participation in their own care – for example, in goal-setting (Baker et al. 2001).

The patient's expectations

There has been a small amount of work published relating to patients' expectations of treatment but more work is needed in this area as well as in the area of felt and expressed patient needs in physiotherapy practice generally.

It appears from a clinical trial investigating acupuncture and massage (Kalauokalani et al. 2001) that patients' expectations may influence clinical outcome independently of the treatment itself. For example, in the study of Kalauokalani et al. (2001) patients who expected to receive greater benefit from massage compared with acupuncture were more likely to experience better outcomes with massage than with acupuncture, and vice versa. This study has implications for future clinical trials and the need to control within research studies for patients' expectations.

Grimmer et al. (1999) investigated expectations of patients with acute low-back pain and found differences between naïve (new) patients and experienced patients. All patients expected to be relieved of symptoms after their first treatment but naïve patients decided to return for more treatments based on the relationship that they had established with the clinician. More experienced patients expected advice to be given during their first consultation (Grimmer et al. 1999). The authors concluded that there is a need for a quality partnership to be established with patients on their first visit, a relationship that patients can trust and value, and a need to determine and interpret patients' expectations, to ensure that patients have enough information to become active participants in their own care and to understand the need for further treatment, if required. Also, it appeared that patients needed enough information to manage their own condition effectively in a time-efficient and sensitive manner (Grimmer et al. 1999).

One study has focused on patients' expectations of chiropractic treatment. Sigrell (2001) found that patients expected the chiropractor to find the problem and explain the problem to them. They also expected to be symptom-free, to feel better after the first consultation and to have been given advice and exercises. In a follow-up study, Sigrell (2002) concluded that patients expected to consult a knowledgeable professional with good communication skills who could provide effective treatment that resulted in a positive outcome.

In a study of satisfaction with physiotherapy among patients with low-back pain, May (2001) identified five dimensions of care that patients found important:

1. the personal and professional manner of the clinician – for example, whether the clinician was skilled, thorough, inspired confidence, friendly and sympathetic and whether s/he listened and was respectful

2. the explanation and teaching which occurred during care, i.e. about the problem itself, the patient's role in care, the treatment process and possible prognosis

3. how much of the treatment was based on a consultative process. Patients valued being consulted on effectiveness of treatment and the treatment being related to the individual's own self-help needs. Patients were concerned about the quality of listening (on the clinician's part) that took place within the treatment sessions, how the clinician responded and what kind of responses the clinician made to patients' questions

4. the structure that shaped access to and the time with the clinician. For example, patients appreciated fast local access to therapy, wanted scope to return to the clinician at a later date following discharge if a flare-up in their condition occurred (an SOS appointment) and wanted enough quality time with the clinician in order to engage with him or her fully

5. the outcome which ensued, i.e. whether treatment was effective and whether the patient gained self-help strategies.

In patients who had undergone hip replacement surgery it was found by Heaton et al. (2000) that patients wished rehabilitation therapy and advice to be tailored to their own specific needs, particularly those with multiple impairments. Patients also felt that they should have the opportunity to carry out their rehabilitation exercises in a supportive environment where clinicians could assess their progress, address their concerns and provide ongoing advice and reassurance.

In a qualitative study exploring the expectations of patients with acute and chronic low-back pain

(Hitchcock G & Moore AP, 2001 unpublished research), the findings demonstrated six key emerging themes. The expectations of both the acute and chronic low-back pain sufferers were very similar. The patients expected:

1. that a diagnosis would be given and the condition would be explained to them fully

2. that advice should be offered, i.e. about how to deal with the problem, how to manage pain states, how to avoid aggravating pain and how to relieve it

3. that a cure would be provided (usually patients had expectations that a cure would be provided early in treatment)

4. that a greater understanding of the clinician's role would be gained

5. that they would be given reassurance about their condition

6. that they would be enabled to set meaningful personal goals for the future.

Several patients, who had all been referred by local general practitioners, did not understand how the role of the physiotherapist integrated with that of the general practitioner or, for that matter, with other health professionals. They did not understand the full clinical remit of the physiotherapist to examine and assess them independently and to offer treatment as they saw fit in liaison with the patient. Some patients felt uneasy as they had been told by their general practitioner that they would be given a certain form of therapy which had then not been offered by the physiotherapist. Patients felt that their confidence was shaken in 'the system', particularly as some believed that only their general practitioner could prescribe or change physiotherapy-related treatments.

Patients in this study were keen to know what they could do to help themselves – for example, what exercises they could do and what activities would be best for them. It was important for patients to be able to set goals and look to the future. Anecdotally, some clinicians feel that their time should be spent on 'hands-on treatment' rather than spending time communicating fully with patients. All the previous studies, however, have offered information which supports the importance of the establishment of a patient–clinician relationship as vital to the maintenance of a stable and effective clinical partnership. In such a partnership, patients' expectations, needs and perspectives on care can be heard, explored and acted upon, and treatment and goals can be planned and developed by mutual agreement. Therefore, it is important that clinicians plan and allocate time for this to occur.

Communication

Rose et al. (1992) highlighted the relief that patients feel when they can talk about the condition with someone who understands their problem. In busy outpatient settings clinicians sometimes fail to allow time for effective communication and it is clear that this can lead to frustration, demoralisation and loss of confidence in the clinician by the patient. It may also lead to poor outcome. Richardson & Moran (1995) asserted that 'appropriate, timely and effective communication with patients can in turn improve the effectiveness of care' and indicated that communication is at the heart of health care delivery because it can enhance dialogue and ensure active participation in decision-making. It can also promote informed choice, and can promote evidence-based health care by ensuring that patients' preferences are noted.

Further, Richardson & Moran (1995) indicated that effective communication with patients can lead to:

- patient empowerment
- enhancement of the quality of care
- improved patient satisfaction
- improved health outcomes
- modification in professional practice in response to patients' needs.

Empowerment

The concept of empowerment is not new in the health promotion literature but has entered the health professional literature only in the last two decades. Defined by Rodwell (1996), empowerment is the process of enabling or imparting power transfer from one individual to another; it includes the elements of power, authority, choices and permission.

The concept has useful attributes for clinicians, which include:

- being a helping process, which enables individuals to change a situation, giving them the skill, resources and opportunities to do so
- it embodies partnership which values self and others
- it aims to develop a positive belief in self and the future
- it encompasses mutual decision-making using resources, opportunity and authority
- it gives individuals freedom to make choices and accept responsibilities for those choices
- it recognises that power originates from self-esteem.

These attributes are essentially the basis of patient-focused care; however, it is not possible for health professionals to empower patients but patients can empower themselves. Patients can be helped towards empowerment by an empowerment process facilitated by health professionals who can provide, firstly, resources, such as information, knowledge, reassurance and therapeutic skills, and, secondly, opportunities, for example a safe physical environment and an open environment in which patients' questions, issues and experiences, needs and expectations can be shared and which can be used by patients to develop a sense of control.

However, for empowerment to be accomplished, patients must possess motivation, participate fully and have a mutual commitment to the process (Labonte 1989).

There may be a range of other factors which influence individuals' abilities to motivate themselves, participate fully and exhibit mutual commitment. These factors may relate to age, gender, ethnicity, previous experiences of health care, the nature and success of the therapeutic relationship and health beliefs. All of these factors should be considered by the clinician in relation to patient empowerment.

Self-efficacy

A further concept which has gained popularity in the health care systems in the USA, Australia and South Africa, and which is beginning to rise in popularity in the UK, is the concept of self-efficacy. Self-efficacy enables a bridge to be built between the person (the patient) and the social world in which the individual must make changes to his or her behaviour in order to maintain or improve the individual's health or disability status (Rollnick et al. 1999).

Self-efficacy is different from self-esteem (which is important for empowerment) as self-efficacy relates to an individual's confidence in his or her ability to make a specific behavioural change. Self-esteem relates more to the individual's general sense of well-being.

Self-efficacy systems are based on the work of Bandura & Walter (1963) who developed a social learning theory based on research. Rollnick et al. (1999) have suggested some practical guidelines for developing self-efficacy based on the work of Bandura (1977) and others:

1. Self-efficacy in individuals varies across situations. Patients can have high self-efficacy in some areas of behaviour, which should be praised and encouraged, but may have low self-efficacy in others where they may need help in finding different approaches in order to gain confidence to change situations. For example, this can apply to a patient with a neuromusculoskeletal lower-limb dysfunction who has mastered crutch-walking in the house and in the gymnasium but now needs to gain confidence in walking on the street.

2. Doing is the best way to enhance self-efficacy, and as many bridges as possible must be built between the clinical treatment setting and the patient's everyday life; sometimes it helps for patients to keep a diary or a record of events so that they can reflect on this and see what their successes have been and what has worked well for them. It can also help for patients to bring a friend or relative to treatment sessions to take part in discussions, and who can then be part of the bridge between the clinical setting and the patient's social setting.

3. People need to have skills to succeed. These skills may be present but may lie dormant; sometimes these skills need to be built up and confidence gained. Such skills could be learning skills, psychomotor skills or interpersonal skills.

4. Feedback needs to be given about deficiencies in the patient's performance so that s/he can improve.

5. People learn best by modelling themselves on others; therefore there is value in patients talking to, and about, friends or other patients who have succeeded in similar tasks. For example, attending self-help groups – such as arthritis support groups – can be helpful (Rollnick et al. 1999).

In some situations self-help groups are run entirely by patients who talk about their experiences and successes in changing their life situations and teach others in similar situations about exercises or activities or adaptations in the home which they have found helpful.

Summary

From the patient-focused perspective, Box 9.1 summarises what needs to be considered in relation to overall patient management.

Readers who wish to know more about changing health behaviours are referred to an excellent text, *Health Behaviour Changes: A Guide for Practitioners* (Rollnick et al. 1999).

Box 9.1

A summary of patient-focused care

Patient-focused care means:

- Building a balanced therapeutic partnership/relationship which consists of trust, respect and understanding for patients' ideas, beliefs, knowledge and values
- Increasing patient autonomy
- Involving patients in decision-making
- Working within the biopsychosocial model of care
- Sharing and dealing with patients' expectations
- Sharing and dealing with patients' needs and encouraging their felt needs to be expressed
- Clinicians should demonstrate good knowledge, therapeutic skills and communication skills, including listening skills
- Clinicians should offer high-quality explanations, education and advice to patients
- Clinicians must offer clear guidance on the physiotherapist's role
- A consultative process within the treatment sessions should be adopted
- A flexible appointment system with SOS appointment availability is important
- Patients should be facilitated to empower themselves
- Self-efficacy should be facilitated
- Clinicians should give time to patient-focused care
- Good outcomes must be achieved
- Professional practice needs to be modified as needed in response to the developing therapeutic relationship

The multifaceted role of the clinician

This chapter has thus far been concerned with the political and professional context of practice and an overview of patient-focused care and its implications for the clinician. It is important that patient-focused care has been addressed early in this chapter as, increasingly, patients are, and should be, the central focus of care and decision-making within our health services and our health practices. The patient's perspective has been presented foremost in this chapter to highlight their importance in the therapeutic relationship. What follows is an overview of the multifaceted role of the clinician within the neuromusculoskeletal field.

The clinician functions within political, managerial service and professional frameworks and every clinician needs to be politically aware of new initiatives in these arenas. They must also know how these initiatives will affect, or have the potential to affect, their practice. Clinicians would be wise to read their professional journals and newsletters and visit NHS, professional body and special-interest group websites on a regular basis in order to keep up to date with initiatives which may affect practice.

The current major influences and considerations for practice which are emphasised in clinical governance procedures are:

- the rise in emphasis on patient-focused care (already addressed in this chapter)
- the requirement for practice to be based on the best available evidence, i.e. evidence-based practice
- the increasing number of treatment modalities becoming available both with and without evidence to support them
- the professional and statutory requirements for all health professionals to engage in continuing professional development
- the emphasis within the health service on efficiency and effectiveness of care as well as cost-effectiveness.

The multifaceted nature of the clinician's role and its complexities were acknowledged by Moore & Jull (2002). The skills of the competent clinician should include those shown in Box 9.2.

Competent application of the fundamental science, art and professional practice in physiotherapy

These skills (Box 9.2) are a fundamental prerequisite to qualification and registration as a physiotherapist in the UK (Health Professions Council 2003b) and therefore are not dealt with here but suffice to say that every clinician has a duty to ensure that skills in these areas are continually refreshed, updated and reinforced (Moore & Jull 2002).

Listening skills and the clinician

The importance of listening to patients' needs, expectations and beliefs has already been addressed in this chapter in relation to the therapeutic relationship. However, it is important here to stress the need

---

Box 9.2

Skills of the clinician

- The ability to apply fundamental science, art and professional practical applications of physiotherapy/physical therapy (a prerequisite for practice and registration)
- Good listening skills
- High-level interpersonal skills, including emotional intelligence and good communication skills
- Education skills, including skills in assessment of learning and evaluation of learning
- High-level clinical reasoning skills
- Skill in the appropriate use of evidence to support practice
- Skill in the use of clinical guidelines for neuromusculoskeletal therapy
- Expertise in examination and assessment of patients with joint, nerve and muscle dysfunction
- Competence and/or expertise in the treatment and management of patients with neuromusculoskeletal dysfunction
- Skills in reflective practice
- Motivation and skills in personal professional development
- Time management skills
- Skills in the use of information technology
- Team-playing/leadership skills

---

for careful listening skills to be applied throughout examination and treatment processes so that appropriate treatment/management strategies can be defined in association with the patient so as to achieve a successful outcome to treatment.

Being a good listener enables the clinician to pick up new avenues of potential fruitful enquiry in the examination process from the odd gesture or a single word spoken or uttered by the patient. In this sense it may be possible to identify that patients have worries and fears and felt needs that they have not yet verbalised, and it gives the clinician the opportunity to help the patient express these issues fully. It may simply be that patients fail to mention facts or symptoms associated with their condition because they feel that such facts or symptoms are either unimportant or unrelated. The good listener will capitalise on these nuances and use them to best effect in clinical reasoning processes (Moore & Jull 2001).

It is imperative that clinicians interpret what patients say in a valid way; hence, the importance of discussion between the clinician and the patient in order to ensure that the interpretation of what has been said is sound and that facts have been clearly understood (Maitland et al. 2005).

Listening skills are an essential part of communication in general (Maitland et al. 2005). Communication consists of two components, verbal, including the tone of voice, and non-verbal (Maitland et al. 2005). It is important for clinicians to recognise their own non-verbal communication as well as being observant of patient's non-verbal behaviours, which, because they are a reflex action, can be more genuine and can reflect more subtly their true feelings.

Clinicians should observe patients carefully, making eye contact and exhibiting an open posture, which makes them more approachable to patients. Clinicians should watch patients' facial expressions carefully as well as their body movements, as they may give much-needed messages about how they are really feeling. Clinicians also need to be aware of their own state of mind as this may influence how they interpret patients' non-verbal communication (Maitland et al. 2005).

Communication

Clear verbal communication is also of vital importance to a successful therapeutic relationship. The clinician must ask questions in a clear and uncomplicated way in order to understand fully patients' symptoms, how they are reacting to the physical examination and what effect treatment is having. The clinician should give clear scope for patients to enter into discussions and voice their opinions, fears, anxieties, needs and expectations. Important pointers in communication are highlighted by Maitland et al. (2005):

- Speak slowly.
- Speak deliberately.
- Keep questions short.
- Ask one question at a time.

The ideal results of the clinician's effective communication with the patient are shown in Box 9.3.

Finally in this section on communication, there follows an example of the importance of ascertaining fully that the patient understands any terminology that is used. There are many terms in the neuromusculoskeletal field which, to the lay person, are very similar – for example, spondylitis, spondylosis, spondylolisthesis, spondylolysis. Patients now have full

> **Box 9.3**
>
> ### The ideal results of effective patient–clinician communication (from Moore et al. 1995, with permission)
>
> - A full understanding of the patient's condition and how it is affecting the patient is gained
> - A full and accurate clinical picture is obtained through the examination process
> - Patients' feelings, needs, expectations, fears and anxieties have been discussed and explored
> - An understanding of patients' confidence in taking responsibility for their condition is obtained
> - Patients know what role the clinician has in their treatment and management
> - Patients understand what neuromusculoskeletal therapy is and what it aims to achieve
> - Patients understand what effects may be expected from treatment
> - Patients understand what their treatment will consist of
> - Patients understand what treatment options there are
> - Patients understand how long treatment will last and how many treatments will be necessary
> - Patients understand what part they have to play in their treatment and home management, both during treatment and after discharge

access via the internet to health information and so it is essential to ensure that they have the right terminology and have understood fully the meaning. An example from practice highlights the issues. A patient, having assumed as a result of a rushed conversation with his general practitioner that he had ankylosing spondylitis, came to treatment in a worried and tormented fashion having consulted the medical literature. He had heard the term 'spondy' and no more and had assumed on coming across 'ankylosing spondylitis' that he was suffering from a progressive disease. The patient was much relieved on hearing that actually the general practitioner had diagnosed the condition as spondylosis (Moore & Jull 1997).

Interpersonal skills

Interpersonal skills include listening and communication components: how we relate to individuals depends on our own attitudes, values, beliefs, knowledge and experience, which become fused together in our own personal philosophy and view of life.

Life changes at any time; for example, personal bereavements, divorce, illness and other life events can change our philosophy of life and therefore how we react and relate to other people (Cross et al. 2006). It is important for therapists to recognise how their own interpersonal skills may be affected at any one time and make adaptations by developing necessary coping strategies, if possible, to change their interpersonal skills if they appear to be influencing a therapeutic relationship negatively. Often, voicing issues with a colleague or a mentor can help; this is important as Trede (2000) has indicated how much patients value a good interpersonal relationship with their clinician.

Golemann's (1996) work on emotional intelligence identifies five domains which may be helpful to the practitioner in terms of dealing with other people. First, knowing one's own emotions is important; managing one's own emotions is also important, and motivating oneself to recognise emotions in others are essential attributes, as is being able to handle relationships. Golemann defines emotional intelligence as 'a capacity for recognising our own feelings and those of others, for motivating ourselves and for managing emotions well in ourselves and in our relationships' (Golemann 1998 p. 317).

Application of neuromusculoskeletal examination and clinical skills

The reader is referred to Petty (2011) for details of the application of relevant examination procedures and to the chapters in this text dealing with the treatment and management of joint, muscle and nerve dysfunctions. This section deals with the fundamental principles of patient management only.

The overall examination and treatment processes are depicted in the flow chart in Figure 9.4, created to show the treatment process together with the development of the therapeutic relationship.

Figure 9.4 shows the examination, treatment and discharge continuum. Good communication and interpersonal skills are vital at each stage of this continuum. On the right-hand side of the figure the effective patient–clinician relationship develops into a continuum, with patients empowering themselves and later developing high self-efficacy. On the left-hand side of the diagram, examination and assessment findings are discussed with patients and a contract is drawn up with them (some NHS hospital trusts have standard formats for these). As part of the contract the clinician fully explains the examination and assessment findings to the patient, discusses and agrees

Figure 9.4 • Patient-focused examination and treatment continuum.

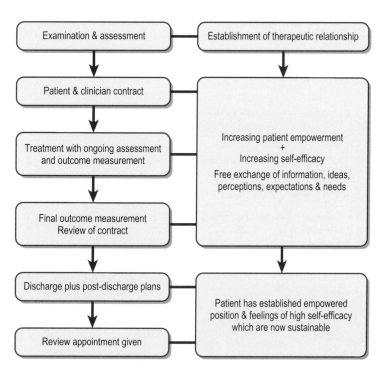

treatment and management strategies and prognosis, including an explanation of treatment options, and finally agrees treatment and management goals with the patient together with suitable circumstances for discharge and how the overall outcome of treatment will be measured. At the end of treatment, when discharge is agreed, a follow-up (SOS) appointment may also be agreed (if offered within the clinician's home department's framework). The contract should be fully documented and signed by both the patient and the clinician.

Treatment

Treatment approaches can be summarised as in Figure 9.5, which depicts a multimodal physiotherapy approach to treatment. Treatment is carried out in the context of the patient's background, social circumstances, expectations, values, attitudes, beliefs and expressed needs and preferences and also within the clinician's code of practice, expertise and preferences for treatment modalities (which may relate to the clinician's physique, size, shape and personal physical ability or dysfunction).

The patient–clinician relationship is integral to the multimodal approach, and management aims at developing coping and management strategies with the patient to facilitate the development of self-efficacy and 'to bridge the gap' between the clinical and social environments. It also includes emphasis on pain relief and rehabilitation of dysfunctional states. Pain-relieving strategies have already been dealt with

earlier in this text but include manual therapy, electrophysical procedures, therapeutic exercise and education and advice with respect to pain-relieving postures and activities. Information on what pain-provoking activities to avoid, and enhancing the understanding of the problem and how modalities/the medication being used by the patient may help in pain relief, are also important. Also included in this aspect of treatment is the development of coping strategies with the patient for the management of pain at home by the use of exercises, positioning and the use of ice therapy and other modalities as appropriate.

Rehabilitation may include therapeutic exercise to affect muscle, joint and nerve and may be aimed at strengthening muscle tissue, mobilising joints and soft tissues to restore range of movement, re-education of muscle function in order to stabilise joints or regions of the body and re-education of muscle activity in active joint movement in functional activities.

Rehabilitation may also include ergonomic advice, for example with regard to seating postures, sleeping surfaces and working postures. Biomedical intervention includes the detailed analysis of movement and dysfunction and re-education to normality. This is often undertaken in a laboratory-based setting where movement analysis equipment is freely available.

Education within the context of rehabilitation should include home management programmes; for example, exercises and activity programmes which will enable patients to continue their

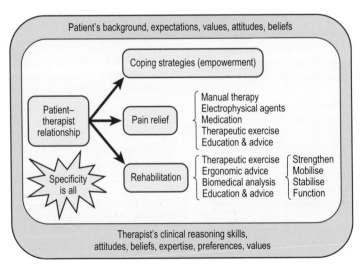

Figure 9.5 • A multimodal physiotherapy/physical therapy approach.

rehabilitation at home during the treatment phase and after discharge if necessary.

The important feature here is that treatment must be made specific to the patient's condition as identified in the examination and assessment components of the management programme; in other words, the specificity of approach is all-important.

Initially, it is necessary to decide what symptoms/ signs are predominating and, if pain predominates, then pain is usually treated first and a pain-relieving modality may be used. The pain-relieving modality, however, must be applied accurately to an appropriate joint or soft tissue and applied so as to produce relief of pain, taking into account the severity, irritability and nature of the condition (Petty 2011).

As the condition improves, the technique that has been used for pain relief may be applied more forcefully or the technique may be changed for another following reassessment of signs and symptoms as perhaps pain no longer predominates and the need now to increase joint range predominates. The need for specificity in the application of treatment cannot be overstated.

It is important also to note the positive effect that the patient's psychological processes may have on descending nerve pathways. In the treatment setting, painful conditions will be approached often using a local technique, which is used to influence sensory input; this, in turn, will also affect descending nerve pathways. Therefore, it can be seen that the patient-focused nature of care, together with specificity of treatment, can have potentially strong influences on the patient's pain levels. It is essential that the choice of treatment modality be made in a rational, scientific and clinically reasoned way and that changes to treatment are equally made on this basis, only and when a change is required or is necessary.

Care of the patient

Every health professional has a statutory duty of care to the patient (Health Professions Council 2003a). This implies that they must act in the best interests of the patient. They must respect the confidentiality of patients, keep their own professional knowledge and skills up to date, act within the limits of their knowledge, skills and experience, and maintain proper and effective communication with patients. They must also obtain informed consent to give treatment (which implies full discussion and consultation with the patient), keep accurate records of patients, carry out duties in an ethical way and behave with integrity and honesty.

Informed consent

Informed consent has been defined as 'a voluntary decision made by a sufficiently competent or autonomous person on the basis of adequate information and deliberation to accept or reject some proposed course of action, which will affect "him or her"'(Gillon 1986, cited by Singleton & McLaren 1995 p. 104). Alternatively, informed consent has been described as 'the voluntary or revocable agreement of a competent individual to participate in a therapeutic or research procedure based on adequate understanding of its nature, purpose and implications' (Sim 1986 p. 584). Sim (1996) believes that informed consent can be analysed into four elements, each of which should be present to a satisfactory degree if consent is valid. These elements are depicted in Figure 9.6.

Disclosure in this context means that the clinician must fully explain the intended interventions, their possible benefits and possible risks but also give information on possible alternative treatments. The clinician must also ensure that the patient has

Figure 9.6 • The elements of informed consent (from Sim 1996, with permission).

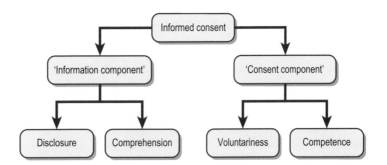

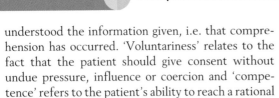

understood the information given, i.e. that comprehension has occurred. 'Voluntariness' relates to the fact that the patient should give consent without undue pressure, influence or coercion and 'competence' refers to the patient's ability to reach a rational autonomous decision.

Patient care in the context of informed consent relates directly to clear accurate communication and the establishment of an effective therapeutic relationship.

Many hospital departments have standard consent forms and procedures for gaining consent and the reader is referred to Sim's (1996) article and to their own clinical governance departments for more local information on informed consent.

Patient comfort

Patients' comfort during the examination and treatment session is of paramount importance to their confidence in the clinician, in their treatment and their ability to relax during treatment. Comfort is also likely to have an impact on the outcome of treatment. Comfort can be assured by ensuring that the patient's privacy is respected, i.e. screening the patient's cubical or ensuring that body parts are adequately covered, and also that the treatment area is as private as possible and that the patient is not inhibited in discussions with the clinician by fear of being overheard when discussing sensitive issues.

Physical support should always be given for areas of the body being treated or examined. For example, using adequate pillows for the head and neck and positioning joints in a supported and facilitatory position for treatment; nose holes in hydraulic plinths can be uncomfortable for some patients and a small face towel folded under the forehead can help to reduce this discomfort.

It is essential to ensure that there is adequate heating in treatment areas if the outside temperature is cold and to ensure that good ventilation is available when the weather outside is very warm; this is particularly the case when patients are undertaking exercise. It is also important to ensure that lighting is sufficient for the needs of the clinician and also for the patient's needs, particularly for elderly patients, and especially if they need to read information booklets, fill in outcome measures and consent forms and the like.

All positions for examination and treatment should be safe and comfortable and should facilitate examination and treatment processes. Clinicians should respect patients' preferences for treatment positions; for example, there are some patients who cannot lie flat, perhaps because of a cardiac problem, and in such cases treatment positions need to be modified accordingly.

Accuracy of treatment

It is essential to ensure that treatment is applied as accurately as possible. It is important always to reassess signs and symptoms during and after each treatment session. Accuracy relates to all aspects of the treatment application and dose.

Dosage and frequency of treatment

The frequency of appointments, i.e. how often treatment should be applied, is sadly underresearched. Anecdotally, it may be that treatment should be frequent enough so that changes resulting from treatment can be assessed. In this way other activities carried out by the patient between appointments are kept to a minimum and helps prevent a confusing clinical picture (Maitland et al. 2005).

Daily treatment may often be preferable when symptoms are severe but not irritable; however, daily treatment may be too much when symptoms are severe and irritable, in which case treatments once or twice a week may suffice. In essence, the dosage and frequency of treatment must be guided by individualised examination findings. Often, clinicians will apply a short session of treatment directly after examination and assessment has taken place and then the patient may be seen the next day in order to assess the effect of the treatment. The frequency of treatment can then be judged by the clinician in discussion with the patient, having assessed the initial reaction to treatment.

Caution must be exerted with patients who believe that the more the treatment hurts the better, and a thorough explanation to the patient of how treatment works and is best applied in painful states is helpful here.

The response to treatment between individuals is variable; some patients achieve full recovery while others do not respond. There is a need in the short term to extend neuromusculoskeletal research in order to develop a better classification or profile of patients who respond to certain modalities (Jull & Moore 2002).

Appropriate dosages of treatment are also under-researched. We know little of what dosage or treatment leads to the best outcome of care (Jull & Moore 2002). Closer investigation of dosage of treatment is required but until this research is available clinicians are best advised to treat each patient on an individual basis and be guided by presenting signs and symptoms at all stages.

Settings for treatment

Treatment should take place only where adequate facilities for examination and treatment are available. A private treatment cubical is most appropriate for individual hands-on treatment sessions, while a gymnasium or laboratory setting with appropriate instrumentation may be better for muscle re-education treatments, for example when using biofeedback or diagnostic ultrasound imaging.

Choice of treatment/technique

Treatment must be chosen specifically to manage the presenting dysfunction, i.e. there must be specificity in all treatments. For example, if a painful joint condition exists a pain-relieving modality should be applied. The technique or modality chosen will depend on what is deemed to be most appropriate by the clinician in discussion with the patient, taking into account the patient's past experiences and preferences. If mobilisation is the chosen modality then it should be applied specifically to relieve pain, not to increase joint range, although, in relieving pain, joint range may increase as a byproduct of pain relief. If joint stiffness is the main problem then mobilisations or exercise should be applied in a specific way in order to increase range of movement, i.e. performed at the end of range. If, after examination, the clinician believes that joint stability is lacking then stabilisation exercises may be prescribed. In essence, treatment must be applied specifically to influence signs and symptoms that are present; for example, pain, instability, muscle spasm, muscle weakness, joint stiffness, swelling and functional disability. Usually the most profound sign and symptom is targeted first and, as this problem begins to regress, then other modalities may be introduced in order to deal with other symptoms and signs that have now become more prominent. The effect of each modality on the condition can then be carefully assessed before another is added or withdrawn. The use of multiple modalities in a 'scattergun' approach will lead to difficulty in identifying which modality has been effective.

Importantly, clinicians must be guided by their clinical reasoning skills and not by blind application of inappropriate evidence. Simply because a patient has presented with a named syndrome, for example low-back pain, clinicians should avoid the temptation to use lumbar stabilisation exercises as a treatment modality. Lumbar spine stabilisation exercises are used when there are signs and symptoms present suggesting that this treatment approach may be beneficial (because evidence exists for the benefit of such exercises in a certain group of patients suffering with low-back pain: Moore & Petty 2001). Where there are clear indications of signs and symptoms related to published research then clinicians should use treatments which have positive evidence to support their use.

The preferences of patients and clinicians are important in the choice of treatment modalities; for example, a patient may in the past have experienced a treatment which is now being suggested. Previously, the patient may have found that the treatment was ineffective, distressing or uncomfortable. In this situation the clinician would be wise to find an alternative treatment or discuss the advantages/effects of the original technique fully with the patient, in order to gain the patient's understanding as to why the choice of treatment appears to be the most advantageous. At this point, and in partnership, the clinician and patient can come to an informed agreement about which modality to use.

The clinician may have particular treatments that s/he believes can be performed better than others; this may relate to the clinician's height, weight, experience and competence in the use of certain modalities, and these are important considerations in the decision-making process about which modalities to use.

Clinical reasoning

It is assumed that the clinician is using clinical reasoning throughout the examination, assessment, treatment and reassessment processes. In the neuro-musculoskeletal field, this has been promoted by Jones (1995), based on the work of Barrows & Tamblyn (1980) and further developed by Edwards (1995); the Barrows & Tamblyn (1980) model focuses on the clinician's activities. The later model by

Edwards adds the patient to the scenario and has been termed cooperative decision-making between the patient and clinician (Figure 9.7). The model is adapted here to include the patient–clinician relationship and the overriding effects of the clinician's attitudes, values, beliefs and expectations as well as those of the patient, together with the patient's expressed needs. In addition, the concept of empowerment facilitated by the cooperative nature of information and explanation-sharing should not be forgotten.

> Knowledge in the clinical reasoning process refers not only to knowledge in particular areas but also to the organisation of knowledge into useful and useable entities.
>
> Jones (1995 p. 20)

Cognition refers to the processes of thinking and includes the synthesis and analysis of information and the testing of working hypotheses relating to patient information. This includes confirming or disconfirming strategies, which actively plays a profound role in knowledge acquisition on behalf of the clinician, hence the close relationship between knowledge and cognition.

> Jones (1995 p. 19)

'Metacognition refers to the clinician's ability to think about their own thinking' (Jones 1995 p. 19), which becomes more possible the more clinical expertise one has. This expertise can only be gained through clinical experience, during which clinical reasoning involves reflection in action and reflection about action (Schon 1987a). Metacognition refers to thinking about what you are doing as you are doing it,

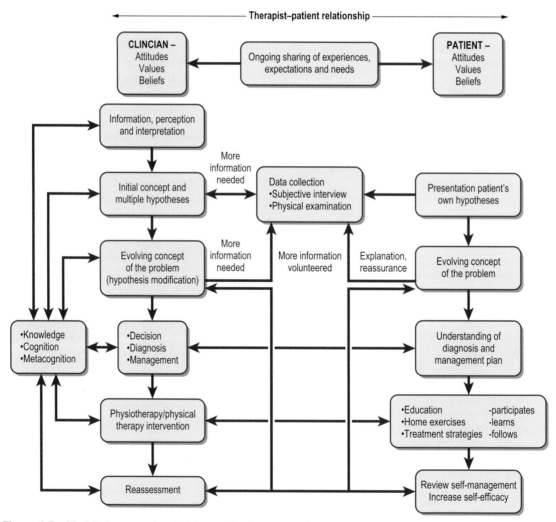

Figure 9.7 • Model of cooperative decision-making between patient and clinican (Meichenbaum D, Turk D C 1987 Facilitating treatment adherence. Plenum, New York. With kind permission of Springer Science and Business Media.).

i.e. when clinicians encounter a problem they engage in a process of critical analysis which then allows them to modify or adapt their practice, or correct their practice until a solution is found. A more detailed explanation of clinical reasoning is to be found in Jones (1995) and Higgs & Jones (1995).

Jones (1995) indicated a number of factors which affect and influence clinical reasoning. There are external factors, which include the patient's needs, expectations, values and beliefs, professional and institutional directives, community needs and expectations and the availability of resources and funding. There are also internal factors relating to clinicians, such as personal values and beliefs, general and local domain-specific knowledge and the individual's cognitive and reasoning strategies (Jones 1995).

The reader is referred to earlier chapters in relation to domain-specific knowledge in the neuromusculoskeletal areas of muscle, joint and nerve and to the companion volume to this text (Petty 2010) for practical application of the clinical reasoning process.

Jones's theoretical model of clinical reasoning has been supported by research by Doody & McAteer (2002), who examined the clinical reasoning activities of expert and novice therapists in an orthopaedic outpatient setting.

Evidence-based practice

In relation to knowledge gained by the clinician necessary for clinical reasoning the reader's attention is now turned to the concept of evidence-based practice which, as discussed earlier in this chapter, has gained momentum in the UK since the Secretary of State for Health's white paper (1998). This paper indicated that treatment undertaken within the NHS should be supported by evidence which is routinely applied.

Evidence-based practice has been variously defined. The definition of Sackett et al. (1996) emanates from evidence-based medicine: 'evidence-based medicine is the conscientious, explicit and judicious use of current best evidence in making decisions about the care of individual patients' (Sackett et al. 1996 p. 71). This definition has been frequently used; however, it has been adapted by Bury & Mead (1998), acknowledging the individuality of the clinician's expertise and also acknowledging the shortage of strong evidence to support all aspects of the physiotherapist's work at the present time. Their definition is as follows 'Evidence-based practice is

the conscientious, explicit and judicious use of current best evidence in making decisions about the care of individual patients, integrating individual clinical expertise with the best available external clinical evidence from systematic research' (Bury & Mead 1998 p. 11).

Evidence-based practice lies within a framework of evidence-based health care, which includes evidence-based policy-making, evidence-based commissioning, evidence-based management, evidence-based practice itself and evidence-based patient choice (Bury & Mead 1998). Increasingly, clinicians are being confronted by patients who are freely and copiously accessing information and evidence on health care practices and treatments via the internet and other media, and this can only help to increase the patient's autonomy and aid informed discussion between the clinician and the patient. Many organisations, for example the NHS and the Chartered Society of Physiotherapy, now offer lists of web-based and paper-form information for patients in order to provide a basis for their choices and decision-making.

Currently, best evidence refers primarily to high-quality scientific research derived from valid and rigorous research. The strength of evidence is shown in Box 9.4. Also coming to the fore currently are meta-analyses which are, in fact, analyses and summaries of the data emanating from a series of high-quality randomised controlled trials. As more research is carried out into physiotherapeutic modalities the number of meta-analyses published in this field will increase.

The judicious use of evidence is key here – the evidence above relates largely to high-quality published

Box 9.4

Hierarchy of strength of evidence (from Bury & Mead 1998, with permission)

I   Strong evidence from at least one systematic review of multiple well-designed randomised controlled trials

II Strong evidence from at least one properly designed randomised controlled trial of appropriate size

III Evidence from well-designed trials without randomisation, single group pre–post, cohort, time series or matched case-controlled studies

IV Evidence from well-designed non-experimental studies from more than one centre or research group

V   Opinions of respected authorities, based on clinical evidence, descriptive studies or reports of expert committees research work. However, there are other sources of evidence available which must be taken into consideration before treatment is applied, for example:

- clinical experience and expertise of clinicians
- the views of experts in the field
- established practice in health settings
- beliefs and values of the patient and clinician based on previous experiences
- expectation of patients based on information from published sources, other people and intrinsic needs
- information from the clinical examination and assessment procedures using rigorous clinical reasoning procedures
- the patient's preferences for treatment
- clinicians' preferences for the use of specific treatment modalities (Bury & Mead 1998).

Bury & Mead (1998) have usefully defined the steps necessary in carrying out evidence-based practice:

- Define the question arising from practice that needs answering.
- Find the evidence.
- Critically appraise the evidence.
- Implement relevant findings into practice.
- Evaluate the impact on practice.

The implementation of evidence-based practice demands high-level skills on the part of the clinician in the appraisal of literature and research; the clinician must also marry this appraisal with all other sources of evidence, as described above. The eventual choice of treatment should, as mentioned earlier, be fully discussed with the patient.

It is important that clinicians use their clinical reasoning skills in order to identify accurately and precisely the nature of the patient's problem so that they can then define the appropriate clinical question for which evidence must be found. There is no excuse for clinicians resorting to the use of evidence which is not appropriate for the individual patient under care and his or her condition. There must be clear indications for the use of evidenced treatment from the patient's clinical picture. Moore & Jull (2000) and Moore & Petty (2001) make this point very strongly.

Despite the agreement among clinicians that research is important in the development of professional practice, in the past there have been a number of reasons for lack of use of evidence by clinicians. These reasons have included: lack of understanding of statistics, lack of access to evidence, conflicting results in research papers, methodological problems in the research processes, lack of replication of studies and poor generalisability of results. In addition, clinicians cited insufficient time available to access evidence, inadequate facilities for the use of evidence-based practice and feeling isolated from colleagues (influencing their confidence in using new evidence and resistance to change in treatments by medical staff) (Metcalfe et al. 2001).

It has also been noted that attendance at short courses is a popular form of continuing professional development for clinicians in the neuromusculoskeletal field, but many short courses are offered without any reference to research underpinning the concepts involved (Turner & Whitfield 1999).

Clinical guidelines

Since the evidence-based practice movement began there has been a rapid development of clinical guidelines within a number of health disciplines and within different countries throughout the world. As a result, clinical guidelines are proliferating; for example, guidelines for the management of whiplash-associated disorder and for low-back pain are currently under development within the UK and will sit alongside other already existing guidelines available in other countries. Guidelines for the management of low-back pain already exist in the Netherlands and in other countries. It may be essential, however, that individual national guidelines be developed owing to differences in scope of practice, funding arrangements for health care, cultural differences in the population and national differences in health beliefs and values.

Clinical guidelines have been defined by Mann (1996) as 'systematically developed statements, which assist clinicians and patients in making decisions about appropriate treatment for specific conditions'.

The key features of guidelines are that they are based on the best available evidence, which has been appraised and evaluated systematically. Guidelines deal with specific interventions for specific client populations. A systematic process is used to decide who will be involved in the development of guidelines; development often involves experts in the field, patient representatives and, increasingly, other relevant professional groups (Mead 1998). It is suggested that readers obtain up-to-date clinical guidelines from their own professional body in the subject areas that are of most relevance to their own practice. Professional body websites will have full details as to how to access them.

As with all evidence, guidelines have to be interpreted and used judiciously, and there may need to be a consensus among clinicians as to how they may be interpreted locally to ensure that all are clear as to the implications of the guideline implementation for their own practice.

Educational skills and the clinician

Educational skills within the role of the clinician have been mentioned throughout this text, and education and advice offered by the clinician have been seen throughout this chapter as key to the therapeutic partnership and mutual patient–clinician understanding. It is also important in helping patients to empower themselves and in potentially developing their self-efficacy.

In the main, clinicians deal with adult learners, who are well described by Knowles (1983); the education of adult learners will be the key area of concentration here. Where children are attending for treatment parents will often be involved in the educational experiences; therefore, the principles of adult learning will apply but the concept of children's education is beyond the scope of this text. In a qualitative study, Trede (2000) investigated the approaches of physiotherapists to education about low-back pain and found that, in a sample of eight physiotherapists who were interviewed in the study, the majority adopted a didactic and clinician-centred approach to patient education. Patients were also interviewed in this study, and Trede concluded that an 'open' patient–clinician relationship is needed in order to encourage dialogue, action and reflection on progress and to ensure that misunderstandings and unrealistic expectations do not occur. Trede (2000) further summarised the components of clinician- and patient-centred approaches to education, as shown in Box 9.5.

Trede (2000) concludes that patients valued a good interpersonal relationship with their clinician as the most effective learning tool.

For details on developing educational skills, see Cross et al. (2006).

As Knowles (1983) has indicated in his theory of adult education, adults as learners see themselves as self-directed and responsible individuals. They possess an accumulation of experiences which are a resource for their own learning and for that of others (including, in the case of the patient, the

---

Box 9.5

Components of clinician- and patient-centred approaches to education (after Trede 2000 pp. 430–431)

Clinician-centred	Patient-centred
Teaches medical facts	Actively listening to the patient
Predicts and controls problems	Displaying a positive attitude to the patient
Symptom of diagnosis sets the scene	Providing technical, factual and counselling support
Listening to patients is of low priority	Providing opportunities for patients to learn independently
Planning is done for patients	Planning exercises with the patient
Patients are necessarily compliant	

---

clinician). Adult learners are motivated to learn when they perceive that the activity is directly related to their own life tasks, and their interests tend to focus on problem-solving rather than on abstract content or theory. For example, teaching structural anatomy in patient education programmes is not the most useful way of facilitating learning in adult patients – they would much prefer to know where their pain is coming from and how to get rid of it!

There are many factors which can affect learning (Cross et al. 2006) but one of the strongest factors is the learning style that suits learners as individuals. The particular learning style which a learner prefers influences the way in which that individual approaches study and the way s/he thinks. Learning styles are related to personality and have nothing to do with intelligence levels. In the clinical setting, if the clinician and patient have different learning styles which are incompatible, then tensions and misunderstandings may arise. Honey & Mumford (1986) identified four learning styles with their own characteristics (Box 9.6).

It is important for clinicians to be aware of their own and their patients' learning styles; the characteristics shown in Box 9.6 will help individuals to define their preferred learning style and then educational events can be adapted accordingly.

Ewles & Simnett (2003) have identified some principles for the education of patients.

Box 9.6

Description of learning styles (adapted from Honey & Mumford 1986)

Activists

- involve themselves fully, without bias, in new experiences
- enjoy the here and now, and are happy to be dominated by immediate experiences
- are open-minded, not sceptical
- are enthusiastic about anything new
- rush in where angels fear to tread
- like brainstorming problems
- become bored with implementation and longer-term consolidation
- are gregarious, and involve themselves with others
- seek to centre all the activities around themselves

Reflectors

- like to stand back to ponder experiences, are thoughtful
- observe from many different perspectives
- collect data, chew over before coming to conclusions
- tend to postpone reaching conclusions
- are cautious, leave no stone unturned
- prefer to take a back seat in meetings and discussions
- enjoy observing people in action

- listen to others
- adopt a low profile
- have a slightly distant, tolerant, unruffled air

Theorists

- integrate observations into logical theories
- think problems through step by step
- assimilate disparate facts into a cohesive whole
- tend to be perfectionists
- like to analyse
- tend to feel uncomfortable with subjective judgements
- tend to be detached, analytical and rational

Pragmatists

- are keen on trying out ideas, theories and techniques
- positively search out new ideas
- like to experiment
- like to get on with things and act quickly
- tend to be impatient with lengthy open-ended discussion
- are essentially practical, and like making practical decisions
- respond to problems and opportunities as a challenge

Principles for the education of patients

The following is adapted from Ewles & Simnett (2003 pp. 246–248):

- Say important things first; patients will be more likely to remember what was said at the beginning of the session.
- Stress and repeat key points and emphasise what are the important points; repetition can help.
- Give specific, precise advice and remember to relate to patients' own physical, personal and social circumstances.
- Structure information into categories, i.e. give patients headings and categories and deliver material under these headings.
- Avoid jargon, long words and long sentences.
- Use visual aids whenever possible – for example, leaflets, handouts, models, videos and written instructions.
- Avoid saying too much at once – only two or three key points will be remembered from each session.

- Ensure that your advice is relevant and realistic by discussing it with the patient.
- Get feedback from patients to ensure their understanding.
- Assess whether learning has taken place.

In assessing whether learning has taken place it is important to try to choose a method that is appropriate for patients and their learning style, their condition and the information and the knowledge you are trying to assess. For example, the clinician could use question-and-answer sessions, gapped handouts or discussion sessions to assess whether patients have clearly understood all the information necessary for them to participate in their own treatment.

When teaching practical skills, Ewles & Simnett (2003) recommend three stages:

- demonstration by the clinician
- rehearsal by the patient observed by the clinician
- practice by the patient observed by the clinician on a regular basis.

Demonstrations need to be clear, accurate, slow and repeated several times. Again, assessing whether learning has taken place is of paramount importance to ascertain whether patients have grasped what it is necessary for them to learn (Cross et al. 2006).

Obtaining evaluation and feedback on the clinician's personal role as an educator, or of the educational experience that has been provided (Cross et al. 2006), can be very valuable. It is sensible to ask the patient to evaluate both the clinician as an educator and the educational experience that has been provided. Peers can also be helpful in this evaluation, and self-reflection can be very useful. It is important to ask the following questions: What happened? What went well? What could have been improved? How could the experience be changed for the better next time? All learning experiences work best if they are planned carefully and in advance. Again, see Cross et al. (2006, Chapter 11) for details.

Home exercise programmes

The importance of good-quality teaching in relation to home exercises cannot be overestimated. It is essential that patients who require home exercises are shown how to do these correctly and that an assessment be made regularly as to how effectively the exercises are being undertaken and what effect they are having.

In relation to home management programmes readers should be aware of issues surrounding the terminology associated with patients responding to agreed/prescribed home management programmes. There are three options: compliance, adherence and concordance. In the 1980s compliance was a popular term in medicine; it reported patients' observable actions in carrying out the practitioner's instructions. Sackett & Haynes (1986) defined compliance as the extent to which the patient's behaviour coincides with the clinical prescription, and this makes it a term which is very practitioner-oriented. 'Adherence' has been used interchangeably with compliance for several years (Kroll et al. 1999), but has implied patient passivity because patients were expected to 'stick' to the practitioner's instructions. The word 'concordance' is being increasingly used as it describes 'unity or the state of being of the same opinion or feeling' (from the Latin *concorde*, meaning 'of one mind': Oxford

English Dictionary 1996). The term 'concordance' appears to fit well with the concept of patient-focused care.

Because terminology is currently changing, much of the previously published work relates to compliance or adherence and therefore the terms for these studies have been expressed as used by the authors concerned.

According to Meichenbaum & Turk (1987), there are many variables which appear to relate to non-adherence, including personal variables in relation to the patient, disease variables, treatment variables and relationship variables, i.e. variables within the patient–clinician relationship (Box 9.7).

Therefore it is important that clinicians, in building their therapeutic relationship with patients, ensure that these factors are minimised wherever possible in order to increase conformance. Jensen & Lorish (1994) assert that, for a treatment plan to be successfully followed, patients must choose to do so, they must know when to carry out the plan, they must have the psychomotor skills to perform the plan and they must remain motivated to see the plan through until the problem resolves. Further, Jensen & Lorish (1994) indicate that the clinician must understand patients' perspectives, motivational factors and their belief systems in order to facilitate change in the patient's behaviour needed to incorporate the treatment plan into their everyday lives. In a study of patient compliance with general practitioner/physicians' instructions, Falvo et al. (1980) indicated that patients were more likely to be compliant the more they perceived that the physician gave them explanations and showed concern for them.

Langer (1999) felt that minority populations were being treated by clinicians who were insensitive to patients' cultural norms, and referred to the impact that this may have had on health service use. Langer (1999) asserted that lack of awareness of cultural issues increases social distance, breaks down communication and precipitates misconceptions between minority patients and their health care providers and that this can lead to opportunities for increasing dissatisfaction and non-compliance.

Finally in this section, Friedrick et al. (1996) found that exercises learnt only by brochures, without being monitored by a physical therapist, were carried out properly in only one-half of the patients in their study, which appeared to result in fewer improvements in impairment.

Box 9.7

Factors related to treatment non-adherence (from Meichenbaum & Turk 1987, with permission)

Personal variables (patient)

Characteristics of the individual
Sensory disturbance
Forgetfulness
Lack of understanding
Conflicting health benefits
Competing sociocultural concepts of disease and treatment
Apathy and pessimism
Previous history of non-adherence
Failure to recognise need for treatment
Health beliefs
Dissatisfaction with practitioner
Lack of social support
Family instability
Environment that supports non-adherence
Conflicting demands (e.g. poverty, unemployment)
Lack of resources

Disease variables

Chronicity of condition
Stability of symptoms
Characteristics of the disorder

Treatment variables

Characteristics of treatment setting
Absence of continuity of care
Long waiting time
Long time between referral and appointment
Timing of referral
Absence of individual appointment
Inconvenience
Inadequate supervision of professionals
Characteristics of treatment
Complexity of treatment
Duration of treatment
Expense

Relationship variables

Inadequate communication
Poor rapport
Attitudinal and behavioural conflicts
Failure of practitioner to elicit feedback from patient
Patient dissatisfaction

Clarity of written information is highly important, and for those readers wishing to develop written materials for patients the following sources may be helpful: Duman (2003) and the Plain English Campaign (www.plainenglish.co.uk).

Measurement of outcome

Throughout treatment, the clinician will assess the outcome of care in terms of the assessment of salient signs and symptoms, and sometimes by utilising a valid, reliable and sensitive measure of outcome. Sometimes clinicians use a measure of outcome at the beginning of treatment and then again at discharge in order to ascertain improvements in the patient's condition. Sometimes clinicians choose to use measures of outcome regularly throughout the treatment process.

In physiotherapy, a measure of outcome has been defined as 'a test or scale administered and interpreted by physical therapists that has been shown to measure accurately a particular attribute that is of interest to patients and therapists and is expected to be influenced by an intervention' (Mayo 1994 p. 145).

It is important that physiotherapists use measures of outcome that are appropriate to the condition being treated and the patient concerned, i.e. in terms of ethnicity and language abilities.

It is equally important that physiotherapists choose measures of outcome which measure changes in the signs and symptoms that are being targeted by treatment. For example, if pain is predominantly being targeted in treatment, then a measurement of pain should be used – and used at an appropriate time in treatment to reflect the changes that have occurred. The tendency to levy a raft of outcome measures which are designed to measure attributes that are not being specifically targeted by treatment must be avoided; for example, the use of a functional measure when only pain has so far been targeted during treatment is unhelpful and can lead to demoralisation of the clinician and the patient when changes do not occur. Some functional changes may occur as a result of a byproduct of pain management but functional improvement may not be optimal by the time major pain relief has occurred; therefore, it appears obvious that different outcome measures should be used at different stages in the treatment process, reflecting progression of, and changes in, patient–clinician responsibilities and the nature of the modalities being used.

The main issues surrounding outcomes are as follows. First, their validity: in other words, does the measure record what it is intended to measure? Second, their reliability, i.e. can the measure be repeatedly used uniformly when administered on one or more occasions or by one or more raters? Third, is the measure sensitive/responsive, i.e. does the measure of outcome have the ability to detect true changes in the patient's situation over time? Is it sensitive enough to measure the subtle changes that sometimes occur in patients undergoing neuro-musculoskeletal therapy (Hicks 1999)?

A wide variety of measures of outcome are available:

- physical measures
- pain scales/questionnaires
- psychological well-being profiling questionnaires
- general health status measures
- self-efficacy measures
- disability measures
- quality-of-life measures
- functional ability measures
- patient-generated indexes
- patient satisfaction questionnaires
- life satisfaction and moral questionnaires
- multidimensional measures.

For details of an overview of a number of measures of outcome relevant to neuromusculoskeletal therapy, see Cole (1994), Liebenson & Yeomans (1997) and the extensive works by Bowling (2001a, b) on measuring disease and health.

In addition, national physiotherapy/physical therapy professional body websites contain details of recommended measures of outcome. As with research evidence, it is important that clinicians apply a critical and analytical eye on any proposed measure of outcome and assess the validity, sensitivity and reliability for its use in their own clinical situations. As can be seen, if applied correctly, outcomes are vitally important for measuring the results of health care. Bearing in mind the Department of Health initiative with regard to the use of quality metrics it is important that all musculoskeletal therapists engage with any data collection systems in their locality.

Clinical audit

In relation to the quality of health care, one of the ways of measuring the quality of the service provided is to measure performance against set standards and then analyse the results. This process is known as clinical audit. Standards to be measured need to be agreed locally or nationally, as does the topic for the audit. Audit is useful in evaluating the process of care, and feedback from audit activities to both departmental staff and individual clinicians can be important in improving practice. Clinical audit can be very important in itself in facilitating the use of evidence-based practice (Buttery 1998). Clinical audit has been defined as 'a clinically led initiative which seeks to improve the quality of outcome and outcome of patient care through structured peer review, whereby clinicians examine their practice and results against agreed standards and modify practice where indicated' (NHS Executive 1996). Again, recent government initiatives in the UK indicate the need for all health professionals to collect data concerning health care delivery in a rigorous and strategic way.

Usually, audit is guided by a cycle of events that comprise:

- agreement of guidelines, protocols or standards
- implementation of guidelines, protocols or standards
- assessment by data collection and analysis of compliance of the guidelines, protocols or standards
- agreement of changes in the guidelines, protocols or standards, if required
- implementation of agreed changes in guidelines, protocols or standards (Buttery 1998).

Personal professional development

Readers of this book may be novice practitioners and may be aiming to improve both their cognitive and practical skills and aspiring to becoming expert practitioners. There are many models of expertise available. These include clinical problem-solving, knowledge in clinical reasoning, the Dreyfus model of skill acquisition and the model of reflective practice; these models are clearly described by Jensen et al. (1999a).

The reflective practice model is growing in popularity in the UK. Schon's work (1987b) has explored how clinicians gain practical knowledge. Schon's theory is that clinicians add to their practical knowledge base not only through experience but also through a process of reflection, which is triggered by the recognition that a situation is not routine. Schon (1987b) believes that there are three processes present in reflection:

1. initial doubt and perplexity if the situation has been identified as non-routine but problematic (what is going on?)

2. questioning the thinking or action that has caused the problematic situation (how did I get here?)

3. working for problem resolution by trying new actions (what can I do to resolve the problem?).

Professionals are believed to learn by experience by using reflective enquiry, to think about what they are doing and what worked and what did not work as they were doing it. Patients can also learn by reflective activities.

Brockbank & McGill (1998) have defined reflection as 'the creation of meaning and conceptualisation from experience'. It is important that all clinicians avoid clinical stagnation and learn to develop continuously from their clinical experiences. Readers may find the following texts helpful in developing their expertise and capitalising on their own professional knowledge: Jensen et al. (1999b) and Higgs & Titchen (2001). In addition, individuals may seek out the opportunity to engage with 'clinical supervision', defined as an enabling process 'defining opportunities for personal and professional growth' (Butterworth & Faugier 1992). Bond & Holland (1998) have further described clinical supervision as an interaction between a supervisee and one or more peers in order to promote professional development through reflection and which is characterised by:

- regular protected time for facilitation of indepth reflection on professional practice
- an interaction that is facilitated by one or more experienced colleagues with expertise in facilitation
- facilitation of time and venue for the provision of frequent ongoing sessions led by the supervisee's agenda
- an enabling process that permits supervisees to achieve, sustain and develop creatively a high quality of practice through means of focus, support and development
- a reflective process, which permits the supervisees to explore and examine the part they play in the complexities of the events within the therapeutic relationship as well as the quality of their practices
- a lifelong learning experience that should continue throughout the practitioner's career, whether s/he remains in practice or moves into management, research or education.

Much more information on clinical supervision can be found in Cutcliffe et al. (2001).

Clinical supervision is a concept frequently used in the nursing profession to facilitate postregistration professional development of individual nurses. It is becoming more widespread in use as more hospital trusts in the UK seek new ways of improving the quality of health care delivery and methods of enabling lifelong learning in their workforces using their existing in-house expertise and experience.

Overall management of patients

In summary, the following are guidelines for clinicians for the overall management of patients:

- Make treatment and overall management patient-focused.
- Ensure that all clinical work falls within professional, local service and national health service-related guidelines for good practice and quality improvement.
- Work within a biopsychosocial model of care.
- Work towards patient autonomy through clinical partnership.
- Ensure that patients have the opportunity to develop an empowered position.
- Facilitate patient self-efficacy wherever possible.
- Undertake multimodel patient management within the framework of the patient–clinician relationship.
- Ensure that coping strategies, pain relief and rehabilitation strategies are addressed within overall patient management.
- Base treatment choices on sound, careful and comprehensive clinical reasoning processes, working within the Edwards (1995) cooperative decision-making model.
- Examination and treatment procedures should be carefully undertaken, accurate in application and specific to the patient's background and condition, bearing in mind the patient's needs, expectations and preferences.

Examination should:

- allow the building of the therapeutic relationship
- ensure a full understanding of the patient's condition, how it is manifesting and how it is affecting the patient

- determine how the condition should be approached with respect to treatment
- determine exactly what the patient's expectations and needs are in relation to his or her background circumstances
- indicate what, if any, contraindications are present in relation to choice of treatment
- help to determine what the likely outcome of treatment will be.

Treatment should be:

- specific to fulfil the stated aims of treatment
- fully discussed with the patient
- accurate in its application
- applied with frequency and a dosage appropriate to the patient's needs and the manifesting signs of the symptoms
- accompanied by the acquisition of informed consent which should be gained as necessary
- based on goals agreed with the patient at the start of treatment
- inclusive of some form of education or advice to facilitate patients' understanding of their problem, their treatment, their home management and their possible coping strategies
- inclusive of patient learning, which should always be assessed and evaluated to ensure that full understanding has taken place
- assessed for outcome and goal achievement, both formally and informally, at appropriate points in treatment, which will vary according to the patient's condition. More than one measure of outcome may be appropriate if the patient's condition and treatment is multifactorial
- aimed at aiding patient empowerment and self-efficacy
- modified, progressed, interrupted and ceased according to the behaviour of the patient's signs and symptoms, with the therapist using a full range of clinical reasoning skills
- based on the best available evidence
- accompanied by a self-care or self-management programme to enhance and continue the effects of treatment. These programmes should be aimed at pain relief and enhancing all other aims of treatment.

With regard to discharge:

- It should take place when agreed goals have been reached or are likely to be achieved in the short term by the patient's home management strategy.

- The opportunity for a follow-up appointment should be given to all patients if permissible within the home department's administrative system.

With regard to multidisciplinary working:

- As with all areas of practice, clinicians must ensure that they engage fully in communicating, liaising and working alongside the rest of the multidisciplinary team.

Finally, all clinicians should indulge in reflective practice during and after each interaction with a patient in order to improve their knowledge, experience and expertise and to ensure continuing professional development. Individuals and clinical departments may give some thought to adopting a system of clinical supervision in order to maximise reflective practice.

Summary

This chapter has emphasised the need for patient-focused care and has highlighted the facets of care in which patients can and should be involved. It has attempted to show how making patients more of a central focus of care can lead to improvements to the quality of health and improve the outcome of treatment. The specificity of treatment has been shown to be of paramount importance based on the integration of high-quality, cognitive and practical skills which are enmeshed with the concepts of evidence-based practice and the use of clinical guidelines and clinical audit. Finally, the need for continuous professional development and the role that reflective practice and clinical supervision can have in the development of the practitioner's expertise have been overviewed.

The reader is left with an adapted quotation to reflect upon:

> If you really want to help somebody, first of all you must find them where they are and start there. This is the secret of caring. If you cannot do that, it is only an illusion, if you think you can help another human being. Helping somebody implies your understanding more than they do, but first of all you must understand what they understand. If you cannot do that, your understanding will be of no avail. All true caring starts with humility. You the helper must be humble in your attitude towards the person that you want to help. You must understand that helping is not dominating, but serving. Caring implies patience as well as acceptance of not being right and of not understanding what the other person understands.

Kierkegaard (1849)

References

Baker, S.M., Marshak, H.H., Rice, G.T., et al., 2001. Patient participation in goal setting. Phys Ther 81 (5), 1118–1126.

Bandura, A., 1977. Towards a unifying theory of behaviour change. Psychol. Rev. 84, 191–215.

Bandura, A., Walter, R.H., 1963. Social learning and personality development. Thinehart and Winston, New York.

Barr, J., Threlkeld, A.J., 2000. Patient practitioner collaboration in clinical decision-making. Physiother. Res. Int. 5 (4), 254–260.

Barrows, H.S., Tamblyn, R.M., 1980. Problem based learning: an approach to medical education. Springer, New York.

Bond, M., Holland, S., 1998. The surface picture: the development value of clinical supervision in skills of clinical supervision for nurses, chapter 2. Open University Press, Buckingham.

Bowling, A.A., 2001a. Measuring disease – a review of disease specific quality of life measurement scales, second ed. Open University Press, Milton Keynes.

Bowling, A.A., 2001b. Measuring health – a review of quality of life measurement scales, second ed. Open University Press, Milton Keynes.

Bradshaw, J., 1972. Concept in social need. New Society 19, 640–643.

Brockbank, A., McGill, 1998. Facilitating reflective learning in higher education. Open University Press, Buckingham.

Brody, D.S., Miller, S.M., Lerman, C., et al., 1989. Patient perception of involvement in medical care: relationship to illness, attitudes and outcomes. J. Gen. Intern. Med. 4, 506–511.

Bury, T., Mead, J., 1998. Evidence based healthcare: a practical guide for therapists. Butterworth-Heinemann, Oxford.

Butterworth, A., Faugier, J. (Eds.), 1992. Clinical supervision and mentorship in nursing. Chapman and Hall, London.

Buttery, Y., 1998. Implementing evidence through clinical audit. In: Bury, J., Mead, J. (Eds.), Evidence based healthcare. Butterworth-Heinemann, Oxford.

Chartered Society of Physiotherapy, 2002. Rules of professional conduct, second ed. Lansdowne Press, London.

Cole, B., 1994. Physical rehabilitation outcome measures. Canadian Physical Therapy Association, Ontario.

Collins Thesaurus, 1995. Harper Collins Glasgow.

Cross, V., Moore, A., Morris, J., et al., 2006. The practice educator – a reflective tool for CPD and accreditation. John Wiley, Chichester.

Cutcliffe, J.R., Butterworth, T., Proctor, B. (Eds.), 2001. Fundamental themes in clinical supervision. Routledge, London.

Department of Health, 2000. The NHS plan. The Stationery Office, London.

Department of Health, 2008a. The next stage review – our NHS, our future. Department of Health, London.

Department of Health, 2008b. Framing the contribution of Allied Health Professionals – delivering high-quality care. Department of Health, London.

Department of Health, 2008c. High-quality care for all. Department of Health, London.

Doody, C., McAteer, M., 2002. Clinical reasoning of expert and novice physiotherapist in an outpatient orthopaedic setting. Physiotherapy 88 (5), 258–268.

Duman, M., 2003. Producing patient information. Kings Fund, London.

Edwards, I., 1995. Unpublished paper cited by Jones M: Clinical reasoning pain. Man. Ther. 1 (1), 21.

Ewles, L., Simnett, I., 2003. Promoting health – a practical guide, fifth ed. Scutari Press, London.

Falvo, D., Woehlke, P., Deichman, N.J., 1980. Relationship of physician behaviour to patient compliance. Patient Couns. Health Educ. 2 (4), 185–188.

Friedrick, M., McErmak, T., Maderbacher, P., 1996. The effect of brochure use versus therapist teaching on patient performing therapeutic exercise and on changes in impairment status. Phys. Ther. 76 (10), 1082–1087.

Gillon, R., 1986. Philosophical medical ethics. John Wiley, Chichester.

Golemann, D., 1996. Emotional intelligence. Bloomsbury, London, p. 43.

Golemann, D., 1998. Working with emotional intelligence. Bloomsbury, London.

Grimmer, K., Sheppard, L., Pitt, M., et al., 1999. Differences in stakeholder expectations in the outcome of physiotherapy management of acute low back pain. Int. J. Qual. Health Care 11 (2), 155–162.

Health Professions Council, 2003a. Standards of proficiency. Health Professions Council, London.

Health Professions Council, 2003b. Standards of conduct, performance and ethics. Health Professions Council, London.

Heaton, J., McMurray, R., Sloper, P., et al., 2000. Rehabilitation and total hip replacement: patients' perspectives on provision. Int. J. Rehabil. Res. 23, 253–259.

Hicks, C., 1999. Research methods for clinical therapists, third ed. Churchill Livingstone, Edinburgh.

Higgs, J., Jones, M. (Eds.), 1995. Clinical reasoning in the health professions. Butterworth-Heinemann, Oxford.

Higgs, J., Titchen, A. (Eds.), 2001. Practice knowledge and expertise in health professions. Butterworth-Heinemann, Oxford.

Hoff, B., 1982. The Tao of Pooh. Mandarin, London, p. XIV.

Honey, P., Mumford, A., 1986. The manual of learning styles. Printique, London.

Jensen, G.M., Lorish, C., 1994. Promoting patient cooperation with exercise programmes: linking research theory and practice. Arthritis Care Res. 7, 181.

Jensen, G.M., Gwyer, J., Hack, L.M., et al., 1999a. Expertise in physical therapy. Butterworth-Heinemann, Boston.

Jensen, G.M., Lorish, C., Sheppard, K.F., 1999b. Understanding patient receptivity to change. Teaching for treatment adherence. In: Sheppard, K.F., Jensen, G.M. (Eds.), Handbook of teaching for physical therapists. Butterworth-Heinemann, Boston.

Jette, A., 1994. Physical disablement concepts for physical therapy research and practice. Phys. Ther. 74, 380.

Jones, M., 1995. Clinical reasoning and pain. Man. Ther. 1 (1), 17–24.

Jones, M., Edwards, I., Gifford, L., 2002. Conceptual models for implementing biopsychosocial theory in clinical practice. Man. Ther. 7 (1), 2–9.

Jull, G., Moore, A.P., 2002. What is a suitable dosage of physical therapy treatment? Man. Ther. 7 (4), 181–182.

Kalauokalani, D., Cherkin, D.C., Sherman, K.J., et al., 2001. Lessons from a trial of acupuncture and massage for low back pain. Spine 26 (13), 1418–1424.

Kierkegaard, S., 1849. The sickness unto death. (translation from Danish by Hannay A. D.). Penguin Books, London.

Knowles, M., 1983. The modern practice of adult education from pedagogy to androgogy. In: Tight, M.M. (Ed.), Adult learning and education. Croom Helm/Open University, London, pp. 53–70.

Kroll, T., Barlow, J.H., Shaw, J., 1999. Treatment adherence in juvenile rheumatoid arthritis. Scand. J. Rheumatol. 28 (1), 10–18.

Labonte, R., 1989. Community and professional empowerment. Infirm. Can. 85 (3), 23–28.

Langer, N., 1999. Culturally competent professionals in therapeutic alliances enhance patient compliance. J. Health Care Poor Underserved 10 (1), 19–26.

Liebenson, C., Yeomans, S., 1997. Outcomes assessment in musculoskeletal medicine. Man. Ther. 2 (2), 67–73.

Maitland, G.D., Hengeveld, E., Banks, K., et al., 2005. Communication in Maitland vertebral manipulation. seventh ed. Butterworth-Heinemann, Oxford, pp. 1–24.

Mann, T., 1996. Clinical guidelines: using clinical guidelines to improve patient care within the NHS. Department of Health, London.

May, S.J., 2001. Patient satisfaction with management of low back pain. Physiother. J. 87 (1), 4–19.

Mayo, N., 1994. Outcome measures or measuring outcome. Physiother. Can. 46 (3), 143–147.

Mead, J., 1998. Developing, disseminating and implementing clinical guidelines. In: Bury, T., Mead, J. (Eds.), Evidence based healthcare – a practical guide for therapists. Butterworth-Heinemann, Oxford, pp. 162–181.

Meichenbaum, D., Turk, D.C., 1987. Facilitating treatment adherence. Plenum, New York.

Metcalfe, C., Lewin, R., Wisher, S., et al., 2001. Barriers to implementing the evidence base in four NHS therapies. Physiotherapy 87 (8), 433–441.

Moore, A.P., Jull, G., 1997. Editorial. Man. Ther. 2 (3), 121–122.

Moore, A.P., Jull, G., 2000. Editorial: fads and fashion. Man. Ther. 5 (4), 197–256.

Moore, A.P., Jull, G., 2001. Editorial: The art of listening. Man. Ther. 6 (3), 129.

Moore, A.P., Jull, G., 2002. Editorial: reflections on the musculoskeletal therapists multifaceted role and influences on treatment outcome. Man. Ther. 7 (3), 119–120.

Moore, A.P., Petty, N.J., 2001. Editorial: evidence based practice – getting a grip and finding a balance. Man. Ther. 6 (4), 195–264.

Moore, A., McQuay, H., Gray, J.A.M. (Eds.), 1995. Evidence based everything. Bandalier 1 (12), 1.

Neistadt, M., 1995. Methods of assessing clients' priorities: a survey of adults' physical dysfunction settings. Am. J. Occup. Ther. 49 (5), 428–436.

NHS Executive, 1996. Clinical audit in the NHS. Using clinical audit in the NHS: a position statement. Department of Health, London.

NHS Executive, 1999. Continuing professional development quality in the NHS. Department of Health, London.

NHS Executive, 2000. Meeting the challenge: a strategy for the allied health professionals. Department of Health, London.

Oxford English Dictionary, 1996. Oxford University Press, Oxford.

Petty, N.J., 2011. Neuromusculoskeletal examination and assessment – a

handbook for therapists, fourth ed. Elsevier, Edinburgh.

Richardson, K.E., Moran, S., 1995. Developing standards for patient information. Int. J. Health Care Qual. Assur. 8 (7), 27–31.

Rodwell, C.M., 1996. An analysis of the concept of empowerment. J. Adv. Nurs. 23, 305–313.

Rollnick, S., Mason, P., Butler, C., 1999. Health behaviour changes, a guide for practitioners. Churchill Livingstone, Edinburgh.

Rose, M., Klenenman, L., Atkinson, L., et al., 1992. A comparison of three chronic pain conditions using the fear avoidance model of exaggerated pain perception behaviour. Res. Ther. 21 (4), 409–416.

Sackett, D.C., Haynes, R.B., 1986. Compliance with therapeutic regimes. Johns Hopkins University Press, Baltimore.

Sackett, D.L., Rosenberg, W.M.C., Gray, J.A.M., et al., 1996. Evidence based practice: what is it and what it isn't. BMJ 312, 71–72.

Schon, D., 1987a. Educating the reflective practitioner. Phys. Ther. 70, 566–577.

Schon, D., 1987b. Educating the reflective practitioner. San Francisco, Jossey Bass.

Secretary of State for Health, 1997. The NHS: modern and dependable. NHS Executive, London.

Secretary of State for Health, 1998. A first class service. Quality in the new NHS. NHS Executive, London.

Sigrell, H., 2001. Expectations of chiropractic patients: the construction of a questionnaire. J. Manipulative Physiol. Ther. 24 (7), 440–444.

Sigrell, H., 2002. Expectations of chiropractic treatment: what are the expectations of new patients consulting a chiropractor and do chiropractors have similar expectations? J. Manipulative Physiol. Ther. 25 (5), 300–305.

Sim, J., 1986. Informed consent, ethical implications for physiotherapy. Physiotherapy 72, 584–587.

Sim, J., 1996. Informed consent and manual therapy. Man. Ther. 1 (2), 104–106.

Singleton, J., McLaren, S., 1995. Ethical foundations of health care. Mosby, London.

Stewart, M., Roter, D., 1989. Communicating with medical patients. Sage Publications, New York.

Swage, T., 2000. Clinical governance in healthcare practice. Butterworth-Heinemann, Oxford.

Trede, F.V., 2000. Physiotherapists' approaches to low back pain education. Physiotherapy 86 (8), 427–433.

Turner, P., Whitfield, T.W.A., 1999. Physiotherapists' reasons for selection of treatment techniques. A cross sectional survey. Physiother. Theory Pract. 15, 235–246.

Waddell, G., Bircher, M., Finlayson, D., et al., 1984. Symptoms and signs: physical disease or illness behaviour. BMJ (Clin. Res. Ed.) 289, 739–741.

Index

Note: Page numbers followed by *b* indicate boxes, *f* indicate figures and *t* indicate tables.